Essentials of Veterinary Surgery

Eighth Edition

W0193295

Essentials of
Veterinary Surgery

Eighth Edition

A Venugopalan BVSc, MS

Formerly Professor and Head
Department of Surgery
College of Veterinary and Animal Sciences
Kerala Agricultural University
Kerala

Oxford & IBH Publishing Co. Pvt. Ltd.
New Delhi
(A Unit of CBS Publishers & Distributors Pvt Ltd)

CBS Publishers & Distributors Pvt Ltd

New Delhi • Bengaluru • Chennai • Kochi • Kolkata • Mumbai
Bhopal • Bhubaneswar • Hyderabad • Jharkhand • Nagpur • Patna
• Pune • Uttarakhand • Dhaka (Bangladesh) • Kathmandu (Nepal)

Essentials of Veterinary Surgery

ISBN-13: 978-81-204-1379-5
ISBN-10: 81-204-1379-2

©2009, 2000, 1994, 1992, 1986, 1982, 1972, 1967, A Venogopalan
Reprint: 2017, 2018, 2019, 2020, 2021

OXFORD & IBH
New Delhi
(A Unit of CBS Publishers & Distributors Pvt Ltd)

CBS Publishers & Distributors Pvt Ltd
204 FIE, Patparganj Industrial Area, Delhi 110 092
E-mail: delhi@cbspd.com, cbspubs@airtelmail.in

Ph: 011-4934 4934   Fax: 011-4934 4935   Website: www.cbspd.com
                                                        e-mail: publishing@cbspd.com;
                                                        publicity@cbspd.com

Branches

- **Bengaluru:** Seema House 2975, 17th Cross, K.R. Road, Banasankari 2nd Stage, Bengaluru 560 070, Karnataka
  Ph: +91-80-26771678/79   Fax: +91-80-26771680   e-mail: bangalore@cbspd.com
- **Chennai:** No. 7, Subbaraya Street, Shenoy Nagar, Chennai 600 030, Tamil Nadu
  Ph: +91-44-26680620, 26681266   Fax: +91-44-42032115   e-mail: chennai@cbspd.com
- **Kochi:** 68/1534, 35, 36 Power House Road, Opp. KSEB, Kochi 682018, Kerala
  Ph: +91-484-4059061-65,67   Fax: +91-484-4059065   e-mail: kochi@cbspd.com
- **Kolkata:** No. 6/B, Ground Floor, Rameswar Shaw Road, Kolkata-700014 (West Bengal), India
  Ph: +91-33-2289-1126, 2289-1127, 2289-1128   e-mail: kolkata@cbspd.com
- **Mumbai:** 83-C, Dr E Moses Road, Worli, Mumbai-400018, Maharashtra
  Ph: +91-22-24902340/41   Fax: +91-22-24902342   e-mail: mumbai@cbspd.com

Representatives

• Bhopal	0-8319310552	• Bhubaneswar	0-9911037372	• Hyderabad	0-9885175004
• Jharkhand	0-9811541605	• Nagpur	0-9421945513	• Patna	0-9334159340
• Pune	0-9623451994	• Uttarakhand	0-9716462459	• Dhaka	01912-003485
• Kathmandu	977-9818742655			(Bangladesh)	
(Nepal)					

Printed at Chaman Enterprises, Daryaganj, Delhi, India

This book is most respectfully dedicated
to my teachers in Veterinary Surgery

Dr. M.N. MENON
former Professor of Surgery in the Madras Veterinary
College and who since retired as the Animal Husbandry
Commissioner to the Government of India;

and

Dr. E. R. FRANK, Dr. J. E. MOSIER,
Dr. J. S. LARSEN and Dr. F. W. OEHME
of the Kansas State University, Manhattan,
Kansas, U. S. A.

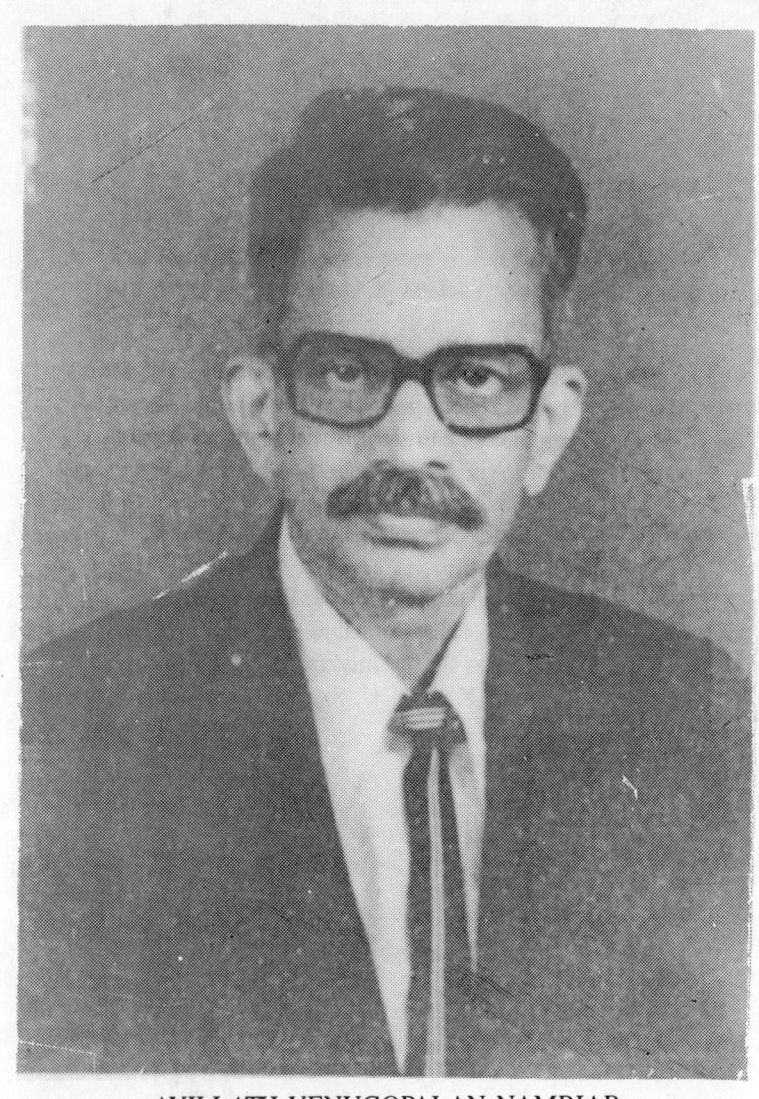

AYILLATH VENUGOPALAN NAMBIAR
(Born on May 26, 1928)

FOREWORD

The book "Essentials of Veterinary Surgery" by Professor A.Venugopalan is a successfully planned work to fill a long-standing need for a textbook in Veterinary Surgery for Undergraduate students. This can also quite effectively serve as a practising guide to field veterinarians.

Great progress has been made in the field of Veterinary Surgery during the past few years. The intention of the author is not to gather all these advancements and the results of modern research in this small volume, but to give the various theoretical aspects and practical approaches as required for the academic programme of undergraduate students in Veterinary Surgery. I believe that this book will be useful to a very great extent to the postgraduate students as well. The presentation is simple, straightforward and lucid. The author has brought in his long years of experience as a teacher in Veterinary Surgery to make the book authoritative and informative. Professor A. Venugopalan deserves warm appreciation for this effort.

I am sure, this book is bound to be very popular both with the students and teachers of Veterinary Surgery.

Dr. M. Krishnan Nair
Dean,
Faculty of Veterinary & Animal Sciences,
Kerala Agricultural University,
Mannuthy

PREFACE

This book *Essentials of Veterinary Surgery* is intended for the B.V.Sc. degree students of Indian Universities. It gives a comprehensive idea about the various topics dealt with in the undergraduate syllabi. The notes that I had prepared and used during my career as a teaching staff of the Department of Surgery in the Kerala Veterinary College served as the basis for this publication.

One of the constant complaints of undergraduate students is that almost all textbooks and reference books available on the subject of surgery are too voluminous, so that from the examination point of view it is difficult to grasp the subject in its essentials within the very limited time available.

I have, therefore, tried to state facts in as concise a manner as possible, laying stress on fundamentals. The subject is dealt with in a systematic and classified manner, avoiding complicated explanatory details, so as to make it intelligible to the average student.

I need not say that it is impossible to contain the vast subject of Veterinary Surgery in a small book of this kind. The list of references given at the end of the book should be consulted whenever additional information is required.

I have furnished, besides the number of *"subjective-type"* questions in each chapter, a few models of *"objective-type"* at the end of the book. This, I hope, will make it more examination-oriented.

College of Veterinary & Animal
Sciences, Mannuthy.

A. VENUGOPALAN

CONTENTS

PART II—REGIONAL SURGERY

PART III—OPERATIVE SURGERY

Part I

General Surgery

CHAPTER 1

Introduction

The meanings of some of the commonly used terms are explained in this Chapter.

Surgery is a branch of medical science which deals with the treatment of injuries or diseases by manual procedures or operations with the hand. It is synonymous with the word "Chirurgia" (Pronounced as: KI-RUR-JIA). The Greek word "Cheir" means hand; and "ergon" means work.

Veterinary Surgery is surgery practiced on animals.

Orthopaedic Surgery is that branch of surgery which is "specially concerned with the preservation and restoration of the function of the skeletal system, its articulations and associated structures." (Definition by the American Board of Orthopedic Surgery).

Antiseptic Surgery is surgery conducted with the use of antiseptic agents to control bacterial contamination.

Aseptic Surgery is surgery carried out practically free of bacterial contamination so that infection and suppuration are avoided.

Conservative Surgery is surgery wherein every attempt is made to preserve or restore a disabled part, rather than its removal, e.g., correction and immobilisation of a fracture in a limb rather than amputation of the limb.

Radical Surgery is surgery by which the root cause or source of a disease condition is removed or rectified, e.g., radical surgery for neoplasm, radical surgery for hernia.

Minor Surgery is surgery which is relatively simple to perform, having no risk on the life of the patient and requires the services of no assistant. e.g., opening of a superficial abscess, wound dressings, inoculations, superficial neurectomies and tenotomies.

Major Surgery is surgery which is relatively more difficult to perform than minor surgery, is time-consuming, involves risk on the life of the patient, and requires the help of an assistant. e.g., caesarian section, mammectomy, thoracic surgery, brain surgery.

Emergency Surgery is surgery which is to be performed urgently to avoid further complication of the disease process or to save the life of the patient.

Elective Surgery is surgery which can be postponed without endangering the life of the patient.

Cosmetic Surgery in veterinary practice is surgery done either to improve the appearance of an animal, or to satisfy the fancy and sentiments of the owner. e.g., trimming of the ears, docking of the tail, etc.

Reconstructive Surgery is surgery done for the correction of deformities or malformations. e g., surgery for cleft palate, contracted tendons, etc.

Plastic Surgery is surgery which is performed for the repair of defects or for correction of deformities, either by direct union of parts or by transfer of tissues from one part to another.

Exploratory Surgery is done to arrive at a diagnosis or for the confirmation of a diagnosis.

Experimental Surgery is the systematic investigation of a surgical problem.

Clinical Surgery is surgery taught with the presence of the patient, so that the objective symptoms and the treatment given can be actually observed by the student.

Clinic (Hospital): An institution in which medical attention is given to patients.

Surgical Anatomy is anatomy of a limited area or region referred to or explained in the proper description of a surgical operation.

Systematic Anatomy is the study of individual organs under a particular system. e.g., anatomy of the liver, anatomy of the respiratory system, anatomy of the locomotor system.

Surface Anatomy is the study of configurations of the surface of the body, especially in relation to their underlying deeper parts.

Topographic Anatomy (Regional Anatomy) is anatomy of certain related parts or divisions of the body.

Surgical Bacteriology is the study of the micro-organisms concerned, e.g., surgical bacteriology of wounds.

Surgical Pathology is a branch of pathology which deals chiefly with the effects produced upon the animal body by a surgical condition.

Trauma is an injury (external violence) inflicted to a part of the body or to an organ by some outside agent.

Physical Trauma is an injury inflicted by a physical agent. e.g., by striking against a hard object.

Chemical Trauma is an injury inflicted by some chemical agent. e.g., by strong acids, alkalies, etc.

Fever is a condition in which there is an elevation of the body temperature due to a disease.

Pyrexia simply means an elevation of body temperature (which may or may not be due to a disease).

Note the difference between *fever* and *pyrexia.*

History (Anamnesis): The Greek word anamnesis literally means "a recalling." In Veterinary terminology, "anamnesis" or "history of a case" means the information gathered concerning the patient about its condition prior to being attended to by the veterinarian, with regard to symptoms exhibited, environments and housing, feeding, defecation, urination, etc., including details of previous treatment, if any.

Incidence (Occurrence) denotes the occurrence of a disease with reference to susceptibility, periodicity or frequency; or with reference to species, age group, or locality. e.g., broken knee is of common occurrence in horses; the incidence of splint is more common in young horses; Urethral calculi is of common occurrence in Andhra Pradesh.

Etiology is the study as to the causation of a disease.

Predisposing Causes are causes which may not actually produce the disease, but which will render the animal liable to the attack of the disease.

Exciting Cause of a disease is a factor which will lead to the production of a disease.

Symptom (Sign) is a change in the condition of the patient indicative of some abnormality. Symptoms may be spoken of as physical symptoms, functional symptoms, pathognomonic symptoms, etc.

Physical Symptom is an objective evidence or sign of a disease.

Functional Symptom is an evidence of deviation from the normal action of a part or organ.

Pathognomonic Symptom is a symptom that surely establishes the diagnosis of a disease.

Diagnosis is the determination of the nature of a disease.

Differential Diagnosis is the comparative study of the diagnostic features of closely related diseases, in order to differentiate a disease from the others resembling it.

Clinical Diagnosis is diagnosis based on symptoms shown and on laboratory tests conducted during the life of the patient.

Post-mortem Diagnosis is diagnosis based on examinations on the body and internal organs after death of the patient.

Lesion: Any pathological alteration in tissue due to disease or traumatic injury is called a lesion.

Lesions visible to the naked eye are called *gross lesions* or *macroscopic lesions* and those that are detectable only through microscope are called *microscopic* or *histologic lesions*.

Sequela is a lesion resulting from prolonged existence of the disease, as a consequence of the disease.

Prognosis means a forecast as to the prospect of recovery from disease.

Remedial Treatment (*Curative treatment*) is the treatment which is specifically intended to cure the disease.

Palliative Treatment is treatment which may not cure the disease but affords some relief to the patient.

Symptomatic Treatment is treatment designed to suppress or diminish the untoward symptoms.

Expectant Treatment is treatment designed only to relieve the untoward symptoms, leaving the cure to nature.

Physical Therapy: The therapeutic use of physical agents other than drugs is physical therapy. It comprises the use of physical, chemical and other properties of heat, light, water, electricity, massage, exercise and radiation.

Aphorism: A concise statement of a principle in any science.

Blood Pressure: There are 3 commonly recorded blood pressures, namely, (1) Systolic pressure, (2) Diastolic pressure, and (3) Mean blood pressure.

Systolic pressure is the maximum or peak pressure developed by the contraction of the heart.

Diastolic pressure is the lowest point in the pressure curve and represents the pressure during diastole.

Mean blood pressure is a measure of the degree of filling of the circulatory system at a given period of time. It is slightly less than the average of the systolic and diastolic pressures and it follows more closely the diastolic pressure curve than the systolic pressure curve.

Anorexia means a total loss of appetite. It is not correct to use this term for partial loss of appetite, for which the appropriate word is *inappetence.*

Nystagmus is exhibited by a rythmic movement of the eyes in a particular direction followed by movement in the opposite direction. (Lateral nystagmus, vertical nystagmus, etc.).

Dorsal recumbency (Supine position) refers to the animal lying on its back touching the ground.

Ventral recumbency (Prone position) is when the animal is lying with its chest and abdomen touching the ground. (Prone position in human anatomy means lying with the face downward; and when the term is refered to the human hand it means having the palm turned down.)

Left lateral recumbency is when the animal is lying on its left side.

Right lateral recumbency is when the animal is lying on its right side.

The terms *proximal* and *distal* are used to describe the relative distances of a limb from its attachment to the body; for example, the arm is proximal to the forearm and the shank (metacarpal region) is distal to the forearm.

Plantar (Palmar/solar) surface of the foot means the lower surface of the foot.

Dorsal surface of the foot means the anterior surface of the foot.

Abduction of a limb is the movement away from the midline of the body.

Adduction of a limb is the movement towards the midline of the body.

Circumduction of a limb is the combination in sequence of the movements of flexion, extension, abduction and adduction.

CHAPTER 2

Reasons for Surgery

The reasons for doing a surgical operation may be any one or more of the following:

(i)   To save the life of an animal, e.g., surgery in the case of an acute intestinal obstruction.

(ii)   To prolong the life of an animal, e.g., removal of a malignant tumour.

(iii)   To hasten recovery from an injury, e.g., splinting of fractures, suturing of wounds.

(iv)   For elimination of a disease process, e.g., extraction of a diseased tooth, removal of a benign tumour.

(v)   For cosmetic reasons, e.g., trimming of ears, docking.

(vi)   For correcting deformities or malformations (Reconstructive surgery), e.g., correction of a congenital deformity like cleft palate (Staphylorraphy or suturing cleft palate), contracted tendons in calves and foals, cryptorchidism.

(vii)   For the replacement of a part by an artificial one, e.g., artificial eye, artificial limb, prosthetic hip

(viii)   On economic reasons or to make an animal socially acceptable, e.g., castration, spaying, dehorning, debleating of sheep, debarking of dogs.

(ix)   To aid in diagnosis of a suspected pathological process, e.g., exploratory laparotomy.

(x)   For investigation in research work (Experimental surgery), e.g., salivary fistula, gastric fistula.

CHAPTER 3

Tenets (Principles) of Halstead

These are the principles of modern surgery first laid down by Halstead (1852—1922).

1. *Gentle handling of tissues.* The tissues should be handled gently. Rough handling, use of blunt cutting instruments, unnecessary clamping of tissues with forceps, etc., cause additional trauma.

2. *Aseptic surgery.* Surgery should be performed under aseptic conditions.

3. *Anatomical dissection.* The dissection of tissues during surgery should be very discretionary. No muscle, nerve or vessel should be cut unnecessarily. To ensure this, the surgeon should possess an adequate knowledge of anatomy. To approach a deeper structure, it is very often possible to separate relevant muscles rather than cut the muscles. When a muscle is to be cut (as in the case of an amputation), it might be better to cut it at its tendinous portion rather than at its belly, to minimise bleeding. In certain situations, it is better to separate the muscle fibres and get through the muscle in order to reach a deeper structure instead of cutting through the muscle. Main nerve trunks should not be cut, as far as possible, during dissections; they may be carefully shifted aside.

4. *Control of haemorrhage.* Bleeding should be controlled at every stage during dissection. (See methods page 437)

5. *Obliteration of dead space.* The creation of so called *"dead space"* or vacant cavities should be avoided while closing the wound after surgery, because blood and exudates will collect there. (Such dead spaces might occur after removal of a tumour, removal of mammary gland, etc., if not properly sutured. Sometimes packing the cavity is desirable to avoid dead space.)

6. *Use of a minimum quantity of suture material.* Sin

suture materials are foreign bodies, only the minimum essential quantity should be used.

7. *Avoidance of suture tension.* Sutures should not be very tight on the edges of the wound; otherwise the blood supply to the edges is obstructed and causes delay in the healing process. The interference to blood supply at points where the edges of wound are crushed by the sutures may cause local necrosis facilitating sutures to cut through the tissue resulting in wound disruption.

8. *Immobilisation.* Immobilisation or preventing excessive movement of the wounded area is very important for healing to take place normally. Sutures. adhesive tapes. bandages. plaster casts. etc., help immobilisation by artificial means.

CHAPTER 4

Suture Materials

A suture is a thread used for uniting wound edges. Nylon, silk, cotton, catgut, stainless steel suture, etc., are some of the common suture materials used. The term "suture" is used for denoting a pattern of suturing also, e.g., interrupted suture, continuous suture. Lembert's suture.

The purpose of suturing a wound is to bring the edges of the wound close together, so that healing may take place quicker.

However, sutures are helpful only if other conditions necessary for primary healing are satisfied: (1) the wound should be fresh; (2) it should not be infected; (3) it should be free from haemorrhage; (4) there should be no obstruction to blood supply to the edges of the wound; (5) there should be protection from interference and infection; and (6) there should be no necrotic tissue.

The suturing of a septic wound is not indicated because it will result in accumulation of pus and may also facilitate growth of anaerobic bacteria.

Qualities of a Suture Material

The qualities desirable in a suture material are mentioned below.

1. *Tensile strength.* Tensile strength is the ability of a suture material to withstand breakage on stretching it. Tensile strength or "knot-pull-limits" is measured and expressed in terms of kg. or lb. by some manufacturers.

2. *Functional strength.* The functional strength of a suture material is the strength that it maintains in tissues when used as a suture. (It is called the tensile strength "in vivo".)

When a knot is tied in a suture there is some loss of strength of the suture material due to rubbing and bending. Inside the tissues. the absorption of moisture and various tissue reaction may reduce the strength. The type of suture material chosen must be such that it retains enough functional strength until healing is complete.

3. *Non-capillary.* Capillary action of a suture material is the capacity to absorb fluids and spread it along its length like the wick of a lamp. This property enables the suture material to absorb serum, exudates, pus, etc. A suture material should preferably be non-capillary.

4. *Non-reactivity.* It should not produce chemical or biological reaction in tissues.

5. *Should be tolerated by tissues.* The suture material should be non-irritant and must be tolerated by tissues.

6. *Flexibility and elasticity.*

7. *Easy to handle.* A suture material which is very stiff (like stainless steel) or one which is unduly pliable like cotton are inconvenient to handle. Hence it should be only moderately stiff and flexible.

8. *Knotable.* Should have the capacity to retain secure knots (knot-holding-power).

9. *Easily sterilisable.*

10. *Uniformity.* It should have a uniform thickness.

11. *Smooth surface.* A smooth surface is desirable for the suture material because it will reduce friction.

12. *Monofilament.* Suture material having single filament is better than a suture material made up of more than one filament.

13. *Absorbability.* An absorbable suture material is preferable in buried sutures.

The Suture-holding Power of Tissues

The suture-holding power of tissues depends upon the kind of tissue, its bulk or quantity held within the suture, the direction in which sutures are placed, and the distance between sutures.

Among soft tissues facia has the maximum suture-holding power and fat tissue the least. The holding power of muscle depends on whether sutures are placed across or parallel to the muscle fibres. When placed across the fibres, the holding power is better than when placed parallel to the fibres. If sutures are placed far apart, proper apposition of wound edges may not take place. But if they are placed too close together, the holding power of tissue diminishes. Therefore, an optimum distance between sutures should be maintained. Skin sutures are usually placed 3/8 inch (about 5 to 6 mm) apart. In the case of hollow visceral organs like intestines, sutures are placed as close as 1/8 inch (about 2 mm) apart to prevent leakage of contents.

Classification of Suture Materials

Suture materials may be classified into two broad categories namely, Absorbable sutures and Non-absorbable sutures.

ABSORBABLE SUTURES

Absorbable sutures are sutures which get absorbed by the tissues after a variable period of time. The absorption takes place by phagocytosis and enzymatic action.

1. *Catgut.* Catgut is the most commonly used absorbable suture. It is made out of the elastic sub-mucosa of sheep intestines. The absorption of catgut in tissues can be delayed by treating it with chromic acid. Catgut is therefore available as "plain catgut" and "chromicised catgut". The chromicised catgut is less irritating to tissues than plain catgut and also is more slowly absorbed. According to the degree of chromicising the following types are available.

Type	Degree of chromicising	Approximate number of days taken for absorption
Type-A	Plain	10 days
Type-B	Mild chromic	15 days
Type-C	Medium chromic	20 days
Type-D	Extra chromic	40 days

Among those listed above, medium chromic (Type-C) is the most commonly used. Plain catgut is used in tissues which heal rapidly, e.g., for suturing parietal peritoneum, ligaturing vessels, etc.

Chromic catgut is used in tissues which heal more slowly, e.g., for suturing muscle. Catgut is available in sealed glass tubes with some fluid preservative.

Since contact with water reduces the strength of catgut, it has to be properly preserved. Depending on the preservative used catgut is available either as *boilable* or *non-boilable* catgut. Boilable catgut is preserved in Xylol, or in solution of Toluene 99.75% plus Phenyl mercuric acetate 0.025%. These tubes can be sterilised by boiling, autoclaving, etc. Boilable catgut is somewhat stiff. To soften it, it is to be soaked in sterile water or normal saline before use.

Non-boilable catgut is supplied in tubes containing 90 to 95% alcohol and so it cannot be sterilised by boiling. Alcohol is a preservative for catgut but when preserved in lower concentrations of alcohol the strength is reduced because of proportionately higher water content. The minimum concentration of alcohol recommended for purpose of preserving catgut is 85% (Oehme, 1974, pp. 56).

Catgut is available in different thicknesses as follows:

Size No.	Diameter in millimetres (*Average*)
000 000 0 (i.e., 7/0)	0.04
000 000 (or, 6/0)	0.08
000 00 (or, 5/0)	0.14
000 0 (or, 4/0)	0.20
000 (or, 3/0)	0.25
00 (or, 2/0)	0.30 ⎫ Peritoneum, bowel wall (small
0 (or, 1/0)	0.40 ⎭ animals) and ligaturing vessels
1	0.48 ⎫ Muscle, facia (S.A.); Ligature larger
2	•0.50 ⎭ vessels.
3	0.60—Facia, muscle (L.A.).
4	0.70
5	0.80—Rumen, uterus, abdomen (L.A.)
6	0.90
7	1.02

Size No. 2/0 and 1/0 are suitable for sutures on peritoneum and bowel wall in small animal surgery and for ligaturing vessels, etc. Size No. 1 and 2 are commonly used for sutures of muscle, facia, etc. in small animal surgery.

In large animal surgery, Size No. 1 and 2 are used for ligaturing larger vessels; No. 3 for facia, muscle etc; No. 5 for rumen, uterus, abdomen, etc. (Oehme, 1974, pp. 56).

Qualities of catgut as a suture material. Possesses adequate functional strength. Easy to handle. Gets absorbed. It being slightly elastic, does not cause strangulation of tissues due to tightening of sutures. Some of the disadvantages of catgut are that it is costly, and that it may be prematurely absorbed in certain individuals who are extra-sensitive to catgut before healing is complete.

The absorption of catgut depends on many factors. The absorption is relatively slow in muscle and rapid in mucous membrane; it is quicker in animals having protein deficiency. In the presence of infection and suppuration as well as in individuals who are hyper-sensitive to catgut, the absorption is very fast. Chromicising slows the rate of absorption.

2. *Kangaroo tendon.* This is another absorbable suture material prepared out of the tendons taken from the tail of kangaroo. Being very strong, kangaroo tendons are useful for suturing joint capsules, hernial openings etc.

3. *Facia lata.* An absorbable suture material made out of facia lata of the bovine. Available in tape-like pieces it is preserved like catgut in glass tubes. This is only rarely used. Facia lata can be collected (usually from slaughter houses) and stored as follows. With usual aseptic precaution the skin over the thigh is reflected. The facia lata is cut and removed in half inch broad tape-like pieces. These pieces are transferred into glass tubes containing physiologic saline solution, incorporated with penicillin 200,000 units and streptomycin 0.25 grams per 10 cc. After thirty minutes the liquid is decanted off and the tube is sealed and kept in a refrigerator at −10°F. When needed for use the tube is broken and the facia is put in sterile physiological saline at room temperature.

4. *Cargile membrane.* This is a thin sheet of tissue made out of bovine caecum used to cover surfaces from which peritoneum has been removed. Not in general use.

5. *Polyglycolic acid suture material.* This is a new synthetic absorbable suture material. It is strong, non-collagenous and non-toxic (Oehme, 1974, pp. 56).

NON-ABSORBABLE SUTURES

These sutures do not get absorbed by the tissues. When used as outside sutures they are removed after healing is completed. If allowed to remain in tissues they get encapsulated.

1. *Silk*. This is a non-absorbable suture commonly used. It is cheap, easily available, easy to handle, easily sterilised by boiling and is well-tolerated by tissues. Silk is available in size numbers 0 to 14. A disadvantage of silk is that it is capillary.

2. *Silk worm gut*. This is prepared out of the silk sacs of the silkworm. It is actually "unborn silk". Available as short strands of 12 to 16 inches it has a smooth surface and is non-capillary.

3. *Cotton*. This is very cheap suture material. It can be sterilised by boiling. It is less irritating to tissues than silk or catgut. But like silk the capillary action is a disadvantage.

4. *Linen*. This is made out of superior quality cotton. It has good tensile strength.

5. *Nylon*. This is a synthetic product. It is non-capillary, strong, and has a smooth surface. It is somewhat stiff and therefore a little difficult to handle and to put secure knots. While using nylon, special knots called "nylon knots" should be put since ordinary surgical knots of nylon become loose very easily.

6. *Horse hair*. It is a cheap suture material. Non-capillary, flexible, easily sterilised by boiling it causes little tissue reaction. But it is not very strong.

7. *Umbilical tape*. This is cotton tape suture about one-eighth inch wide and is used to tie the umbilical cord of the new born. It is available in reels in plastic containers.

8. *Dermal suture*. This is a non-absorbable suture used for skin suture. It is silk coated with tanned gelatin or other protein substance. The protein coating prevents ingrowth of granulation tissue into the suture material and also makes it non-capillary. It is not available.

9. *Pagenstecher*. This is linen coated with proteinlike substance, available in glass tubes (like catgut). Though non-absorbable, they are used in gastro-intestinal surgery. It is not available.

10. *Vetafil*. This is a non-absorbable suture made out of a synthetic fibre. It is a patent product. It is non-irritant, non-capillary and easy to handle. Sizes commonly used are medium (diameter 0.2 mm) heavy (0.3 mm), extra heavy (0.4 mm) and special (1.1 mm).

11. *Stainless steel wire*. S.S wires of different sizes are used for suturing. They are very strong and are chemically inert. They

do not lose strength by wetting and are easily sterilised by boiling, autoclaving, etc. Also they are non-capillary and non-irritant. Its disadvantages are: 1) Being stiff, difficult to handle; 2) May cut through tissues; 3) Knots are insecure unless carefully placed; 4) Sharp ends may prick through tissues; 5) Continuous sutures may break into fragments when subjected to constant movement and therefore it is better to put interrupted suture only.

12. *Wires of tantallum, silver* etc., are similar to stainless steel wires, but are costlier.

13. *Aluminium wire.* It is more flexible than stainless steel.

14. *Wound clips.* Michel wound clips are sometimes used for skin sutures. The clips are made of a malleable metal. They are applied with special forceps and compared to sutures can be applied far more quickly. They do not enter into the wound and do not leave recognisable scars. But they are not strong enough to hold wound edges under tension and can be easily removed by the patient.

15. *Pin sutures.* Ordinary pins can be used for keeping skin edges together.

16. *Prolene.* Good synthetic material. non-irritable.

Choice of Suture Materials

All suture materials being foreign bodies, cause some tissue reaction. Non-absorbable sutures remain in tissue without causing reaction. provided they are sterile. Absorbable sutures get absorbed from tissue gradually by phagocytosis. The relative intensity of tissue reaction caused by different suture materials are illustrated below:—

Catgut	Maximum
Natural fibres like cotton	Less
Synthetic fibres, braided	
(i.e., containing more than one filament)	Lesser
Synthetic fibres, single strand	
(i.e., containing only one filament)	Least

In suturing wounds suspected to be heavily contaminated or where there is possibility of infection absorbable sutures are sometimes preferred, since the non-absorbable sutures persist in tissues and harbour the bacteria. For hollow organs like uterus, bladder, etc., absorbable sutures are preferred. Absorbable sutures (chromic catgut) are used for biliary tract and urinary tract to avoid any chance of leaving a portion of the suture to act as a focus for calculi formation.

Non-absorbable sutures are preferred in places where much tension is expected. Single strands are better as they cause lesser irritation to tissues, but knots are less secure with it than with multi-filament suture material.

Silicon-coated nylon is used for vascular surgery so that only the minimum tissue reaction is caused.

Steel, nylon and such other non-elastic and strong suture materials are used for uniting facia, tendon, etc.

Principles of Tying a Knot

(a) Knots placed in suture should be secure and maintain the suture in proper tension.

(b) Portions of suture material that have been crushed by clamps or artery forceps should not be included in a suture or a knot as the suture may break off at that point.

(c) While placing a knot, the sawing effect between the suture strands should be avoided as it will weaken the strands.

(d) The knots should be tight enough not to untie; but suture should not be excessively tight to cause strangulation, except in the case of haemostatic sutures.

(e) The completed knot should be small and compact. In buried knots the cut ends should be short so that the quantity of suture (which is a foreign body) left inside is minimum.

Types of Knots

There are innumerable types of knots. Only a few of them which are of interest to the surgeon are listed below. Students are advised to consult original references cited for more detailed description, especially for the figures.

1. *Square knot.* The first loop of the square knot is made by making a simple throw by turning around one of the two ends (say, end A) of the suture material around the other end (say, end B); and it is tightened carefully so that the ends do not cross and are pulled with equal tension. The second loop of the square knot is made by making what is called a reverse throw by taking the end B around A, unlike during the first throw. Here also the ends should not cross and should be pulled with equal tension.

A square knot may contain more than two throws to make

it more secure; in which case, each throw will be a reversal of the former.

2. *Half-hitch.* This is an incomplete knot. One end of the suture material is taken around the other to form loop. But when this loop is tightened, one end is pulled with greater tension than the other. (Unlike while placing a square knot.) It may also be noted in this connection that if one of the two ends of the square knot is unduly pulled, it will turn itself into a half-hitch and will become insecure.

3. *Granny knot.* In the granny knot, the first throw is made similar to the first throw of the square knot. But the next throw is made without reversing the ends.

Note. Students are advised to practice with a piece of thread to study the differences between square knot and granny knot and also the half-hitch.

4. *Surgeon's knot.* In the surgeon's knot the first loop is made by taking two turns of one of the suture ends against the other; and the second loop is similar to that of a square knot. Because of the additional turn in the first loop, it is not likely to get loosened in the process of placing the second loop. The surgeon's knot is more secure than a square knot. But it consumes more time, the size of the knot is larger, and hence places more suture material in the tissues. Some surgeons, therefore, prefer the square knot repeated twice or thrice to a surgeon's knot. Another disadvantage of surgeon's knot is that it fails to exert adequate tension if used for ligaturing small vessels, because of the additional turn and increased bulk of the first throw.

5. *Double surgeon's knot (Double reef knot).* It is recommended when using suture materials that are likely to slip. (e.f.,] nylon). This is actually a surgeon's knot plus a third throw, similar to the second throw. It is also called a *"Triple knot"* or *"Reinforced surgeon's double slip"* or *"Reverse knot"*, or *"Nylon knot"* or *Surgeon's knot with square knot.* This is a surgeon's knot with an additional square knot.

Methods of Tying the Final Finishing Knot to End a Continuous Suture

There are different methods of doing this, and will be demonstrated in the class. Also see Mayer *et al.*, 1959.

Buried Knots

In a sub-cuticular suture, the knot is buried and is not visible outside. The suture thread is passed through one of the edges of the skin starting from the sub-cutis upwards and is returned through the other edge in a reverse manner (i.e., from above downwards) so that the knot can be placed at the starting point of the suture in the sub-cutaneous space. When the next suture is placed the first knot is automatically covered by the tissues. In a continuous sub-cuticular suture also the beginning knot is placed in a similar manner and gets covered when the suture is tightened. The finishing knot also can be buried with a little care.

Questions

1. Indicate the suture material you would prefer to use for each of the following, explaining the reasons for your choice and also mentioning the disadvantages, if any:—
a. Subcutaneous facia b. Laparotomy along linea alba in bovine c. Closure of hernial ring in inguinal hernia in bitch·d. Hernial ring, ventral hernia, cow·e. Subcuticular suture·f. Suture of bone fragments.

2. What is the major advantage of a surgeon's knot? Compare it with a square knot.

CHAPTER 5

Suture Patterns, Instruments and Technique

The suture patterns are broadly classified into interrupted sutures and continuous sutures. Special sutures used for various purposes like tension sutures, tendon sutures, suture for vessels, nerve sutures, etc., may also fall in one of these two categories. Clip sutures, pin sutures, safety pin sutures, etc., belong to a different type, but may be compared to interrupted sutures.

Suture patterns may further be classified as: (1) Apposition sutures, (2) Inversion sutures, (3) Eversion sutures, (4) Purse-string suture (tobacco-pouch suture), (5) Tension suture (relaxation suture), and (6) Other miscellaneous sutures.

Examples under the various categories are listed below. Students are expected to draw diagrams of each by referring to any of the books cited, and also practice with a needle and thread.

Interrupted Sutures

When the wound is sutured by a number of independent sutures, they are called interrupted sutures. Generally speaking, interrupted sutures are preferable to continuous sutures because even if one suture in the line is broken or untied the others may not be affected. But interrupted sutures are more time-consuming. require more suture material. and the large number of bulky knots is a disadvantage.

1. *Simple interrupted sutures.* It is the most commonly used suture for the skin. The suture penetrates one edge from outside and goes to the other edge pierces it from underneath and comes out on the skin of the other edge, the knot is tied and the excess suture material is cut off distal to the knot,

The suture when tied is at right angles to the line of incision. It goes across the line of incision. The knot should be on one side and not on the line of incision. The point of piercing of each edge is usually one-eighth inch (2 to 3 mm) from the line of incision. It will be more convenient to start the suture from the distal edge and then go through the proximal edge. See that the skin edges are not inverted while the suture is being tied; it may be just apposition: or. if not. slightly everted.

The distance between sutures varies, but usually three-eighth inch (0.6 c.m.) is sufficient.

2. *Mattress suture* (*Horizontal mattress suture; Interrupted horizontal mattress suture; Four-stitch interrupted suture; U-suture*). This suture is preferable to simple interrupted suture where tension is expected. It is actually a relaxation suture (tension suture) also, in addition to being an apposition suture. If it is tightened, eversion of wound edges also can be brought about.

The suture is started like a simple interrupted suture but it returns to the same edge of the wound travelling in a U-shaped manner, and is tied. When tied, the exposed pieces of the suture are seen parallel to and on either side of the line of incision.

3. *Mattress suture through rubber tubing.* When the tension expected is too much, and the sutures are likely to cut through the skin, it is desirable to pass the exposed portions of the mattress suture through small pieces of rubber tubing kept parallel to the edges.

4. *Cross-mattress suture* (*X-mattress suture*). Here the exposed portion of mattress suture is passed to the opposite edge diagonally (instead of at right angles to the suture line), presenting the appearance of "X". The concealed portion is parallel to each edge.

The advantage is that it brings about better apposition than a simple horizontal mattress suture described above.

5. *Interrupted inverted mattress suture.* Here the exposed portion of the suture is seen across the line of incision and the concealed portion runs parallel to the line of incision. Suture is not made to pierce through the mucous coat in a hollow organ but runs through the muscular coat.

6. *Halstead suture.* This is actually a double interrupted Lembert's suture using a single thread which is reversed to the

same side and tied.   It is different from a simple horizontal mattress suture.

7. *Vertical mattress suture.*   Unlike in the horizontal mattress suture, the exposed portions of the suture on either side of the incision are at right angles (vertical) to the line of incision instead of being parallel.

The suture pierces the skin of the one edge from outside about 0.5 to 1.0 cm away from the line of incision and pierces the opposite edge at an equal distance from below upwards. It then pierces the skin of the second side close to the line of incision and reverses to the original side, and the knot is tied. The tightening is done to bring about just apposition of edges and not eversion.

Vertical mattress sutures also have the capacity for withstanding tension and are even better than horizontal mattress sutures in this respect. They cause less interference in the blood supply to the edge than the horizontal sutures.

The disadvantages are that it is more time-consuming and uses more suture material in the tissue.

8. *Donati's vertical mattress suture.*   This differs from an ordinary vertical mattress suture slightly. The suture material is exposed in only one of the two edges because in the other edge it is intracutaneous.

9. *Crushing (or, Gambee) suture.*   This is a special type of apposition suture suitable for intestinal anastomosis. The passage of suture through the two cut ends of the intestine facing each other, is as follows, starting from serosa of one edge to the serosa of the other edge : From the serosa to the lumen: prick mucous membrane close to the edge and come out through the muscularis. Next penetrate through the corresponding muscularis of the opposing edge and into its lumen and prick mucous membrane of that lumen slightly away from where it entered: come out through serosa: and the two ends of the suture are tightened and tied. When this is done the mucous edges are slightly inverted, and the remaining portions of the edges are only brought into apposition. Crushing suture is preferable to ordinary inversion sutures when the lumen of the bowel to be united is small. As the edges are not fully inverted, the lumen is not obstructed. (Do not confuse the name "crushing" with "Cushing" on next page.)

Continuous Sutures

In a continuous suture a series of stitches are made up of the same continuous thread so that only the first and last stitches are tied. The advantage of a continuous suture is that it takes less time than interrupted sutures covering the same distance. However, the *disadvantages are*: damage to the suture anywhere along its length makes it loose and the wound may disrupt; a continuous suture is not as good as an interrupted suture in places exposed to much tension; and if not carefully placed, proper apposition of edges may not be obtained.

1. *Simple continuous suture (Furrier's suture).* This is started as a simple interrupted suture and the subsequent stitches are continued with the same thread till the final knot is tied. The running suture pass through the *tissues* at right angles to the edges and the *exposed portion* of the suture go diagonally to the line of incision.

Useful for peritoneum, muscles, etc., but not usually recommended for skin as perfect apposition of edges may not be brought about.

2. *Continuous lock stitch (Blanket stitch; Ford inter-locking suture; Reverdin s continuous suture).* The "locking" is brought about by passing the needle and thread through each loop of the simple continuous suture before it is tightened. The stitches hold the tissues in better apposition because of the "locking".

3. *Continuous Lembert's suture.* This is an inversion type suture used for hollow viscera like intestines. Sutures pass through serosa and muscular and sub-mucous coats, but *not* through the mucous membrane. The suture runs at right angles across the line of incision through the tissues; and the exposed portion of the suture runs diagonally, so that the adjacent portions of suture passing through tissues are parallel to each other.

4. *Connell suture.* It is an inversion suture. The suture passes through each edge alternatively. It penetrates through all coats of a hollow organ including the mucous membrane in the case of bowel. When tightened, the suture thread is hardly visible outside, except at the knots. During the process of placing, the portions of suture that are visible are at right angles to the line of incision and those that are within the tissue of either edge are parallel to the line of incision.

5. *Cushing suture.* Similar to Connell suture the only diffe-

rence is that cushing suture do not penetrate the mucous coat and enter the lumen.

6. *The Parker-Kerr suture* is a cushing suture which is used to close a stump. It is first passed around the forceps holding the stump, and then the forceps is withdrawn and the suture is tightened and tied. It can also be used as a temporary stay suture without knots in intestinal anastomosis, to close each of the segments of intestines temporarily.

7. *Modified cushing (Guard's suture)*. Similar to Cushing's but is extended beyond the two commissures at the starting and ending of the suture, imagining an extended line of incision. The advantage is better efficiency in preventing leakage of contents.

8. *Continuous inverting mattress sutures*. Connell and Cushing sutures are examples of this.

9. *Schmieden's suture*. This is a continuous suture for the intestines which should always be covered by a continuous Lembert or Cushing suture because the suture partially enters the lumen. The suture which comes out through the serous surface of one edge during the course of placement goes over to the mucous surface of the other edge and comes out through the serous surface of that edge. The advantage of Schmieden's suture is its quick placement.

10. *Continuous everting mattress suture*. This is indicated when the edges of a skin suture are to be everted by a continuous suture. The pattern of running the suture is somewhat similar to a Connell suture, with the important difference that unlike Connell the exposed threads are parallel to the line of incision while those buried in tissue run across the edges.

11. *Continuous sub-cuticular (sub-epidermal) suture*. The suture is similar to a continuous horizontal mattress suture except that it does not come outside the skin. Instead, the bites are taken in the inner layers of the skin (the sub-cuticular layers). If the suture is not to be removed, absorbable suture is used and the beginning and ending knots are buried. The opposing *surfaces* of the two edges can be brought about in good apposition, and the patient need not be brought to the hospital again for suture removal. Since the suture is not exposed, there is less chance of the patient interfering with it.

If non-absorbable suture material is used, removal after healing can be facilitated by keeping the knots exposed (instead of buried). To remove the suture, snip the suture at the knot at one end and pull off by the other end.

12. *Shoe-maker's stitch* (*Cobbler's stitch*). There are three different methods for applying this suture as explained below. It causes eversion of the edges, and the suture on either side seen from outside, in the completed stage, is parallel to the line of incision. The degree of eversion can be adjusted by the degree of tightening and by the distance from the line of incision.

(a) The suture material is threaded by a separate needle at each end of it. One of the needles pricks through both edges of the wound at the starting point and the length of the suture thread is adjusted equally on both sides. The two needles one after the other are then taken through the same points of both edges for the next prick, but from different directions. The suture ends are pulled and tightened. The process is repeated for subsequen' pricks and finally the two ends are knotted.

(b) Another method is by using a long needle with a handle and with eye close to its tip called *Shoe-maker's needle* or *Cobbler's needle*. The needle without suture is passed through the edges at the starting point, and then threaded and pulled back. The length of suture on either side is adjusted equally. Make the next prick with the threaded needle and afterwards remove the suture end from the eye. Introduce the other end of suture through the eye of the needle and pull back the needle. Tighten the suture ends to make the first grip of the stitch. Continue the procedure up to the end of the incision and knot the ends.

(c) In a third method, using the Shoe-maker's needle or Cobbler's needle, the suture thread is passed through both edges of the wound and its length is adjusted almost equally on both sides. The needle carrying the longer end of the suture is again passed through both edges of the wound for the next prick. The thread brought by the needle on the opposite side is held with the fingers and the needle alone is drawn back from tissues. This leaves a loop of suture material within the fingers. Next step is to trace the other suture end at the starting point and pass it through the loop held within the fingers. Hold the two ends of the suture material (i.e., one carrying the needle and the other free end that has been passed through the loop of opposite side), separately and pull them to tighten the loop. The process is repeated to the whole length of the wound and finally the two ends are tied to make a knot. It will be noted here that there are two components of the suture thread, namely, one carried by the needle and forming a loop at every prick and the other free component which commonly passes through these loops. It is necessary to tighten them after each prick.

TENSION SUTURES (RELAXATION SUTURES)

A tension suture or relaxation suture is used to relieve tension on the edges of the wound. Sometimes they are used to relieve tension on another set of sutures already placed. Many of them may be grouped under a special type of interrupted sutures, but it is more convenient to study them separately.

1. *Quill suture and Stent suture.* These are vertical mattress sutures in which pieces of quill or gauze, are incorporated on either side.

2. *Far-near and Near-far suture.* These are sutures going very deep into tissues besides the skin. For purposes of explanation, imagine two points on the skin at right angles to the line of incision, on each of the skin edges. Let us mark them as A and B on one side and C and D on the other side. Points A and D are the points far away from the line of incision; and B and C are the near points.

The suture entering the tissues through A comes out through C on the other side (hence called "far-near"), and then the suture reverses through points B and D (hence "near-far"), and is tied.

3. *Far-far and Near-near suture.* This name also indicates the course of passage of the suture thread through the two edges of the wound successively.

4. Deeply placed simple interrupted sutures may be used as a relaxation suture to support another set of sutures.

5. Mattress sutures already described are also used as tension sutures.

BONE SUTURES

Stainless steel wire may be used to suture broken fragments of bone in a fracture.

1. *Circlage.* The wire is taken around the bone fragments. The disadvantage is the possibility of necrosis of bone due to

pressure on the periosteum.

2. *Hemi-circlage*. This ensures less pressure on the periosteum. One or two holes are drilled into each opposing fragment and the suture wire is passed through the holes and tied.

TENDON SUTURES

There are different methods of doing this. The underlying principles are that the suture cutting through the tendon should be prevented; and that the cut surfaces of the tendon should oppose each other and should be brought as close together as possible without much tension on them, if not in close apposition.

The cutting through of suture through tendon tissue is prevented by "weaving" the suture through each piece for a variable distance, or by passing it through the thickness in one or more "cross-wise" pattern.

The opposing of cut ends is assured by pricking the suture needle through *corresponding* points of the two cut surfaces.

SUTURES FOR VESSELS

These are everted sutures to bring the innermost tunic (endothelial layer) of the cut ends of the vessel into close contact. Two or three stay sutures may be placed as a preliminary to putting the sutures.

NERVE SUTURES

Nerve sutures are not likely to be successful unless done carefully under an operating microscope to guide the nerve fibres correctly. They do not have any practical value in veterinary surgery.

Another Classification for Suture Patterns

Suture patterns may also be classified as 1) Apposition sutures, 2) Inversion sutures, 3) Eversion sutures, 4) Purse string sutures (Tobacco-pouch sutures), 5) Relaxation (Tension) sutures, and 6) Miscellaneous sutures.

1. *Apposition sutures*. These sutures bring about apposition of the edges of the wound. They are commonly used for wounds on skin, muscles, oesophagus, etc. Examples are simple interrupted suture, simple continuous suture or Glover's

suture, continuous lock stitch or Blanket Stitch, Pin suture and sub-cuticular suture.

2. *Inversion sutures.* In these sutures the edges of the wound are inverted and brought together. They are indicated in hollow visceral organs which have a serous outer coat, like stomach, intestines, uterus, etc. When sutured the serous surfaces of either edge come in contact. The serous exudation from these surfaces coagulates and provides a seal along the suture line. Inversion sutures are therefore very efficient in preventing leakage of contents from the interior of the viscera that is sutured.

Examples are Lembert's suture. Czerny's suture. Connel's Suture. Cushing suture. etc.

Lembert's suture passes through the serous, mucular and submucous coats but not through the mucous coat. Lembert's may be of the interrupted or continuous patterns. The individual stitches are as close as one-eighth inch so as to prevent leakage of contents.

Czerny's suture is a double row of Lembert's sutures, one row covering the other.

3. *Eversion sutures.* The edges are everted, e.g., certain skin sutures and sutures uniting cut ends of vessels.

4. *Purse-string suture (Tobacco-pouch suture).* This suture is used to narrow the lumen of a hollow organ, or to close its stump during surgery. Also employed for constricting anal and vulvar openings after reduction of prolapse of rectum/vagina/uterus etc.

5. *Relaxation sutures (Tension sutures).* Examples are interrupted sutures used as relaxation sutures; Quilled suture; Button suture (similar to quilled suture but using buttons instead); Mattress sutures; Vertical mattress suture; "Near-and-far" sutures; Tension suture passed through rubber tubes kept over and across the incision; Tension sutures tied over gauze roll placed over line of incision; etc.

Miscellaneous Sutures

Figure-of-eight-suture. Figure-of-eight suture for laparotomy which may be used to close laparotomy wound in large animals. The suture starts from one of the skin edges, goes to muscular and parietal peritoneal edges of the opposite side, and then to corresponding peritoneo-muscular edge of opposite side penetrating it from within outwards, crosses over diagonally to opposite skin edge and comes out through it, and the two ends are knotted.

This suture can also be put as a double suture if the end emerging from the skin surface is reversed again through the tissues before placing the knot; in the case of the double figure-of-eight suture the knot comes on the same side where the suture was started.

When properly placed and tightened, a single figure-of-eight suture has an *outside appearance* of a simple interrupted suture and the double figure-of-eight suture may look like a horizontal mattress suture, even though their internal arrangements are different.

(ii) *Retension suture.* Used to retain gauze packings inside a wound cavity.

(iii) *Staple-type suture.* In which one edge is placed over the other and sutured.

(iv) *Overlapping or sliding stitch.* One edge overlaps the other. Used for closing certain hernial rings.

(v) *Various tendon sutures.* Co-apting sutures, suturing splayed tendons, etc.

Instruments Used for Suturing

The chief instruments used in suturing are suture needles and needle holders (needle forceps). Tissue forces to hold edges during suturing, scissors to cut suture ends, wire-shears while using wire-sutures, etc., are the accessory instruments.

Suture needles are available in different shapes, e.g., straight, half-curved, half-circle, three-eight circle, etc. Generally speaking curved needles are better suited for suturing deeply placed tissues.

The tip or end of the needle may be either smoothly tapering (round-bodied and tapering) or cutting or having sharp cutting edges (i.e., the cross section of the tip is triangular).

The eye of the needle may be circular or oval or rectangular. It may be close to one end of the needle or away from it, or in the centre, etc. Eyeless needles or atraumatic needles are also available. In an atraumatic needle the suture material is attached firmly with the needle.

A round-bodied straight needle with smooth tapering end is suitable for delicate tissues like mucous membrane, peritoneum, liver, etc., which tear very easily.

A straight needle with cutting tip is used for skin, tendon, facia, etc., which are tough and not very deeply situated.

Half-curved needle has one half of its body straight and the other half gradually curves toward the tip so that the point is at 45 degrees with the proximal half of the body.

Half-circle needle is similar to a semi-circle. It penetrates tissues almost at 180 degrees and are suitable for deep-seated tough tissues.

Mayo needle is a strong half-circle needle with a cutting tip and a square eye. Specially suitable for penetrating tough tissues that are located deeply.

Suture Technique

1. *Analgesia.* This is necessary only in the case of very sensitive and restless animals. Local analgesic solution is injected subcutaneously in the form of weals along the edges by introducing the inoculation needle through the wound itself.

2. *Use of Needle Holder.* (needle forceps, Needle-holding forceps). When needles of small size are used it is more convenient to use a needle holder. The needle holder should be clamped away from the eye of the needle. Curved needles should be held at the tip of the jaws of the forceps as otherwise the shape of the needle might get altered.

3. *Use of tissue forceps.* Tissue forceps are used to hold the edges of a wound while suturing. This should be done gently without causing excessive trauma.

4. *Avoid excessive tension on sutures.* If there is much tension on sutures they may cut through tissues or may interfere with blood supply to the edges of the wound. Tension can be minimised with the help of relaxation sutures.

5. *Size of suture material.* Suture material should be sufficiently thick and strong enough to withstand tension. Thinner sutures are preferable to excessively thick ones provided they are strong enough.

6. *Method of placing knots.* Knots must be tight and compact as otherwise they are likely to become loose and suture will give way. The pattern of knot ordinarily recommended is the *Surgeon's Knot.* The *Nylon Knot* and *Triple Knot* are advisable while using stiff suture materials. The ordinary *Granny Knot*

should never be used in surgery. A forceps or needle holder may be used for placing knots.

7. *Length of the cut ends* of the suture (after tying the knot) need not be longer than one-eighth to one-fourth of an inch. But if they are very short the knot may become loose and open.

8. *Method of opening a tube of catgut.* Place the tube inside a rolled up towel and hold it at either end with hands. Break the tube by bending. The glass pieces are discarded. The catgut is pulled and stretched before being used for suture.

9. *Handling the suture.* Remember that while suturing, the loose portion of the suture should not be allowed to drag along but should be gathered in the hand; as far as possible do not crush the suture by holding with forceps while placing knots; if a portion is crushed with forceps do not use that part for further suturing; and do not pull the suture excessively as it will lessen its strength.

10. *Method of threading the needle.* A convenient method of threading the needle is done by holding the suture tip within two fingers and pressing the needle eye to it.

11. *Removal of sutures.* While removing sutures the soiled portion of the suture should not be allowed to pass through the tissues. First, clean the area with spirit and apply a good antiseptic (Tr. Iodine) over it. Hold the suture and gently lift it so that a little of its buried portion is exposed. Cut at this newly exposed part and draw out the suture. After removing the suture, an alcoholic solution (Tr. Iodine) is applied over the area to seal the small openings on the skin left by the suture.

LIGATION

A ligature is a suture material used for tying vessels. Ligation of blood vessels is done in almost all surgical operations. Ligation of large vessels should be done in such a way that the ligature will not slip. For such vessels a transfixing ligature is preferable.

Questions

1. What are the suture materials commonly used for suturing wounds? Which material would you recommend for internal sutures? Why?

2. Enumerate the advantages and disadvantages of a good suture material giving examples wherever necessary.

3. Write short notes on: i) Suture materials, ii) Suture patterns, iii) Rules in suturing and factors that influence healing, iv) Ligation of vessels.

4. Give a full account of the type of sutures and suture materials used in cattle and dogs. What are the causes of disruption of sutures in such operations?

5. Describe the methods of suturing adopted for surgical wounds and discuss the choice of material used in each group of situation depending on the depth of tissue involved.

6. Write a short essay on suture materials and their choice with reference to the various methods of suturing and the uses to which suture materials are put in veterinary surgical practice.

CHAPTER 6

Wounds

A wound is a break in the continuity of soft tissues caused by trauma.

Wounds may be broadly classified into two categories, viz., Closed wounds and Open wounds.

Closed Wounds

A closed wound is a wound in which there is no break in continuity of skin (or mucous membrane), but the underlying tissues are damaged to a varying degree, e.g., contusion, bruise, haematoma.

Contusion. A contusion is produced by blunt objects and results in damage to subcutaneous tissues without breaking the continuity of the skin surface. Contusions are classified into first, second and third degrees according to the extent or severity of the injury.

Bruise. A bruise is a mild degree contusion. It is character-ised by rupture of capillaries in the skin giving rise to a reddish blue or purplish colouration of skin (Echymosis). (The colouration of skin, however, is not appreciable in animals with deeply pig-mented skin.)

Haematoma. A heamatoma is a collection of blood in an abnormal cavity. It is usually caused by injury to a superficial vein. Haematomas are frequently seen subcutaneously or sub-mucously. The common seats of haematoma in various species are:

Cow: (1) Mammary vein. *Cause*: Chance of rubbing against hard ground, butting by the calf. (2) Vaginal mucous membrane. *Cause*: Injury during copulation.

Bull: Haematoma involving the penis. *Cause* : Injury during copulation.

Horse: Spur vein or external thoracic vein. Likely cause of injury by the rider.

Dog: (1) Ear flap. (2) Vaginal mucous membrane. *Cause*: Injury during copulation.

Open Wounds

An open wound is a wound in which there is break in the continuity of skin. Open wounds are classified into the following categories.

Incised wounds. Incised wounds are caused by sharp cutting instruments, such as knives, scalpels, fragments of glass etc. An incised wound tends to gape, the extent of gaping depending upon the elasticity and tension of the surrounding tissues. Its edges are regular and there is comparatively less injury to cells. It bleeds freely and may be painful. If the edges are in apposition and the wound is protected from infection it heals by first intention.

2. *Lacerated wounds.* A lacerated wound presents torn and uneven edges. Sometimes the skin may be more or less extensively injured and it may be lifted over a wide area from underlying tissues.

3. *Punctured wounds.* Punctured wounds are caused by sharp pointed objects like nails. They have a relatively small opening and may be very deep. Infection or foreign particles might have been carried deep into the wound. The opening is inadequate for drainage. Example: Punctured wounds on foot due to gathered nail.

4. *Penetrating wounds.* These are deep wounds communicating with cavities like abdomen, thorax, joints, larynx, trachea, etc. Example: Stab wounds.

5. *Perforating wounds.* A perforating wound has two openings, one of entrance and the other of exit, e.g., perforating wounds of neck, leg, thorax, abdomen, head etc. (*Note*: The terms "perforating wounds" and "penetrating wounds" are sometimes used synonymously.)

6. *Gunshot wounds.* These are produced by various types of fire arms. The point of entrance of the bullet is marked by a smaller opening on the skin but the course of the bullet in deeper tissues exhibits more extensive damage.

7. *Abrasions.* Abrasions are wounds in which the superficial layers of skin only are removed.

8. *Avulsions (Evulsions).* An avulsion is a wound in which

there is actual loss of tissue. Examples: evulsion of hoof, evulsion of horn.

2. *Aseptic wound.* It is a surgical wound made under aspetic conditions wherein the chance of bacterial contamination is practically avoided.

10. *Contaminated wounds.* A contaminated wound is a wound in which micro-organisms are present. Strictly speaking, all wounds other than aseptic wounds are contaminated wounds.

Infected wounds (Septic wounds). An infected wound is a wound in which micro-organisms have invaded the tissues and have started multiplying and producing toxins. (A contaminated wound may become infected after a *"lag period"* of six to eight hours.)

11. *Granulating wounds.* A granulating wound is a wound which is showing tendency to heal.

12. *Ulcerating wounds.* An ulcerating wound is a wound which has no tendency to heal.

Symptoms

The symptoms resulting from wounds may be described as local, general, and remote. *Local symptoms* include haemorrhage, pain, gaping of the lips of the wound and the phenomena of repair. *General symptoms* comprise those of febrile disturbance, and vary according to the virulence of the infecting organism and the degree of injury to the tissues and the toxaemia.

Remote symptoms are observed on a part away from the wound. Examples: abscess formation in a dependent lymph gland; paralysis or loss of sensation to a dependent part or neuritis extending along the course of a nerve involved in the wound.

Healing of a Wound

Healing of a wound may take place by any of the following methods, viz., first intention healing (primary union), second intention healing, mixed intention healing, third intention healing and healing under a scab.

1. *First intention healing (primary union).* In first intention healing the narrow space between the edges of the wound is at first filled with blood clot. The capillaries and fibroblasts grow into this from the edges and healing is completed in about five to fourteen days. The scar tissue formed in first intention

healing is very little. By about the third day, proliferating capillaries appear in the wound. And by about the fourth day, fibroplasia also is evident. Until fibroplasia starts, the wound has little tensile strength. Sufficient tensile strength is obtained by ten to fourteen days.

For primary healing to take place, the following conditions are to be satisfied. The wound should be clean and fresh. It should be free from infection. It should be free from bleeding. There should not be any foreign bodies and there should be only the minimum of dead cells. Must have good blood supply to its edges. The part should be given rest (immobilisation). In wounds involving different layers of tissue the edges of the respective anatomical layers should be in proper alignment and apposition.

2. *Second intention healing (healing by granulation).* Second intention healing is by "replacement of tissue". It happens in wounds having extensive loss of tissue and in wounds whose edges are widely separated. The granulation tissue consisting of budding capillaries and fibroblasts grow from the edges and the bottom of the wound to fill up the gap. The granulation tissue is a highly vascular tissue. It is velvety in appearance, soft, moist and pink. It is called granulation tissue because of the granular appearance presented by the numerous budding capillaries. These capillaries grow up and anastomose with each other forming a network. The fibrous tissue also proliferates and the fibres are interlaid among the capillaries. With this growth of fibrous tissue and capillaries coming up to the surface of the wound, the surface epithelium also grows from its borders and makes healing complete. At a later stage the fibrous tissue contracts, causing constriction and obliteration of most of the newly formed capillaries, thereby giving the characteristic pale colour of scar tissue or cicatrix. Healing by second intention takes fourteen to twenty-one days. Large wounds with extensive loss of tissue may take about six weeks or more.

3. *Mixed intention healing.* Mixed intention healing is the healing of a wound partly by first intention and partly by second intention. This happens when a sutured wound has partially disrupted.

4. *Third intention healing* (Healing by secondary suture). Third intention healing takes place when the granulating surfaces

of an extensive wound, which may otherwise heal only by second intention, are united by sutures so as to bring about quicker healing.

5. *Healing under a scab.* This type of healing occurs in superficial wounds like abrasions. The exudate present in the wound dries up and forms a scab. Underneath this scab the healing process (granulation) takes place and when it is complete the scab automatically separates and is cast off.

Factors Responsible for Delayed Healing of Wounds

The factors responsible for delayed wound healing may be summarised as follows.

1. *Bacterial infection.*
2. *Foreign bodies in the wound.* Foreign bodies like metallic or glass pieces, thorns, suture material, dead tissues, etc., increases exudation and delays the reparative process.
3. *De-vitalisation of tissues.* Devitalised tissues provide good media for bacterial growth. They also exhibit poor reparative capacity.
4. *Desiccation of tissue.* Desiccation of tissue due to prolonged exposure to air causes devitalisation and delays healing.
5. *Haematomas and serum collections.* Haematomas and serum collections provide media for bacterial growth and thereby delay healing.
6. *Improper apposition of tissue, dead space etc.* If there is a wide gap between the edges, healing is delayed. When the cut edge of a particular tissue is united to another tissue, proper healing may not take place, (eg., apposition of a skin edge with a muscle edge). If there is interposition of tissue between the edges (e.g., portion of omentum protruding through a laparotomy wound) healing is interfered with. "Dead space" (vacant space left between tissue layers) delays healing as this additional space also must get filled up by granulation tissue.
7. *Inadequate blood supply.* Inadequate blood supply from any cause delays healing by causing ischaemia and devitalisation of tissue. Tightly placed sutures and plaster casts interfere with blood supply.
8. *Presence of malignant neoplastic tissue.*
9. *Lack of immobilisation.* Frequent movement of the wounded area causes rupture of the newly-formed granulation

tissue and therefore delays healing.

10. *Chemical and mechanical trauma.* Death of cells or devitalisation of cells may be caused by chemical trauma (like strong antiseptics) or by mechanical trauma (frequent movements, blows etc.) and delayed healing may result.

11. *Old age.* Wound healing progresses slowly in animals of advanced age.

12. *Malnutrition.* Malnutrition, especially protein deficiency, predisposes to delayed healing of wounds.

13. *Vitamin C deficiency.* Vitamin C is necessary for the formation of intercellular substance and the maturation of pre-collagen of connective tissue. Therefore a deficiency of this vitamin interferes with proper healing.

14. *Vitamin K deficiency.* Vitamin K is concerned with coagulation of blood. Deficiency of vitamin K predisposes to bleeding and formation of haematomas and serum collections and thereby delays healing.

15. *Deficiencies of other vitamins.* Vitamins A, D, thiamin, riboflavin, pantothenic acid, etc. also cause delayed healing of wounds.

16. *Dehydration, water-logging, oedema etc.* are other factors that might delay the healing of wounds.

Healing and Regeneration Capacities of Different Tissues

1. *Skin.* Skin has good capacity for healing, provided the edges are in apposition.

2. *Mucous membrane.* Wounds on mucous surfaces like mouth, vagina, conjunctiva etc. heal very rapidly.

3. *Serous membrane (Mesothelium).* The healing on serous surfaces is quick. When a large area is involved, small islands of cells grow here and there and unite with each other to fill up the gap.

4. *Muscle.* Muscle tissue is not regenerated, but is replaced by fibrous tissue.

5. *Connective tissue.* Connective tissue has great capacity for regeneration.

6. *Tendon.* The elastic tissue of tendon is not regenerated but is replaced by fibrous tissue.

7. *Adipose tissue.* Adipose tissue, which is only a modified connective tissue is generated.

8. *Neurons.* Neurons (nerve cells) once destroyed are not regenerated. But nerve fibres regenerate depending on the severity of the injury, if the neutron is intact.

9. *Hyaline cartilage* is not regenerated, but is replaced by connective tissue.

Treatment of Wounds

(a) *Contusions* (See page 653)

(b) *Haematomas* when small get absorbed. Otherwise they may have to be opened and treated.

The first step in the treatment of *open wounds* is control of bleeding.

(c) *Aseptic incised wounds* and fresh, noninfected wounds are sutured whenever practicable, to bring about healing by first intention.

(d) *Contaminated and infected wounds* (*septic wounds*) are treated on the following general principles:

1. *Control of bleeding.* Bleeding is controlled and ligaturing large vessels, if any.

2. *Cleaning of the wound.* The hair around the wound are clipped, taking care to see that the cut pieces of hair do not enter the wound. The wound and surrounding areas are irrigated with mild, non-irritant, antiseptic lotion for removing dirt and dead tissue. The following lotions are commonly used: Perchloride of mercury lotion (1 in 1000) and Acriflavin lotion (1 in 500). Eusol lotion contains eupad 1 in 40. (Eupad is a mixture of bleaching powder and boric acid.) Hypertonic saline solution (5 to 10%) is also used for irrigating wounds; it is good for removing dead cells and discharges.

If the wound is fresh suturing may be attempted. Suturing should not be done if there is infection or foreign bodies as this will cause accumulation of discharges.

Wounds that are not sutured may be irrigated daily or on alternate days. Application of normal blood serum to the wound is reported to have beneficial effects on the tissue resistance and phagocytosis. Lactoserum (milk serum or whey) also has the same effect as blood serum.

In wounds of feet warm antiseptic foot-baths (10% Formalin) may be given.

3. *Control of infection.* After irrigating the wound it is covered with a moist antiseptic pad or an antiseptic powder or ointment to prevent further infection. Moist antiseptic pad is prepared by soaking cotton wool in antiseptic lotions. Antiseptic powders commonly used are boric acid, eupad (bleaching powder+boric acid), Iodoform, BIPP (bismuth subntiras (1 Part)+Iodoform (2 Parts)+liquid paraffin sufficient to make a paste), sulphanilamide powder etc. Ointments commonly used are boric ointment, penicillin ointment, streptomycin ointment, chloromycetin ointment, terramycin ointment, etc. If there is infection, antibiotics are also given orally or parenterally in addition. In treating wounds of horses a prophylactic dose of antitetanus serum (1500 to 3000 units) is always recommended because of their great susceptibility to tetanus. Application of very strong antiseptics to a wound should be avoided as it will destroy the granulation tissue and delay healing. When the wound is healing normally, as indicated by the presence of healthy granulation tissue, an emollient mildly antiseptic ointment or an oily dressing like sulphanilamide-shark liver oil is the best.

4. *Providing drainage.* (Sterilised gauze/Capillaty tubes/Perforated tubes.) If there is exudation and discharge, the wound should not be sutured. If it is very deep it is advisable to keep a fenestrated rubber tube in the wound for drainage. A deep wound with narrow external opening may have to be enlarged for providing adequate drainage. If the external opening of a deep wound is not in a position suitable for drainage, a counter-opening may be made in a dependant part and a seton may be passed through it.

5. *Immobilising a wounded area.* If proper immobilisation (vide page 10) is not provided, healing is delayed and there is likely to be formation of excessive granulation tissue (*"exuberant granulation"; "proud flesh"*). Exuberant granulations are usually seen on wounds below the knee and hock. The excess growth of granulation tissue protruding through the wound should be suppressed for proper healing to take place. For this purpose, powdered caustic (like copper sulphate or potassium permanganate) is applied over the wound and pressure bandages is put. When the bandage is changed after about 48 hours, a superficial

layer of the granulation tissue that has been destroyed by the caustic also comes away with the bandage. This treatment is repeated 2 or 3 days until the excess granulations are completely removed. If the growth of granular tissue is too much and cannot be suppressed like this with the use of chemicals, it may have to be removed surgically. (See also addendum on page 654).

TREATMENT OF PUNCTURED WOUNDS

A punctured wound is not sutured because it might contain foreign particles and bacteria carried deep into it. The narrow external opening may have to be enlarged to provide drainage. Antibiotics are indicated because these wounds are specially conductive to bacterial growth. In the case of punctured wounds of the foot it is customary to cauterise with shoe-nail made red-hot, followed by antiseptic dressing. In the case of a suppurating penetrating wound on the foot, the horny tissue close to the wound may be pared off to facilitate drainage.

TREATMENT OF AVULSION OF HOOF AND AVULSION OF HORN

If the bleeding is severe a tourniquet is applied for about half an hour to control it. Then the wound is cleaned with an antiseptic lotion like perchloride of mercury. Placing a moist antiseptic pad soaked in the lotion a bandage is applied. The bandage is removed the next day and afterwards the wound is dressed with an oily dressing or ointment (sulphanilamide—shark liver oil, boric ointment, penicillin ointment, etc.). This dressing is repeated on alternate days. After a few days, growth of a thin layer of horn tissue can be recognised on the wound surface. At this stage the wound may be smeared with a protective layer of tar. The horny tissue develops completely within a few months.

DEBRIDEMENT* (EXCISION OF THE WOUND)

Debridement is a method of treating a wound containing lot of damaged tissue. debris and foreign matter by excision around its sides and depth. It can also be resorted to in treating a badly lacerated wound. The superficial portion of the wound containing contused and de-vitalised tissue is completely cut and removed

Technique: First cover the wound cavity with a padding of

*Pronounced : De-bred-maw, or Debrima.

cotton wool dipped in an antiseptic solution. Clip the hair and sterilise the surrounding skin. With aseptic precautions, carefully cut around the wound and completely excise the damaged areas of the wound. The new fresh wound that results after wards may be sutured. if possible. to bring about primary healing. Even if suturing is not possible. it will still heal quicker than the original wound containing debris.

Complications of Wounds

The following are some of the complications resulting from wounds: 1) Severe haemorrhage leading to shock; 2) traumatic neuralgia; 3) traumatic emphysema; 4) venous thrombosis and embolism; 5) traumatic fever; 6) erisipelas; 7) septicaemia and pyaemia; 8) gas gangrene; 9) tetanus; 10) other infections; and 11) adhesions between adjacent structures during the healing process of the wound.

1. *Haemorrhage.* Bleeding from a wound is normally arrested by the coagulation of blood. Coagulation may not take place easily if the wounded vessel is large. Deficiency of vitamin K or calcium may interfere with the formation of clot. Continuous haemorrhage may be due to certain hereditary conditions like haemophilia, or due to diseases like leucaemia, diseases of liver, heart or blood vessels. When there is continuous bleeding from a wound it may lead to *shock. Syncope* (fainting) is a condition wherein there is cerebral anaemia and unconsciousness due to a sudden fall in blood pressure or active vasomotor depression. There is also muscular relaxation and cardiac and respiratory inhibition. In animals excessive bleeding may cause syncope. (In man syncope is also caused by a sudden emotional reflex.)

2. *Traumatic neuralgia.* Severe pain along the course of a nerve is spoken of as neuralgia (hyperesthesia). Traumatic neuralgia means neuralgia as a result of traumatic injury. Traumatic neuralgia may be primary or secondary. When the neuralgic pain is present ever since the wound was produced, the condition is spoken of as *primary neuralgia.*

If the neuralgic pain starts only after a few days, due to subsequent infection of the wound or due to pressure from cicatrical contractions, it is referred to as *secondary neuralgia.*

Treatment: The wound should be cleaned with an antiseptic

lotion. An anodyne and antiseptic dressing (like idoform) should be applied. Warm, moist fomentation and administration of sodium salicylate are also indicated.

3. *Traumatic emphysema.* Emphysema is caused by the infiltration of the tissue spaces with air. It is a common complication of punctured wound of the respiratory tract (e.g., nasal cavities, trachea) and alimentary canal (e.g., rumen, caecum). It is also noticed in punctured wounds of the axilla and groin and periarticular tissues. During movements of the affected part, air gets into the wound and then spreads into the surrounding subcutaneous tissues giving rise to an emphysematous swelling. The condition is recognised as a soft, painless, crepitating swelling. It is usually harmless and the air gets absorbed in a few days. When air from the digestive tract is responsible for emphysema, there is chance of infection. Traumatic emphysema involving an extensive area may cause general discomfort and dyspnoea.

Treatment: Apply pressure and try to expel the air through the wound. The wound may be enlarged, if necessary, to let out the air. When the wound is situated in the axilla or groin, give rest to the animal to avoid movement of the area so that further entry of air into the wound will be prevented.

4. *Venous thrombosis.* Venous thrombosis may result due to injury to a vein at the site of the wound. The thrombus may break down and parts of it may be carried in the blood stream as emboli. These emboli, when sufficiently large, may even cause death by obstructing important vessels like the pulmonary artery. They may also carry infection from the site of the wound (septic emboli) and bring about general septicaemia.

5. *Traumatic fever.* The rise of body temperature noticed as a result of severe traumatic injuries (e.g., wounds) is known as traumatic fever. Fever noticed after major surgical operations is called post-operative fever. The rise of temperature is due to the reaction of the tissues to the trauma. Traumatic fever is characterised by high temperature, a pronounced leucoytosis and neutrophilia. The temperature ordinarily comes down within one or two days. But sometimes it may persist for longer periods if there is bacterial infection. In such cases treatment with antibiotics and sulphonamides becomes necessary.

6. *Erisipelas.* Erisipelas is caused by the infection of the wound with streptococcus. It is noticed in the horse and dog.

The disease is seen in three forms, viz., cutaneous, phlegmonous and gangrenous forms. In the *cutaneous* form of erisipelas there is diffuse, hot painful swelling of the skin which spreads rapidly. This may be accompanied by lymphangitis and lymphadenitis. There will also be rise of body temperature as in the case of traumatic fever. In the *phlegmonous* form of erisipelas diffuse suppurating lesions are seen and in the *gangrenous* form extensive areas of gangrene are noticed. Erisipelas is a serious condition and may become fatal if not treated.

7. *Septicaemia and pyaemia.* These are characterised by profound depression in the general condition of the animal and febrile disturbances. Antibiotics, sulphonamides, etc., may be used for treatment.

8. *Gangrenous septicaemia (Gas gangrene).* This condition is produced by the infection on the wound with gas producing organisms. It is not a common condition but has been recognised in the horse, dog, pig and ruminents. Hot, painful, oedematous swelling develops surrounding the wound. The swelling spreads very rapidly. Later on putrefactive changes are noticed giving rise to foetid gas and greyish red discharge. There is high rise of temperature initially followed by a subnormal temperature. Prostration and general symptoms of toxaemia also become evident. The condition is incurable once the symptoms have developed. Use of antibiotics and administration of polyvalent anti-gangrene serum may be tried.

9. *Tetanus.* Tetanus is a disease caused by the infection of the wound by Clostridium tetani. Cl. tetani is an anaerobic organism which multiplies in the wound and produces a toxin. The toxin gets absorbed into the body and affects the nerve centres giving rise to tetanic convulsions. Wounds caused during castration and docking are particularly liable to get infected. The disease develops only after a few days. (This period varies from three days to three weeks.) Sometimes the wound might have healed by the time the symptoms of the disease are noticed.

10. *Other infections.* Wound may get infected with many other organisms besides those mentioned above, (e.g., Actinomycosis, Actinobacillosis, Botryomycosis, Sporotrichosis, Black quarter, Anthrax, Farcy, etc.).

11. *Adhesions.* An open wound involving injuries to

muscles and tendons may, during the healing process, form adhesions between the wounded surfaces that are in contact. Such adhesions cause difficulty in the normal movement of tendons and cause lameness.

Maggot Wound (Traumatic Myiasis)

The Greek word "Myia" means "fly" and Myiasis means a condition caused by infestation of the animal body by flies or their larvae (maggots).

Maggot infestation of wounds or ulcers is called "Traumatic myiasis" or "Maggot wounds".

Myiasis may be primary or secondary, depending on the species causing it.

The *Primary myiasis* causing flies deposit eggs on the edges of abrasions and small wounds of warm-blooded animals, and have the habit of breeding only in wounds. The larvae (maggots) hatching out from the eggs burrow deep into tissues and enlarge the wound cavity. The maggots of primary myasis *feed on living tissue.*

The *secondary myiasis* causing flies could complete their life cycle without the maggot stage in wounds of warm-blooded animals. When infesting wounds, these maggots *feed only on necrotic tissue and exudates* and do not burrow deep into flesh.

Primary myiasis causing flies are as follows.

(1) Lucilia cuprina (Green bottle fly; Copper bottle fly). Most important in Kerala.

(2) Lucilia sericata;

(3) Calliphora erythrocephla and C. vomitoria. (Common in Kerala) (Blue bottle fly);

(4) Phormia terrae-novae;

(5) Phormia regima. (Phormia species not common in Kerala.)

Secondary myiasis causing flies are as follows.

1. Chrysomia bezziana and C. chloropyga (Bluish-green bottle fly). Most important in Kerala.

2. Sarcophaga haemorrhoidalis (Flesh fly). Very common in Kerala.

3. Musca domestica (Common house fly).

Life cycle. The eggs deposited on wounds hatch out in about one day. The larvae take about six days to complete their growth and they drop out into the soil to pupate. From pupal stage to adult fly takes eight days to twenty one months, deperding on temperature. Average time taken for complete life cycle from egg to fly is twenty one days.

Prognosis: *Primary* myiasis without treatment for two weeks or more can cause death of the animal in seasons when flies are numerous, due to repeated and intensive infestations. It is more dangerous in sheep, goat and horse than in cattle. Wounds treated within four days after infestation usually recover, though it may take about a month.

Secondary myiasis easily responds to treatment.

Sometimes, primary myiasis attracts flies causing secondary myiasis and primary and secondary myiasis may, therefore, be seen in a case simultaneously.

Treatment: Maggots that are superficial are removed with a forceps and a gauze dipped in chloroform, turpentine or camphor-in-oil, is allowed to remain in wound for about twenty-four hours. The gauze is removed and by that time most of the maggots might have been killed. Remove using forceps and repeat if maggots have not been completely removed. The drug should be dropped deep to come in contact with the maggots. Thereafter treat the wound like an open wound, if all maggots have been removed. Fly-repellents like neem-oil may be applied over the wounded area.

A major disadvantage with the use of above drugs are that they are very irritant and painful. A better idea will be to use some of the patent preparations like "Loraxane (ICI)" which contains insecticide Lorexane plus antiseptic Proflavine. An alternative dressing suggested for maggot wounds is the daily application of a paste of well-ground, *fresh* Anona leaves which is claimed to-be fly-repellant and antiseptic. (See also page 654)

Note: Maggots ingest necrotic tissue and keep the wound in an alkaline medium, unlike bacteria which thrive better in an acidic medium.

SURGICAL BACTERIOLOGY OF WOUNDS

Infections getting through wounds are called "*Surgical infections*". The application of the knowledge of bacteriology for the diagnosis and treatment of surgical infection is called "*surgical bacteriology*".

The bacteria concerned in most surgical infections are the following:

1) Staphylococcus, 2) Streptococcus, 3) Bacillus coli, and 4) Bacillus pyocyaneus.

1) *Staphylococcus.* The types commonly seen are: Staphylococcus aureus, S. albus, and S. citras. Infections due to staphylococci are characterised by the production of *frank pus*. They appear in the form of abscesses containing thick, creamy pus. Septicaemia and pyaemia also may be caused.

2) *Streptococcus.* Streptococcal infections do not usually give rise to frank pus. The inflammation is in the form of cellulitis and has a tendency to spread and involve extensive areas. The area is swollen but there is no abscess formation as in the case of staphylococcal infection. The discharge is thin, watery and scanty. The affected tissue may at times undergo necrosis.

3) *Bacillus coli.* B. coli is a normal inhabitant of the alimentary tract. Infections due to B. Coli usually give rise to a *thin, watery pus with offensive odour*.

4) *Bacillus pyocyaneus.* This organism is usually seen in mixed infections. The pus produced by B. pyocyaneus has a *greenish* colour.

Wounds Produced by Bites of Animals

These wounds are deep, caused by penetration of teeth of the animal. They are of special concern because various pathogenic organisms found in the mouth of animals are carried deep into the wound. They also provide conditions suitable for anaerobic bacteria.

Dog bite. There is chance of contracting rabies if bitten by an infected dog. Wherever possible, the dog should be kept under observation for ten days to rule out possibility of rabies. (However, there are reports of people having contracted rabies even after bite by a dog not showing any symptom of rabies. Hence some doctors recommend antirabic treatment in all cases of dog bite.)

The wound should be washed with plenty of soap and water, (It is unnecessary to cauterise with carbolic acid.)

Type of Anti-rabic vaccines available and sources for supply:

1. Phenolised Vacine (s/c or i/m) } Pasteur Institute,
2. BPL (Beta Propio Lactone)   } Coonoor.
   inactivated (s/c)
3. Freeze-dried vaccine   } IVRI, Izatangar
   with diluent 3 cc (s/c)
4. Single dose, prophylactic,   } Hafkin Institute,
   carbolised vaccine (6ml) s/c or l/m } Bombay.
5. "Carbolised prophylactic an-
   tirabic vaccine 20% for dogs".
   6 ml. (only 3 ml. for pups   Public Health
   below six months) s/c or l/m   Laboratory,
6. Curative/Prophylactic 7 to14   Trivandrum.
   days course (5%). (s/c or l/m)
7. "RABISIN" cell-culture vaccine
   (SII, Pune) : One ml l/m or   Serum Institute
   s/c for all species and age, on   of India, Pune
   Days No. 0, 3, 7, 14, 30, and 90.

Species	Duration of treatment	Phenolised Vaccine (s/c)	BPL vaccine (s/c)
1. Man: Adult:	14 days.	10ml.	4ml.
Child:	14 days.	5ml.	2ml.
2. Cat, Dog, Monkey:	7 days.	5ml.	2ml.
3. Calf, Goat, Sheep, Pig, Deer:	7 days.	10ml.	4ml.
4.Cattle, Pony,		20 to	
Horse:	14 days.	30 ml.	10ml.
5. Camel, Elephant:	14 days.	60 to	
		70 ml.	30ml.

2. *Scorpion sting.* (Scorpion bite) Stings of certain varieties of scorpions are sometimes fatal to small animals and the following symptoms are noticed : There is severe pain. burning sensation and weakness immediately after the sting. Within four to six hours there is profuse sweating. gasping and the patient is in almost shock-like state. Within about 10 hours pulmonary oedema develops and vomiting of blood may be noticed. Death may result within two or three days. Treatment is symptomatic. Morphine-atrophine injections are given to relieve pain. Glucose-saline injections.

are given to counteract shock. Cortico-steroids are very helpful in mini.nising the inflammatory reaction.

3. *Snake bite.* There are various types of snakes. Only a very few of them are poisonous. The three poisonous varieties commonly seen in India are the cobra, krait and viper (Russel's viper).

Snake venoms are of two types. The first type of venom is rich in neurotoxins and acts essentially on the *nervous system* e.g., cobra venom and krait venom.

The second is the venom rich in cytolysin and haemorrhagin and acts on the *cardiovascular system,* e.g., viper venom.

Symptoms of snake bite: The bite of a *cobra* or a *krait* is followed by severe pain and local swelling. Necrosis of tissues around the wound starts in about forty-eight hours. There is also muscular weakness, inability to swallow, inability to open the eyes, dribbling of saliva, etc. Later on there is respiratory paralysis on account of the depressent action on the respiratory centre. Allergic reactions like urticaria may be marked. The haemolysis is insignificant in the case of cobra bite.

The venom of *viper* acts on the cardio-vascular system. There is intravascular coagulation of blood, extravasation due to dilatation of capillaries, and also haemolysis. Convulsions also may occur due to haemorrhage in the cerebral cortex. Death results from interference in the circulation, pulmonary embolism and asphyxia. Locally there is pain, swelling, thrombosis and necrosis. At post mortem, haemorrhagic elements, infarctions and blood in serous cavities are noticed.

Treatment: Snake venom invades the system mostly through the lymphatic channels, and not so much through the blood stream. The old methods like use of tourniquet, incision at site and aspiration, are not recommended now. The wound is cleaned and washed with potassium permanganate solution and is treated on general principles. (See also page 651).

4. *Insect bites:* Bites of insects like wasps, bees, certain flies, spiders, etc., give rise to local inflammation and urticarial eruptions.

Treatment: The wound is washed with an alkaline solution (e.g., ammonia). If possible the "sting" of the insect left in the wound should be removed. Urticarial eruptions can be treated with corticosteroids.

5. *Rat bite*. Rat bite gives rise to a type of intermittent fever ("rat bite fever") in man. This is supposed to be due to infection by a spirochete (Spirillum minus) contracted through the bite. However, rat-bite fever has not been reported in animals.

Questions

1. What is a contusion? What are the different degrees of hematomas? Illustrate your answer with suitable examples and explain the frequency with which they are met with in animal practice.

2. Classify wound. What are the possible complications of wounds? Briefly mention the principles of treatment of these complications.

3. What are the essential requirements for first intention healing of a wound? How will you treat a septic wound?

4. Give a general account of the symptoms, prognosis and treatment of abdominal wounds in the horse?

5. Describe the various stages in the healing process of a wound. What are the factors which retard healing of a wound?

6. Describe the special characteristics of incised, lacerated and punctured wounds and discuss the complications met with.

7. Write an essay on healing by second intention. State how it differs from first intention healing. Name the factors which promote healing by first intention in bone repair.

8. Write short notes on: (i) Punctured wounds; (ii) Bier's treatment for wounds; (iii) Haematoma; (iv) Evulsion of hoof in bovine; (v) Avulsion of horn; (vi) Traumatic emphysema; (vii) Traumatic fever.

9. Write an essay on neglected wounds and their complications.

10. What complications are likely to be encountered in the healing of wounds?

11. How would you treat a deep jagged wound at the back of hind pastern of a bullock? What complications might develop and how would you deal with them?

12. Give a brief account of diseases brought about by infections in neglected wounds. What prophylactic and remedial measures you will adopt in such cases?

CHAPTER 7

Shock

Historical Aspects

The word *shock* was presumably used in medical literature during the 18th century and at that time it denoted a gradual and progressive collapse of the functions of vital organs as a result of injury or surgery. There was very little knowledge about the pathogenesis of shock, and the post mortem findings also could not reveal any visible changes in internal organs and offer convincing evidence in cases of death due to shock.

A better understanding of the clinical symptoms of shock was obtained by the end of the 19th century, but still the phenomenon of reduction of blood volume (hypovolemia) was not recognised.

Later, as a result of experimental studies in animals, George W. Crile in 1899 found out the most important features of hypovolemic shock like failure of venous return and low central venous pressure. He also observed improvements in venous pressure and increased cardiac output by administering saline infusions and in cases where this treatment failed, he attributed the failure to exhaustion of the vasomotor centre.

For the next twenty years the phenomenon of shock was explained in two famous theories, namely, *vasomotor exhaustion*, causing pooling of blood in the larger veins and decreased venous return, and *vasoconstriction* causing failure of blood flow to vital organs.

In 1918 Cannon observed the relationship between *low blood pressure* and *arterial blood acidosis* present in shock and he attributed the acidosis to the accumulation of fixed acids (lactic acid) in tissues and found clinical improvements by administering sodium biocarbonate.

Studies by other workers in later years postulated that the severity of shock depended on the magnitude of decrease in blood volume and that in traumatic shock hypovolemia is the essential causative factor and that the toxic factor like histamine was rather insignificant.

Modern studies aimed at measurements of haemodynamic and metabolic factors are in progress but many details of the phenomenon of shock are yet to be revealed.

Definition

Shock is a clinical condition characterised by decreased blood flow to vital organs due to imbalance between size of vascular bed and effective circulating blood volume and the inability of the body tissues to metabolise nutrients normally. The decreased blood flow to vital organs (like kidneys, liver, etc.) is caused by the pooling and stagnation of blood elsewhere in circulation. The defective blood flow to tissues implies incomplete oxygen supply to those tissues and consequent interference with metabolisation.

Classification of Shock

A *modern* classification of shock into four types quoted by MacLean based on etiology and approach to treatment is given below.

    I. Hypovolemic shock due to
        (1) blood loss;
        (2) plasma loss; and
        (3) water loss.
    II. Cardiogenic shock due to
        (1) myocardial infarction;
        (2) arrhythmia;
        (3) tamponade;
        (4) late hypovolemia;
        (5) epidural and general anaesthesia; and
        (6) pulmonary embolism.
   III. Shock characterised by peripheral pooling of blood due to
        (1) loss of tone in *resistance vessels** as may happen in

---

  * The term *resistance vessels* with reference to blood pressure, are the arterioles supplied by the sympathetic nervous system. By inducing sympathetic stimulation, constriction of these arterioles and increase in peripheral resistance can be brought about. Conversely, the depression of sympathetic nervous system, as may happen in spinal anaesthesia, can bring about loss of tone in these resistance vessels and consequent reduction in blood pressure.

spinal anaesthesia; and

(2) trapping of blood in *capacitance vessels*** as may happen in endotoxin shock.

IV. Septic shock due to the failure of cells of vital organs to perform normal metabolic function despite availability of oxygen.

Another classification of shock is into two types, called primary shock and secondary shock.

Primary shock develops immediately after injury and *secondary shock* develops an hour or more after the injury. Primary shock is transient and usually of nervous origin. It is marked by cold sweating, fall in blood pressure and a slow pulse rate. Milder forms of primary shock passes off quickly and severe forms may lead on to secondary shock.

Shock has also been classified as : cardiogenic, vasogenic, haematogenic and neurogenic.

Etiology

(a) DIRECT CAUSES

1. *Severe Haemorrhage*: Haemorrhage brings about shock by directly reducing the volume of blood in circulation. The amount of blood in an animal body is roughly one-thirteenth to one-fifteenth of its live body weight. Severe shock develops if twenty five per cent of this total amount of blood is lost. Shock due to haemorrhage is called *haemorrhagic shock* or wound shock or surgical shock. If the cause of haemorrhage and consequent shock is trauma or external injury, it is called *traumatic shock*.

2. *Trauma*: Severe external violence without haemorrhage can also produce shock and it is also listed under traumatic shock. Extensive tissue damage seems to be the cause of shock in these instances, e.g., crush injuries.

3. *Burns*: Burns involving large areas of the body cause shock mainly due to the effusion of the fluid constituents of blood (plasma effusions into the blisters).

4. Rough handling of viscera during surgical operations.

5. Toxaemia due to bacterial or other toxins.

** The term *capacitance vessels* here implies vessels principally of the liver and splanchnic bed.

6. *Bacterial infection*: The shock resulting from bacterial infection is called bacterial shock or septic shock.

7. Anaphylactic reactions against certain drugs or other foreign proteins. The shock resulting from anaphylaxis is called *anaphylactic shock*.

Note: The term insulin shock refers to a clinical phenomenon due to hypoglycaemia resulting from administration of insulin in high doses.

CLINICAL SYMPTOMS

(1) *General Appearance*: The patient is in a state of severe prostration or collapse. The eyes are sunken and pupils are dilated. Visible mucous membranes are dry, pale and anaemic. Cold sweating (i.e., sweating even though the body temperature is low) may be noticed. In the horse and camel yawning may be observed which is indicative of anoxia.

The animal is not able to raise the head and keep it steady. Vomiting may be noticed. The animal is extremely weak and may be partially or completely unconscious. The extremities are cold. The superficial veins are in a collapsed state due to lack of blood, which is suggestive of peripheral circulatory of impairment.

(2) *Pulse*: It is rapid and imperceptible. Blood pressure may remain unchanged for sometime but later on falls.

(3) *Respiration*: Respiration may be unchanged in the beginning but later becomes shallow and rapid. Sobbing type of respiration may be noticed in the horse and dog. Cheyne-Stoke's respiration may be observed when pain or nervous irritation is present. (Cheyne-Stoke's respiration is an abnormal form of breathing in which the respiratory movements become gradually less and less until they almost disappear; and then after remaining imperceptible for a short time, they gradually increase in depth until they are again exaggerated.)

4. *Urine*: The quantity (volume) of urine passed is reduced (Oliguria). The concentration is very high. Abnormal constituents may or may not be present.

Pathophysiological Changes

1. *General changes in haemodynamics and metabolism*: The most important pathological feature in shock is the interference with cellular metabolism leading to its ultimate failure.

The cell metabolism is directly related to the supply of oxygen and its utilisation by the cells. In hypovolemic shock, the decreased oxygenation of cells is due to the inadequate oxygen supply to the tissues through the blood. On the other hand, in shock due to cellular damage, like septic shock, there is inability of the cells to utilise even the oxygen made available to them. The following haemodynamic and metabolic measurements have been experimentally studied in shock.

(1) Arterial blood pressure.

(2) Pulse rate.

(3) Central venous pressure (CVP) in the right atrium of the heart.

(4) Cardiac index.

(5) Urine flow.

(6) Respone to volume replacement in circulation.

(7) The oxygen content of arterial blood.

(8) Difference in oxygen content of arterial and venous blood.

(9) Arterial blood lactate.

Let us examine how these parameters are influenced in the four types of shock mentioned above, i.e., hypovolemic shock, cardiogenic shock, shock due to peripheral pooling of blood and septic shock.

The *arterial blood pressue* is decreased in all the four types of shock.

The *pulse rate* is increased as a compensatory mechanism, but in cardiogenic shock it may be either increased or decreased depending on the condition of the heart.

The *central venous pressure* (CVP) is decreased in hypovolemic shock and in shock due to peripheral pooling. However, in cardiogenic shock and septic shock, the CVP is increased.

The *cardiac index* is increased in septic shock (Hyper haemo dynamism), whereas in the other three types of shock it is decreased.

The *urine flow* is decreased in all the four types.

The response to volume replacement of circulation or *volume load* is increased only in hypovolemic shock and there is decreased response in the other three types.

The *oxygen content* of arterial blood is decreased in all types of shock.

The *difference in oxygen content* of arterial and venous blood is decreased in septic shock whereas in the other three types it is increased.

The *arterial blood lactate* is increased in all the four types.

2. *RBC Count*: The erythrocyte count in shock is generally increased due to haemoconcentration.

3. *WBC Count*: The leucocyte count is increased.

4. *Blood Volume*: The blood volume in circulation is greatly reduced and this is one of the most characteristic features of surgical shock. The toxins produced by damaged or devitalised tissues circulate in the blood. These are histamine or histamine-like substances and cause extreme capillary dilatation, increased permeability of capillary walls, and reduction in the volume of circulating blood. There is dilatation of capillaries and so many new capillaries that are ordinarily in a collapsed state, begin to take part in circulation and this causes a "pooling" or "sludging" of a major portion of the circulating blood in the capillaries. There is also increased filtration through the capillary walls. Pronounced reduction in circulating blood volume and fall of blood pressure results.

5. *Responses of Cardio-vascular System*: The impulses from the carotid sinus and aortic arch are conveyed through the ninth and tenth cranial nerves (Glossopharyngeal nerve and Vagus nerve) to the vasomotor centre in the medulla whenever there is lowering of blood pressure. Immediate response from the centre is conveyed through the sympathetic system which brings about generalised constriction of arterioles and consequent increase in *peripheral resistance* to circulation. The sympathetic stimulation also increases the rate of heart beat and the force of contraction of the heart. The net result of all these phenomena is a compensatory increase in blood pressure. There is also constriction of the venous walls as a result of the compensatory sympathetic stimulation and blood from large venous reservoirs are squeezed into the general circulation, and thereby increases the effective volume of blood in circulation. Blood from the limbs, bowel and kidneys are diverted to more vital areas. However, the vessels of the heart and brain are relatively little affected by the sympathetic stimulation as compared to those of less vital organs like those of kidneys. This enables more blood to be diverted to the heart and brain as compared to other areas.

6. *Acidosis*: The diminished flow of blood interferes with the removal of acidic metabolic products from the tissues and the decreased secretion of urine contributes to their retention in the body. Consequently acidosis develops.

7. *Ammonia Content of Blood*: There is increase in the ammonia content of blood during shock. This raised ammonia level is caused by anoxia of the kidneys. There is also increased absorption of ammonia through the intestines where it is produced by enhanced bacterial activity. Added to this is the inability of the anoxic liver to metabolise ammonia to urea. Ammonia intoxication is, therefore, caused.

8. *Vitamin-C* content of the tissues, particularly of adrenal cortex, is greatly reduced.

9. The *protein* content of blood is lowered, but as a result of reduced kidney function the non-protein-nitrogen (NPN) content increases.

10. *Potassium Content of Blood*: The increased tissue break down causes negative nitrogen balance and increase in the potassium content of blood (hyperkalemia).

11. *Blood sugar* level in shock is usually higher than normal in the initial stages but later falls to low levels.

12. *Viscosity* of blood is increased in shock due to loss of plasma through capillary walls.

13. *Electrolyte content*: The cation (Na and K) content of tissue cells and intra-cellular fluid is altered. There is escape of K from the cells into the extra-cellular fluid due to the alterations of the structure of cell membrane on account of tissue anoxia.

14. *Endocrine influences*: There are three important endocrine responses in shock, namely, the discharge of Catecholamine from the adrenal medulla and from nerve endings of the autonomic system, the stimulation of anterior pituitary, adrenal cortex and stimulation of secretion of renin by the kidneys, and stimulation of posterior pituitary.

Catecholamines stimulate the heart, constricts arterioles in the skin, kidneys and viscera; dilates arteries in the myocardium, and constricts most of the veins. Catecholamines also stimulate production of glucagon, inhibit production of insulin, and accelerate glucogenolysis from liver and muscles. They also stimulate the production of ACTH from the pituitary.

The production of *insulin* by the pancreas is inhibited during shock, as in any other condition of stress. The production of *glucagon*, a hormone which has actions opposite to that of insulin, and which also believed to be produced by pancreas, is stimulated in shock. Glucagon causes breakdown of liver glycogen into glucose (glucogenesis) and also promotes production of glucose from aminoacids (gluco-neo-genesis).

Hypovolemia causes production of aldosterone by adrenal cortex. Aldosterone is also produced by a direct stimulus on adrenal cortex by the ACTH hormone of anterior pituitary.

The decreased renal blood flow with decreased pressure stimulates production of renin by the kidneys which stimulates production of angiotensin. Angiotensin has vasopressor effect which also promotes excretion of potassium and retention of sodium (sodium bicarbonate).

When there is hypotension, the posterior pituitary produces more of antidiuretic hormone (ADH) which helps to restore plasma volume by retention of water in the body.

15. *Impairment of Circulation*: The normal blood pressure and the volume of blood in circulation are maintained by three main factors; namely, (i) the force of heart beat, (ii) the size of the vascular bed, and (iii) the volume of blood in circulation. In shock the force of heart beat is reduced. The extent of vascular bed is greatly increased due to generalised capillary dilatation and also due to participation of new capillaries in circulation. As a result of these, the blood pressure and blood circulation are impaired.

16. *Vasomotor Reactions*: In the initial stages of shock there is vasoconstriction acting as a compensatory mechanism aimed at maintaining the blood pressure. This vasoconstriction is selective, being more pronounced in the skin and peripheral areas than in vital tissues like brain, liver and kidneys. The object of this selective vasoconstriction apparently is to *divert* more blood to important organs. The ischaemia of the skin also helps to preserve body heat. However, in severe cases of shock these compensatory mechanisms are insufficient to maintain blood pressure and to divert enough blood to vital organs, because of increase in the capillary permeability. (See also irreversible shock discussed at the end of this chapter.)

Treatment

In veterinary practice, the treatment of shock is practically feasible only in early stages of hypovolemic shock and septic shock. The general principles of treatment are mentioned below.

1. *Replacement Therapy*: Prompt replacement of the blood volume is the most important part of the treatment for hypovolemic shock. This is called *replacement therapy* or *substitution therapy*. Whole blood or plasma or various substitute solutions specially prepared for the purpose, may be used for replacement therapy.

Whole blood is preferable in shock due to haemorrhage. Plasma is more desirable in shock due to burns. Injections of normal saline solutions help to make up the volume and also supply the essential electrolytes. Buffered saline solutions containing various electrolytes are available, e.g., Ringer's solution, Lock's solution, etc. The saline solutions may be combined with colloidal substances and amino acids. The fluids used to make up the blood volume are in general spoken of as *plasma expanders* or *plasma extenders*.

Injection of Whole Blood (Blood transfusion). Whole blood is administered intravenously. Either the direct or the indirect method of transfusion may be adopted. Incompatibility of blood between individuals of the same species but belonging to different blood groups, is not generally seen in animals. Therefore blood obtained from any healthy individual of the same species may be used for transfusion.

(a) *Direct method of transfusion*: A blood transfusion apparatus is used for the purpose. The rate of flow from the donor to the recipient can be observed through an interconnecting glass or transparent plastic tube. One disadvantage of this method is that the actual quantity of blood administered cannot be measured.

(b) *Indirect method of transfusion*: In the indirect method, blood is first collected from the donor and is then injected into the recipient. If necessary, the collected blood can be stored and kept for use in an emergency. Coagulation is prevented by the use of sodium citrate or by defibrination.

Sodium citrate converts Ca of blood into a soluble compound, calcium-sodium-citrate and thus prevents coagulation. The quantity of sodium citrate added to blood is at the rate of 1g of sodium citrate in 1 ounce of water of 9 ounces of blood. (This makes about 0.3% of sodium citrate in the blood.)

If the defibrination technique is employed, coagulation of blood is prevented by agitating the drawn blood beyond the normal coagulation time for the species (cattle: 10 minutes, horse: 15 minutes, etc.). Fibrin formed is removed by filtering through a fine piece of sterile muslin and the blood is ready for transfusion.

(c) *Quantity of blood to b*ᵒ *transfused*: Usually *2.5 cc of blood per pound body weight* (5.5cc per kg body weight) is given. The quantity may be increased if the haemorrhage persists.

Plasma: Plasma collected from the same species (homogenous plasma) or from other species (heterogenous plasma) might be used to counteract loss of blood volume.

The plasma from the donor can be collected and stored as follows. Sodium citrate solution is added to the blood to prevent coagulation. Storing in the refrigerator for three to eight days separates the plasma from dog blood. But centrifuging is necessary to separate bovine plasma.

If a suitable broad spectrum antibiotic, e.g., terramycin 1 mg per ml is added as a preservative, plasma can be stored in the refrigerator for about three months.

Plasma transfusion can be given at the rate of *upto 10 cc per kg body weight*. (See also Addendum on page 69)

Injection of Normal Saline or Other Plasma Expanders: The *crystalloid* solutions commonly used as plasma expanders are the following.

(a) Normal saline.

(b) Normal saline with 5% to 25% of glucose.

(c) Ringer's solution (containing NaCl, KCI, calcium chloride and sodium bicarbonate in distilled water).

(d) Lock's solution (containing NaCl, KCI, calcium chloride, sodium bicarbonate and dextrose in distilled water).

An easily available and effective crystalloid solution for treatment of shock is 5% glucose in normal saline with 90 milliequivalents of sodium carbonate added to each litre to adjust the PH of the solution at 7.4. (See also Addendum on page 69)

The quantity of the solution to be administered depends on the quantity of whole blood or plasma lost from circulation.

Usually administration is continued until pulse returns to normal. The quantity to be given may be calculated at the rate of 2 cc to 4 cc per pound body weight of the animal. (about 4 to 8 cc per kg body weight). Half of this calculated amount is administered intravenously and the remaining portion subcutaneously.

When large quantities of fluids are required to be administered (say more than 5.5 cc per kg body weight), the additional fluid should consist of colloids in the form of fresh frozen plasma, albumen or whole blood.

25 to 50 gm of albumin may be added per litre of normal saline.

2. *Ventillation*: Respiratory failure must be checked and proper ventillation provided by administering oxygen. Oxygen may be administered either through an endotracheal tube or by placing the animal in an oxygen chamber. Inhalation of oxygen prevents serious cellular degeneration and metabolic disturbances.

3. *Counteracting Acidosis*: It is advantageous to administer sodium bicarbonate to counteract acidosis. It is essential when larger quantities of fluid are to be administered.

4. *Use of Drugs Acting on Cardio-vascular System*: The object is to improve blood pressure and to stimulate blood flow, although each of the drugs commonly used for this purpose has its own limitations. Some of the drugs are mentioned below.

Adrenaline (epinephrine) accelerates the heart rate, increases systolic blood pressure and moderately increases mean blood pressure. Blood flow to the heart, brain, splanchnic area and skeletal muscle are increased, but circulation in the kidneys, skin and mucous membranes is decreased.

Digitalis is specially useful in older patients and in those predisposed to congestive heart failure.

Drugs like Methoxamine, Norepinephrine, Metaraminol, Dopamine, Isoprotenol and Phenoxybenzamine are not commonly used in veterinary practice.

5. *Counteracting Peripheral Resistance*: The increased pheripheral resistance is not the cause of shock, but only a result of shock. In the treatment for shock, the peripheral resistance is reduced by the replacement of blood volume itself, and the use of vasodilators for this purpose is unnecessary in most of the cases.

6. *Control of Sepsis*: It has been established experimentally that chances of recovery from rather fatal cases of shock is enhanced by supportive treatment with aureomycin or other suitable antibiotics. In this connection, it may also be recollected that when arterial blood flow in the liver is diminished on account of shock, the anaerobic organisms from the digestive tract invade the portal circulation and multiply in the liver. Gram-positive or gram-negative organisms and fungi may be involved, although gram-negative organisms are more commonly associated.

Irreversible Shock

This is a rather old term. Shock is said to be reversible or compensated if the patient is likely to recover from it. Irreversible shock or uncompensated shock is clinically recognised as the failure of the patient to recover in spite of treatment. At this stage no improvement in blood pressure and pulse is noticed even with transfusion therapy. The longer the duration of shock the greater is the chance for irreversibility. The following tissue changes are evident in irreversible shock.

1. *Increase in Capillary Permeability*: The capillary walls become permanently damaged due to toxins liberated in the body and due to prolonged anoxia. Therefore they lose their semi-permeable nature and become permeable to plasma and even whole blood. The re-absorption of fluid from tissue spaces into the blood stream (so as to revive the blood volume) becomes impossible because of the loss of semi-permeability of the capillary wall. Thus the fluid exchange through the capillary walls becomes irreversible.

2. *Reduction in Blood Pressure; Hypoxia/Anoxia; and metabolic derangement.* The blood pressure is greatly reduced due to the reduction in blood volume resulting from increased capillary permeability. Further deterioration in blood pressure is caused by the generalised vaso-dilatation caused by the abnormal release of VDM (vasodilator material) due to the anoxia of the liver.

The blood pressure is influenced by the antagonistic action of two subtances, viz., the vasoexcitor material (VEM) possibly renin produced by the kidneys, and the vasodilator material

(VDM) believed to be apoferritin, produced by the liver. Depending on the overproduction of one of these two substances, there is a proportionate increase or decrease in blood pressure. The release of VEM and VDM happens when there is lack of blood supply to the kidneys and liver respectively. During shock the blood supply to vital organs like brain, liver and kidneys are maintained in an order of priority by minimising blood supply to less vital organs. When the blood supply to the kidneys is reduced in this manner the kidneys release more of VEM in order to raise the blood pressure and improve the circulation. If this is not sufficient to improve blood circulation there is decreased blood supply to the liver also. The anoxia of the liver then begins to release VDM which further reduces the blood pressure and the resulting impairment in general circulation deteriorates the tissue anoxia already present. The semi-permeability of the capillary walls is lost because of the prolonged anoxia. As a result of these tissue changes treatment is not likely to be beneficial in irreversible shock. Saline solutions, plasma or even whole blood administered intravenously may escape into the tissue spaces through the damaged capillary walls.

3. Disseminated intravascular coagulation in septic shock.

Crush Syndrome

The pathological symptoms resulting from extensive crush injuries has been termed as crush syndrome. Crush injuries are caused by the fall of heavy objects.

SYMPTOMS

There is severe pain so long as the part remains crushed under the object. After the object is removed and the weight crushing the body is released, characteristic symptoms are noticed. The part gets swollen enormously and the animal exhibits symptoms of shock. The actual mechanism of crush syndrome has not been well-understood. It is explained as follows:

The crush injury causes damage to the tissues including capillary walls. The devitalised tissues release toxins. So long as the part remains compressed, blood circulation in the area is very limited and therefore the toxins are not absorbed into the general circulation in appreciable quantities. Once the weight is removed the damaged capillaries whose walls have lost the natural tone, begin to dilate enormously, causing a pooling of blood in these vessels There is also increased exudation through capillary walls which is responsible for the swelling. The increased blood circulation in the part also carries with it the toxins, producing toxaemia.

TREATMENT

The sudden inrush of blood into the affected area when weight is released should be prevented by putting a tight ligature or tourniquet proximal to the seat of injury. If a limb is involved and if the injury is severe, amputation of the damaged portion is sometimes advisable. Antihistamines and the general treatment for shock are indicated.

Dehydration

The term dehydration indicates a condition where there is an abnormal reduction in the water content of tissue cells, i.e., a reduction in the intra-cellular fluid. Dehydration may be caused either due to excessive loss of water or indirectly due to loss of electrolytes. It may be : Hypertonic, Hypotonic, or Isotonic.

Dehydration due to loss of water: The water in the animal body consists of intra-cellular fluid and the extra-cellular fluid represented by inter-cellular fluid and blood plasma.

The fluid exchange between these intra-cellular and extra-cellular compartments takes place through the cell membrane and is controlled by the osmotic pressure on either side of the cell membrane. When there is excessive fluid loss from the body (due to haemorrhage, burns, excessive loss through kidneys and sweat, increased pulmonary ventilation, etc.), the osmotic pressure of blood plasma increases the absorption of inter-cellular fluid into the blood stream which in turn results in escape of intra-cellular fluid into tissue spaces and dehydration of tissues.

Dehydration due to loss of electrolytes: The chief ions concerned in the osmotic equilibrium between body fluids are the following.

Na^+, K^+, Mg^{++}, NH^+, H_3^+ . . . . cations;

and Cl^-, PO_4^-, HCO_3^-, SO_4^- . . . . anions.

          (phos- (bicarbo- (sulphate)

          phate) nate)

The extracellular fluid mostly contains Na and Cl whereas the intracellular fluid mostly contains K and PO_4. The electrolytes from the extracellular fluid are lost by excretion through the kidneys, lungs and also due to vomiting, diarrhoea etc. The electrolytes lost in this manner are chiefly Na and Cl.

Loss of electrolytes from the body reduces the osmotic pressure of blood plasma and consequently inhibits the 'osmoreceptors' in the brain. This in turn causes diminution in the secretion of anti-diuretic hormone (ADH) by the posterior pituitary. Lack of ADH removes the normal inhibition on the excretion of water by the kidneys. This results in increased water loss through urine causing dehydration of tissues.

TREATMENT

Administration of electrolyte solutions.

Water intoxication: When excessive quantity of fluid is administered, more than what the kidneys and other excretory channels can cope with, the osmotic pressure of extracellular fluid is lowered. Therefore fluid enters the tissue cells, causing turgidity or 'water-logging' of cells. This has also been called 'water-intoxication'.

Acidosis and Alkalosis

Acidosis is a pathological condition resulting from alteration in the pH of blood plasma. The blood plasma normally has a pH of 7.35 to 7.45 and its carbon dioxide pressure is 40 mm of Hg at 37°C.

An increase or decrease in the CO_2 content or addition of alkaline substances will alter the pH towards the acidic or alkaline side, as the case may be. The exchange of carbon dioxide from blood takes place in the alveoli of the lungs during respiration.

Loss of acid radicals (like Cl), as may happen due to continuous vomiting, results in *alkalosis*; and loss of basic ions (like Na), as may happen in diarrhoea, causes *acidosis*.

Inadequate kidney function and decreased excretion of urine (oliguria) causes acidosis due to retention of acidic metabolic products. Hence acidosis may be due to endogenous causes like defective ventilation of lungs or defective kidney function.

Abnormalities in metabolism may cause metabolic acidosis.

In the normal case compensatory mechanisms operate and the acidosis and alkalosis are corrected, explained as follows.

1. *Respiratory Acidosis*: This is due to retention of carbon dioxide on account of decreased ventilation of the alveoli.

Common causes are depression of respiratory centre by drugs like morphine, injury of the central nervous system, and diseases affecting the lungs like pneumonia, emphysema, etc.

The kidneys try to compensate by retaining bicarbonates, excretion of acid salts, increased ammonia formation etc.

2. *Respiratory Alkalosis*: Increased alveolar ventilation resulting in excessive loss of carbon dioxide brings about respiratory alkalosis, caused by hyper-ventilation of lungs.

Renal compensation takes place by excreting more of bicarbonates, retention of acid salts, and decreased ammonia formation.

3. *Metabolic Acidosis*: There is retention of fixed acids or loss of base bicarbonate due to diarrhoea, starvation or lactic acid accumulation, etc.

Increased rate and depth of breathing is seen as pulmonary compensation. The renal compensation is also seen similar to respiratory acidosis but is slow.

4. *Metabolic Alkalosis*: Loss of fixed acids, accumulation of bicarbonates or potassium depletion, caused by vomiting, excessive intake of bicarbonates or administration of diuretics results in metabolic alkalosis.

Compensatory phenomena include decreased rate and depth of respiration and increased excretion of bicarbonates by kidneys, retention of acid salts, decreased ammonia formation, etc.

TREATMENT

Defective ventilation should be rectified by correcting respiratory difficulties.

Metabolic acidosis can be corrected by administering sodium bicarbonate. Weak alkalinising agents like tri-hydroxymethyl-amino-methane (THAM) may be used in respiratory and metabolic acidosis.

Administration of saline solutions also have a corrective function in both acidosis and alkalosis by replacing electrolyte losses.

Questions

1. Define shock. Describe the clinical symptoms and surgical pathology of secondary shock.
2. Write an essay on the etiology, symptoms and treatment of shock.
3. Write an essay on the vasomotor reactions in shock and explain how these are modified in irreversible shock.
4. What is meant by irreversible shock? Compare and contrast the specific changes noticed in irreversible shock with those seen in reversible shock. Explain why the usual treatments for shock are ineffective in irreversible shock.
5. Define shock. Outline the principles of treatment in haemorrhagic shock.
6. What are the indications for fluid transfusion in surgical practice? Give a brief account indicating the various fluids used and their doses.

Addendum

Note 1: The usual rate for blood transfusion is *fifty drops per minute* so that one bottle is transfused in about four hours. But patients in severe shock will have to be given at a much faster rate. Patients who suffer from cardiac or pulmonary disease or are severely anaemic must be transfused at a much slower rate, as slow as *twelve drops per minute.*

When plasma alone is transfused, no grouping or cross-matching is necessary.

During transfusion of whole blood or plasma, there is always the risk of viral infections getting communicated, which might manifest itself even after ninety days.

Note 2: When fluids are given intravenously as a drip, the usual recommended rate of flow is *forty to seventy drops per minute.* A faster rate will affect cardiac and pulmonary systems and lead to *intravenous shock* ("I.V. shock"). Leave back some portion of the fluid in each transfusion bottle to safeguard against any sediment or particulate matter entering directly into the blood stream.

Chapter 8

Burns and Scalds

Burns and scalds are thermal injuries. A *burn* is an injury caused by hot solids, flame etc. A *scald* is an injury caused by hot liquids or steam. The degree of injury depends on the temperature of the object and its duration of contact with the body. A scald is likely to be more severe than a burn because the hot liquid may penetrate deeper into the tissues.

CLASSIFICATION

Burns are classified into three types according to the thickness of tissue involved, viz., *First degree burn* involving only the epidermis; *Second degree burn* in which the thickness of skin is involved more or less completely but not the subcutaneous fat; and *Third degree burn* in which deeper tissues like subcutaneous fat and muscles are also involved.

SYMPTOMS

Physical Symptoms: The appearance of the burnt area depends on the degree of burn. In *first degree burn* there is diffuse swelling and sometimes vesicle formation. (A vesicle is a small circumscribed elevation of the epidermis containing a serous liquid). The vesicles subside within about a week. In *second degree burn* blisters* are formed by the exudation of plasma. The exudation may continue for thirty-six to forty-eight hours. The blisters are very painful. In *third degree burn* the complete thickness of skin plus subcutaneous fat/muscles/other deeper tissues are involved. The dead area of skin appears brownish black and leathery. There may be a bad odour.

The area surrounding a burn shows oedema and hyperaemia. During healing the dead portions slough off. This sloughing

*A blister is a large-sized vesicle.

is a slow process taking eight to nine weeks. The sloughed tissues are replaced by scar tissue which appears thin, shining and hairless, if hair roots are damaged.

Systemic reactions: There is intense pain and thirst if the lesions are extensive. A varying degree of toxaemia is present. Shock develops if the lesions are extensive and severe, because of the severe pain and due to the reduction in blood volume resulting from plasma loss through exudations. Septicaemia may develop due to secondary bacterial infection.

PROGNOSIS

Prognosis depends more on the extent of the injury (i.e. the area of skin involved) rather than on the degree of burn in a limited area. Shock may result if more than 4% of the skin surface is affected by burns. *Prognosis is unfavourable if more than 50% of the skin surface is involved.* In first degree burn, healing may take place within 10 days and second and third degree burn may take three to four weeks or more.

TREATMENT

Dehydration and shock, if present, must be treated first. Local treatment consists of applying emollients. The blisters may be ruptured to drain the exudate. The dead portion of skin covering the blister is not removed at this stage because by doing so the underlying raw surface will be exposed. If the skin surface is eroded, the exposed areas are protected by astringent, antiseptic and anodyne ointments. Local analgesics may be incorporated in these ointments to control pain. Ointments commonly used are tannic acid ointment, iodoform ointment, etc. Antibiotics ointments like penicillin ointment are also advisable to control bacterial infection. Antibiotics may also be given systemically to counteract septicemia.

Chemical Burns

Injuries caused by chemicals like strong acids and alkalies are referred to as *chemical burns*. The chemical produces localised necrosis of skin and deeper tissues with which it comes in contact. The degree of tissue destruction depends on the strength of the chemical and the duration of contact. The degree of necrosis is severe if the corrosive chemical is not promptly removed. A line of demarcation is seen between the dead and healthy tissues. The devitalised tissues may get infected. After sloughing of necrosed area an ulcer is produced which heals gradually.

TREATMENT

If detected immediately, the chemical may be neutralised by a suitable acid or alkaline solution. Alkalies like sodium bicarbonate and soap solution are used in the case of burns due to acids; acidic solutions like vinegar are used in the case of burns due to alkalies. If suitable acid or alkaline solutions are not available, washing with plenty of plain water may be resorted to. The ulcer produced by the sloughing of necrosed areas is treated on general principles.

Frost Bite

Frost bite is a condition caused by exposure to extreme cold weather. There is destruction of superficial tissues.

Incidence: It is met with in all species of domestic animals. The very young animals and those that are undernourished are more susceptible. In pigs, ears and tail are commonly affected. In poultry, combs and wattles.

Lesions: The degree of severity of frost bite varies from temporary chilling of tissues to freezing and necrosis of a portion of tissue.

SYMPTOMS

In mild cases the skin at first becomes pale and bloodless followed by intense redness, heat, pain and swelling. The hair may fall out and the epidermis may peel off. The inflammation subsides within a few days.

In severe cases the affected part becomes swollen and painful and later on undergoes necrosis. Patches of skin are destroyed in this manner and a clear line of demarcation develops between the affected and normal portions. Sloughing of the dead skin leaves a raw surface.

TREATMENT

The lesions should be treated with mild antiseptics. A preparation containing turpentine, ammonia and chloroform one part each in six parts of a bland oily base is satisfactory for the purpose.

Electric Shock

Electric current passing through the animal body may cause coma and death if the current is sufficiently strong. It may also cause burns locally. Treatment consists of administering artificial respiration, parenteral administration of respiratory and cardiac stimulants, etc., in addition to the treatment of burns.

Lightning Stroke

Animals struck by lightning may die immediately or within a few hours. Rarely they do remain in an unconscious or semiconscious state for sometime and then recover. Some of the recovered animals may show unsteady gait, partial paralysis, etc., due to nervous lesions, while others may be apparently normal. The cause of sudden death is believed to be ventricular fibrillation.

Lesions: The nerve tissue of animals seriously affected with lightning stroke shows on microscopical examination small haemorrhages and degenerative changes. On unpigmented skin the so called *lightning figures* may be seen in the form of dark branching lines.

TREATMENT

Treatment is symptomatic like administration of cardiac and respiratory stimulants, artificial respiration, etc.

If the patient does not die within a few hours after the accident, it usually survives.

Sun Stroke, Heat Stroke, etc.

These are conditions caused by disturbances in the heat regulating mechanisms of the body.

ETIOLOGY

High environmental temperature, high humidity and inadequate ventilation. Sun stroke is caused by direct exposure to sun rays. Excessive physical strain and obesity are predisposing causes.

Heat Stroke is more commonly seen in dogs and horses.

The chief symptoms are deep accelerated breathing and collapse. The symptoms occur suddenly. The rectal temperature may be raised up to 110°F. There is a staring expression in the eyes. Vomiting may also be noticed. The treatment should be prompt as otherwise the condition is likely to be fatal. Cold water should be applied to the body. Small animals like dogs may be immersed in water, if possible. Ice packs are applied to the head. Cold water enemas are also indicated. The rectal temperature should be taken every five minutes and treatment should be modified according to the response shown. Largactyl may be given to lower the body temperature. Large animals should be given a dose of 10 to 15 cc of a 5% solution 1/m per 1000 lb. body weight. Small animals should be given 1.25 cc. of 2.5% solution 1/m per 25 lb body weight. (See addendum on page-653).

Heat Cramps are common in animals doing work in a hot environment and result from deranged electrolite balance due to excessive electrolyte loss, especially through sweat (*acute salt loss*). Draft horses are commonly affected. The chief symptoms are severe muscular spasm and sudden cessation of sweating. Vomiting may be present. The condition is treated by administering cold water through stomach tube. If vomiting is present, physiological saline is given intravenously instead of administration by stomach tube.

Heat exhaustion is seen in draft horses, cattle and swine but only very rarely in dogs. Due to the high environmental temperature the peripheral blood vessels dilate and when this occurs without corresponding increase in the blood volume circulatory collapse results. There is weakness, muscular tremours and collapse. Respiration is accelerated and deep. Pulse is accelerated. The body temperature may or may not be raised. The rise of temperature in any case is not so high as in heat stroke. Cold water should be applied to the body. Cold water with salt may be given orally. Physiological saline is administered intravenously. (See addendum on page-653).

Questions

1. What is the difference between a burn and a scald? Classify burns and describe the surgical pathology and treatment for burns.

2. Write a short note on sun stroke.

CHAPTER 9

Phlebitis

Phlebitis (inflammation of the vein) is caused by any of the following: (1) Trauma, (2) Infection, (3) Extension of an inflammatory focus outside the vein, (4) Toxins.

CLASSIFICATION

Three types of phlebitis have been recognised. They are Adhesive phlebitis, Purulent phlebitis, and Haemorrhagic phlebitis.

In *adhesive phlebitis* thrombus is formed on the inflammed endothelium which may partially or completely block the lumen of the vessel. The perivenous tissues are oedematous and pain is evinced along the vein.

In *purulent phlebitis* the inflammatory symptoms are more marked and abscesses may form along the course of the vein.

Haemorrhagic phlebitis is characterised by repeated haemorrhages due to disintegration of the clot by mechanical interference or infection.

TERMINATION

Phlebitis is accompanied by thrombus formation which may partly or completely occlude the vein. The interference in the venous flow causes oedema of the dependent region, but this may get compensated by the establishment of collateral circulation. If there is no infection the inflammation gradually subsides and the thrombus becomes organised. The inflammed portion of the vessel may appear like a fibrous cord. Infection or mechanical interference may disintegrate the thrombus and cause septic embolism or secondary haemorrhage.

TREATMENT

1. Control the bleeding, if present.

2. Mechanical disturbance of the clot should be prevented to avoid embolism.

3. Counter-irritants may be applied in the dependent region to stimulate collateral circulation.

4. Antibiotics may be given to control infection.

5. In suppurative phlebitis excision of the affected portion of the vein is sometimes advisable. This is done after ligaturing the vessel proximal and distal to the lesion. This is also advisable in haemorrhagic phlebitis when bleeding is severe.

Jugular Phlebitis

Inflammation of the jugular vein sometimes results after phlebotomy. Two forms are commonly met with, namely, Simple phlebitis, and Suppurative or purulent phlebitis.

Blood may escape through the wound in the vein and collect subcutaneously. A local phlebitis results. If infected, it becomes a purulent phlebitis.

The skin wound after phlebotomy instead of healing by first intention discharges a serous or sanguinous fluid. Due to the interference in the venous drainage oedema develops in the lips, face and parotid region. The vein appears stiff and cord-like owing to the presence of thrombus within it. The thrombus formation can be detected by the inability to raise the vein. After a few days and if the infection is not very severe, the clot organises and contracts and the vein can be felt as a hard thin cord. The swelling disappears due to the establishment of collateral circulation.

If the infection is severe, symptoms of purulent phlebitis are evident.

Questions

1. Write an essay on phlebitis with reference to incidence, causes and complications encountered.

2. Write an essay on the symptoms, etiology and treatment of jugular phlebitis in cattle.

Write a short note on Phlebitis.

CHAPTER 10

Lymphangitis

Lymphangitis is the inflammation of the lymphatic vessels.

ETIOLOGY

Simple traumatic lymphangitis is due to streptococcal infection gaining entrance through an open wound. The limbs, usually hind limbs, are commonly affected. Lymphangitis may also be caused by specific diseases like Farcy (Glanders, caused by Pfeiferella mallei), Tuberculosis (Tuberculous lymphangitis), Epizootic lymphangitis (caused by cryptococcus farciminosus), and Ulcerative lymphangitis (caused in the horse by corynebacterium *ovis*). Nodular thickening of the lymphatics and ulceration may be noticed in specific lymphangitis. Examination of the discharge from the ulcers may reveal organisms.

SYMPTOMS

Lymphangitis is usually observed suddenly. In working animals it is seen after a period of rest. (As working horses are usually given rest on Sundays the disease is sometimes noticed on Mondays. Hence simple lymphangitis is popularly called *Monday-morning disease*. The animal is off its feed and dull. Severe lameness, local oedema and sometimes fever, are evident.

CLASSIFICATION

Serous lymphangitis: This is a simple inflammatory condition of the lymphatics and is characterised by oedema resulting from retention of serous exudations (lymph) in tissue spaces and is followed by recovery. But recurrence is common and such repeated attacks may cause fibrous thickening in the affected part (Elephantiasis).

Purulent lymphangitis: Abscesses form along the lymphatics and they rupture causing ulceration. These ulcers may discharge a white or creamy pus.

Gangrenous form: It is recognised by gangrenous patches of varying depth throughout the affected region.

Septicaemic form: It is accompanied by symptoms of septicaemia. The complications accompanying this disease are bursitis, tendinitis; synovitis of the tendon sheaths, etc.

PROGNOSIS

In uncomplicated cases of serous lymphangitis prognosis is generally favourable. In the other forms prognosis is guarded.

TREATMENT

1. Application of liniments and massaging the area to stimulate circulation.

2. Saline purgatives and diuretics to eliminate fluids and toxic products from the system.

3. Potassium iodide internally may hasten the reabsorption of oedematous fluid.

4. Apply Mag Sulph-Glycerin Paste locally. When lymphangitis becomes chronic, fibrous thickenings are caused for which no treatment is effective.

5. Purulent and gangrenous forms will require, besides the treatments suggested above, the treatments for abscess, ulcer or gangrene, as the case may be. Use of sulphonamides, antibiotics, etc., also becomes necessary depending on the virulence and sensitivity of the causal organism.

Lymphadenitis

It is the inflammation of lymphatic glands.

ETIOLOGY

Infection. Streptococcal and staphylococcal infections common. Systemic diseases like strangles may cause lymphadenitis.

SYMPTOMS

There is enlargement of the gland. Sometimes it may develop into an abscess.

TREATMENT
1. Blistering ointments are sometimes helpful in simple inflammation of the gland.
2. Administration of potassium iodide.
3. Administration of antibiotics, sulphonamides, etc., depending on the causal organism.
4. If in the form of an abscess, general treatment for abscess is given. Extirpation of the gland may be necessary.
5. Extirpation of the gland may be advisable in certain cases of chronic lymphadenitis also where in the enlargement persists.

Tumours of Lymphatic Glands
These are usually of a malignant nature. It is better to extirpate them in most cases.

Questions

1. Write an account of non-specific lymphangitis occurring in equines.

CHAPTER 11

Bursatee (Bursati)

Bursatee is a disease affecting the skin and subcutaneous tissue of horses, characterised by the formation of fibrous tumours.

The disease is seasonal in occurrence, prevalent in the rainy season (June-Oct.) and hence the name Bursati.*

ETIOLOGY

Not known. Supposed to be due to the migration of some parasitic larvae.

SYMPTOMS

The disease starts with hot, painful swellings in the subcutaneous and/or submucous tissue. The swellings develop into hard, fibrous masses within a week. After another 15 to 20 days the skin sloughs off leaving an ulcer. A slight, yellowish red, discharge collects on the ulcer. The ulcer when squeezed gives out a hard fibrous core called *Kunkur*. Kunkur is a dense, fibrous mass approximately the size of a pea containing cellular elements including neutrophils, monocytes, etc. There is no pus formation unless there is secondary infection. Caseation does not happen even in very chronic cases. The ulcer becomes covered by scabs within a few days if not exposed to infection. But if infected, they grow to large sizes.

The ulcers usually heal with the onset of winter but may reappear in the next rainy season. The regions frequently affected are: pastern, fetlock, neck, withers and shoulder. Rarely the tumours are noticed on the mucous membranes of the vulva and sheath.

---

* The word *bursat* in Hindi means rain.

TREATMENT
1. Squeeze out the contents of the fibrous tumours.
2. Clean and dress the ulcers with BIPP.
3. Administration of arsenicals and other skin tonics.
[Ref:--*Handbook of Contagious and Infectious Diseases of Animals* published by the Government of India Press, (1944), pp. 66-67].

Questions

1. What is *Bursatee*? Describe the clinical picture and its surgical pathology.

CHAPTER 12

Tumours (Neoplasms)

A tumour (neoplasm) is caused by a purposeless multiplication of living cells.

(The word neoplasm means new growth. Neoplasia means formation of new tissue. A neoplasm is different from inflammatory hyperplasia.)

INCIDENCE

Tumours are more common in carnivora as compared to other animals. Among other animals horse and cattle are more often affected than sheep, pig and goats. Old animals are affected more commonly than younger ones.

ETIOLOGY

The etiology of tumours is not well established. Certain types of tumours are caused by virus, e.g. oral papilloma in the dog and venereal granuloma.

CLASSIFICATION

1. *Clinically* tumours may be classified into two types, viz., Benign or Simple tumours and Malignant tumours. A benign tumour does not recur after removal whereas a malignant tumour does recur.

2. Based on their histological structures tumours may be classified as fibroma, osteoma, etc.

3. Based on the embryonic layer from which the tumour tissue is derived tumours may be classified as epiblast, mesoblast or hypoblast.

Varieties of Tumours

1. CONNECTIVE TISSUE TUMOURS

(i) *Fibroma*: A tumour consisting of white connective tissue fibres. Usually well-capsulated and easy to remove. Common locations are head, neck, shoulder, leg, etc. Nasal polypi seen in the nasal cavity of horse and rarely of cattle are a special variety of fibroma. They may resemble osteoma.

(ii) *Chondroma*: It is composed of cartilaginous tissue.

(iii) *Osteoma*: It is composed of bony tissue and is one of the most common tumours arising from bones of the skull and extremities. Dental alveoli, sinuses of head and mandible are common sites in the horse.

(iv) *Odontoma*: Composed of tooth tissue, i.e., enamel, cementum and dentine.

(v) *Epulis*: Arising from bone and periosteum at the alveolar border.

(vi) *Myoma*: Made up of muscular tissue, e.g. rhabdomyoma affecting the tongue.

(vii) *Myxoma*: A tumour whose structure resembles connective tissue and the vitreous humour of the eye.

(viii) *Lipoma*: A tumour made up of fat cells.

(ix) *Neuroma*: A tumour made up of nerve cells and fibres.

(x) *Glioma*: It is composed of neuroglial tissue.

(xi) *Angioma*: It is made up of lymphatic or blood vessels.

(xii) *Sarcoma*: A *malignant* tumour involving any kind of connective tissue like bone, cartilage, fibrous tissue, etc. Sarcomas are composed of mesoblastic cells in their developmental stage and exhibit proliferative and infiltrating tendencies, e.g., chondro-sarcoma, osteosarcoma, lymphosarcoma, fibrosarcoma, mela-noma, etc. Fibrosarcoma is the most common type of sarcoma found in domestic animals especially horses and mules. It is commonly seen in the form of nodular growths affecting ear, mandible, vagina, penis, maxillary sinus, etc., of horses. Fibromas and fibrosarcomas are common in the pharynx of bovine. Melanoma is tumour composed of melanin pigmented cells. They are usually malignant. Common in old grey horses, red pigs and Ayrshire cattle. Bones of extremities in dogs are commonly affected by osteosarcomas.

2. EPITHELIAL TUMOURS

(i) *Papilloma*: A tumour originating from the epithelium of the skin or mucous membranes appearing in the form of a wart-like growth from the surface, e.g., warts on the skin, oral papilloma, vaginal papilloma.

(ii) *Adenoma*: An epithelial tumour with a gland-like structure originating from glandular epithelium, e.g., adenoma of salivary gland, lymphadenoma involving lymphatic gland, etc.

(iii) *Carcinoma*: A malignant epithelial tumour, e.g., carcinoma of the eye, horn, mammary gland, sheath, etc. Depending on the type of epithelial cell a carcinoma may be called squamous-celled, basel-celled, columnar-celled, spheroidal-celled, mucoid-celled, or embryonal-celled.

3. ENDOTHELIAL TUMOURS

(i) *Mesothelioma:* It develops from mesothelial tissue.

(ii) *Perithelioma*: It develops from tunica adventitia of blood vessels.

(iii) *Psammoma*: A fibrous tumour of brain tissue.

(iv) *Cholesteatoma*: A tumour of crystalline, structure, e.g., cholesteatoma of the brain, tympanum and middle ear.

4. LYMPHOID TISSUE TUMOURS

(i) *Lymphoma*: A tumour made up of lymphoid tissue.

(ii) *Lymphosarcoma*: A malignant neoplasm arising in lymphatic tissue.

5. TERATOMA

A tumour containing disorderly arrangement of tissues and organs, resulting from faulty embryonic differentiation and organisation.

(i) *Dermoid cyst*: A tumour composed of cutaneous tissues.

(ii) *Dentigerous cyst*: A tumour containing tooth, e.g., dentigerous cyst of the temporal bone met with in the horse.

DIAGNOSIS

Papillomas and warts are easily identified by their gross appearance. A *benign tumour* is comparatively slow in growth. It resembles the tissue of origin, is not adherent to overlying skin, and usually do not ulcerate. They do not invade or infiltrate into surrounding tissue. *Malignant tumours* (cancer), viz., **sarcomata** and carcinomata, grow rapidly and give rise to secondary tumours in their vicinity and in other parts of the body as a result of neoplastic elements carried through the blood or lymph stream. Skin is usually adherent to the tumour and may ulcerate. The cells constituting the tumour are immature and are in a state of active multiplication.

PROGNOSIS

A benign tumour is not harmful except when it is large enough to cause mechanical pressure on the surrounding tissues/ organs and interferes with their function. They may be successfully excised (removed) if situated in a place where operation is possible Malignant tumours in the great majority of cases are incurable.

TREATMENT

Removal of tumours may be done by any of the following techniques.

1. *Ligation:* A tight ligature is applied at the base of the tumour so as to cut off its blood supply. The tumour sloughs off within about ten days. Ligation is convenient only in the case of pedunculated tumours. During the process of sloughing the ligature becomes loose so that it may have to be replaced. It is therefore better to use an elastic ligature.

2. *By using red-hot iron:* The tumour is clamped below its base and the red-hot iron is applied distal to the clamp so as to remove the tumour. By this method removal is possible without much haemorrhage.

3. *By using the ecraseur:* The ecraseur is useful specially for removing small pedunculated tumours situated in the pharynx, vagina, etc. The tumour is held within the chain loop and is tightened around the base of the tumour to effect removal.

4. The *wart enucleator* is very useful for removing small tumours like warts.

5. *Chemical caustics* like caustic potash, arsenical paste, nitric acid, acetic acid, etc., may be used for removing small

tumours. Salicylic acid ointment is very effective for warts.

6. *Excision* (surgical removal): The tumour is carefully dissected out from the surrounding tissues. Care should be taken to remove all the tumour cells and at the same time there should not be too much damage to the surrounding tissues. If the surrounding lymph glands are involved, they should also be removed.

7. *Treatment for malignant tumours:* Treatment is useless in the case of malignant tumours because of their tendency to recur. But temporary relief may be afforded by total excision of the tumour. Amputation of the affected part is sometimes advisable when the tumour is situated on extremities like limbs, tail and penis. Combination of Surgery, Radiation and Chemotherapy, as practised in human medicine, are rarely practicable.

8. *Treatment for warts:* Larger warts may be enucleated surgically. The use of "wart vaccine" is found useful in certain cases in the bovine. A 20 to 25 cc of the vaccine is given subcutaneously and is repeated once or twice at weekly intervals. Another vaccine found useful is prepared as follows: Remove a few warts and triturate them in normal saline (1 cc of saline to each gram of wart). Leave at room temperature. Remove supernatant fluid. Heat to 50°C for one hour. Add 5% to 10% phenol-formalin. The dose is 5 to 10 cc S/c. In young animals prognosis is generally unfavourable because warts tend to recur. (3) *Dimethyl sulphoxide* (DMSO) has been successfully used in the treatment of warts. The (medical) DMSO is to be applied undiluted over the warts. Single application usually assures gradual disappearance of warts with no recurrence.

Questions

1. How does a tumour differ from an inflammatory enlargement? Describe the difference in the clinical picture between a benign tumour and a malignant tumour. Give suitable examples of each.

2. What is teratoma ? Write briefly on its incidence with special reference to dogs and calves and give an outline of the treatment advised.

CHAPTER 13

Cysts

A cyst is a sac containing liquid or semi-solid substance. Ordinarily a cyst has an inner lining of secreting membrane. Occasionally a cyst may contain a solid structure like tooth, hair, etc. Examples are dentigerous cyst, dermoid cyst.

Varieties of Cysts

1. Retention cyst arising from occlusion of a duct or gland, e.g., salivary cyst, ranula, honey cyst.
2. Exudation cyst due to accumulation of fluid in a pre-existing cavity, e.g., hydrocele.
3. Congenital cyst present at birth, due to failure of an embryonic cavity to close, e.g., urachal cyst.
4. Cysts developing from misplaced embryonic tissue, e.g., dermoid cyst, dentigerous cyst.
5. Encapsulation cyst formed around foreign bodies and parasites.
6. Degeneration cyst resulting from degeneration of a new growth.

DIAGNOSIS

Cysts are non-inflammatory and slow in development. They have a well-defined periphery. A cyst containing fluid will fluctuate uniformly. If the contents are semi-solid and hard it fluctuates *en masse*. A cyst is easily differentiated from an inflammatory swelling, abscess and haematoma. (See chapters on abscess and wounds.) Exploratory puncture may help confirm the diagnosis.

TREATMENT

1. The cyst is punctured with a trocar and canula or inoculation needle and the contents are evacuated. An irritant solution

like tincture iodine is then injected into the cavity to destroy the lining membrane. During the healing process, the cavity of the cyst may get obliterated.

2. The cyst may, instead of puncturing, be incised to evacuate the contents. This is specially useful when the contents are semisolid or solid.

3. Passing a seton through the cyst.

4. Excision of the cyst is the best method of treatment when it is practicable. The cyst is isolated from surrounding tissues by dissecting around it and is removed just like a tumour. When the cyst is very large and deep-seated, it might be desirable to open the cyst before dissecting it.

Note: See also Chapter 36 for Ranula.

Dentigerous Cyst of the Temporal Bone

A dentigerous cyst is an abnormal tooth developing in an abnormal situation, outside the mouth.

A dentigerous cyst is sometimes seen in the horse, developing on the temporal bone.

SYMPTOMS

A small sinus opening at the base of the ear, giving out a thick discharge.

DIAGNOSIS

A probe passed through the sinus opening will strike the tooth.

TREATMENT

The tooth may be removed surgically. A sufficiently large incision is made to open out the sinus tract leading to the tooth and the tooth is then removed by using a dental forceps or tooth chisel. The sinus tracts are cauterised. The wound is sutured, leaving an opening at its bottom for drainage.

Branchial Cyst (Honey Cyst)

Branchial cyst is a congenital abnormality. It is occasionally met with in the dog.

The cyst results from failure of the branchial arches to fuse (particularly the mandibular and hyoid arches). The cyst develops very gradually and is noticed when the dog attains maturity.

SYMPTOMS

A soft, fluctuating non-inflammatory swelling is seen on the ventral aspect of the neck. Sometime it gives rise to a fistulous opening on the skin. (Branchial fistula.)

TREATMENT

Careful excision of the cyst. The cyst wall should be removed completely as otherwise secondary cysts are likely to develop.

Ranula (Salivary Cyst) See page 299.

Questions

1. What are cysts and how will you differentiate them from other forms of tissue distension or tissue growth?

CHAPTER 14

Inflammation

Inflammation is a purposeful reaction of living tissues to the action of an irritant.

The purposes of inflammation are to destroy and remove the irritant, and to repair the damaged tissues.

Causes of Inflammation

Inflammation is caused due to the irritation of living tissues. The irritant responsible for this may be any of the following types.

1. Trauma, e.g., any external violence.
2. Physical agents, e.g., excessive cold, heat, electricity, irradiation.
3. Chemicals, e.g., acids, alkalies, poisons.
4. Bacteria, viruses, other micro-organisms, parasites.

Symptoms

The five cardinal (fundamental or chief) symptoms of inflammation are *Rubor, Calor, Tumor, Dolar, et functio laesa* (Redness, heat, swelling, pain and disordered function).

Rubor (redness of the affected area) is due to the dilatation of blood vessels and increased blood to flow to the part and possibly also due to bleeding from small blood vessels which might have ruptured. The redness can, however, be observed only if the skin is non-pigmented.

Calor (abnormal heat) is caused by the increased flow of warm arterial blood to the part (hyperaemia) and chemical changes in tissues.

Tumor (swelling) is due to exudation of plasma and other blood constituents into the inflamed area and cellular proliferation. The swelling varies in size according to the vascularity of the area, the degree of injury, kind of tissue, etc. It is obviously less marked in avascular tissues and hard tissues, as compared to vascular tissues and loose areolar tissues.

Dolar (pain) is due to compression of sensory nerve terminals in the area and sometimes due to local neuritis. The intensity of pain varies according to the nerve supply to the region, tenseness and hardness of tissue, etc.

Vascular and exudative changes: There is increased blood flow to the area (hyperaemia) after a short period of vaso-constriction. The irritant causes devitalisation of tissue cells and the damaged cells produce histamin-like substance which cause dilatation of capillaries in the inflammed area. The dilatation of capillaries slows the blood stream and both these changes together encourage exudation of plasma and escape of cellular constituents of blood through the capillary walls. This exudate is called *inflammatory exudate*. The collection of inflammatory exudate causes swelling (*inflammatory oedema*).

Along with the exudation of plasma there is also *emigration of lecocytes* through capillary walls. A varying quantity of erythrocytes also escapes into the inflammatory exudate (*diapedesis of erythrocytes*), especially when damage has been caused to the capillary walls. The blood cells that may be noticed in an inflammed area are neutrophils (Microphages of Metchnicoff), monocytes, lymphocytes, eosinophils, basophils, plasmocytes and erythrocytes. In the first 6 to 24 hours neutrophils predominate. The connective tissue cells present are wandering connective tissue cells (hystiocyte; macrophages of Metchnicoff) and fixed connective tissue cells (fibroblasts).

Inflammation in non-vascular tissues: The phenomena of inflammation are essentially similar to inflammation in vascular tissues; but the vascular and exudative changes are less pronounced or absent. The connective tissue reaction is more marked.

Varieties of Inflammation (Classification of Inflammation)

1. According to the acuteness of onset, intensity of symptoms and duration of course:

(a) *Acute inflammation* (*Exudative inflammation*): Acute inflammation is caused by a severe irritant. The symptoms are very pronounced.

(b) *Sub-acute inflammation*.

(c) *Chronic inflammation*: Caused by mild and frequently

repeated attack of an irritant. The exudative phenomena and other symptoms are not so marked as in acute inflammation. The characteristic feature of chronic inflammation is formation of fibrous tissue.

2. According to the nature of exudate:

(a) *Serous inflammation*: Inflammation of serous membranes like peritoneum and pleura wherein a serous exudate is produced.

(d) *Haemorrhagic inflammation*: When RBCs are present in the inflammatory exudate.

(e) *Fibrinous (croupous) inflammation*: In which the exudate contains large quantities of fibrin. The fibrin coagulates and may cause adhesion between inflammed surfaces presenting a "bread and butter" appearance, e.g., fibrinous pericarditis.

(d) *Purulent (suppurative) inflammation*: It is characterised by the formation of pus.

(e) *Phlegmonous inflammation*: Caused by pyogenic organisms, presenting a semi-purulent or purulent exudate.

(f) *Catarrhal inflammation*: Inflammation affecting principally a mucous surface and which is marked by a discharge of mucous and epithelial debris.

(g) *Membranous or Diphtheritic inflammation*: Affecting mucous surfaces, characterised by the formation of a false membrane, e.g., inflammations caused by Fusiformis necroforus.

(h) Mucopurulent, sero-fibrinous etc.

3. Based on sequelae or tissue changes:

(a) *Adhesive inflammation*: Which brings about adhesion of opposing surfaces.

(b) *Obliterative inflammation*: Inflammation of the lining membrane of a cavity or a vessel which results in adhesion between the surfaces and consequent obliteration of the lumen.

(c) *Hyperplastic (Plastic; Productive; Proliferous) inflammation*: It leads to the formation of new connective tissue in abundance.

(d) *Atrophic (Cirrhotic, Fibroid, Sclerosing) inflammation*: Which results in atrophy and deformity.

(e) *Granulomatous inflammation*: The inflammed tissues resembling granulation tissue. (Granuloma means a tumour-like mass of granulation tissue.) For example inflammations caused by Actinomyce, Micobacterium tuborculosis, etc.

(f) *Necrotic inflammation*: in which there is death of the affected tissue.

4. According to the extent of tissue involved:

(a) *Diffuse inflammation*: Spread over a large area or one which affects both interstitial and parenchymatous tissue.

(b) *Focal*: Confined to a particular spot or area.

(c) *Disseminated inflammation*: Wherein there are a number of distinct foci.

(d) *Interstitial inflammation*: Which primarily affects the stroma of an organ.

(e) *Parenchymatous inflammation*: Affecting primarily the essential tissue elements (parenchyma of an organ).

5. Based on etiology:

(a) *Specific inflammation*: Caused by any particular micro-organism.

(b) Traumatic inflammation that is caused by an injury.

(c) Allergic inflammation caused by substances that are allergic.

(d) *Toxic inflammation*: Caused by toxic substances or inflammation leading to toxaemia.

6. Depending on the location:

(a) *Metastatic inflammation*: One that is produced in a distant part by conveyance of infective material through the blood or lymph.

(b) *Reactive inflammation*: Occurring about a foreign body or focus.

Terminations of Inflammation

In mild cases of inflammation there is *delitescence* (disappearance of symptoms). Other favourable cases terminate in *resolution* after the irritant has been removed or neutralised.

The inflammatory exudate gets reabsorbed through lymphatics and the damaged cellular matters are removed by phagocytosis. The tissue cells are either regenerated or are replaced by fibroconnective tissue. There is apparent resumption of function though there is alteration in the tissue. There might also be fibrous thickening or induration.

When inflammation is produced by pyogenic organisms there is pus formation (*suppuration*) leading to formation of abscesses.

When the inflammation is severe, there is massive death of tissue. This death of tissue *en masse* is called *gangrene*.

Treatment of Inflammation

The cause of inflammation should be removed.

Cold and astringent applications are indicated to suppress inflammatory exudation. Applications of cold water, ice, astringent lotions like white lotion, are commonly used.

Compression and application of pressure bandages are also advisable to minimise the inflammatory swelling.

Warm applications (fomentations) are indicated in severe inflammations where tissues are threatened with gangrene. They induce proper circulation and thereby favour reabsorption of exudates. Fomentations are given in the form of either dry heat or moist heat. Heated bran, sand etc., covered in cloth bundle is used to provide dry heat. Cloth pieces dipped in hot water provides moist heat. Moist heat is more soothening than dry heat.

For superficial lesions application of a local analgesic preparation (like cocainised vaseline) to relieve the pain.

When the congestion due to inflammation is severe, scarification is sometimes resorted to. (The superficial layer of tissue is scraped to induce slight bleeding.) The disadvantages of this method are that it causes additional trauma and also paves the way for possible infection.

For septic inflammations, antiseptic applications and antibiotic therapy are indicated. Bier's hyperaemia may also be tried.

Cortisone and its allied preparations are extensively used as anti-inflammatory agents. They are excellent for alleviating the symptoms but may have no remedial value.

Questions

1. What treatment would you adopt for an acute inflammation of a vascular area?

2. Write a short essay on inflammation.

CHAPTER 15

Suppuration and Abscess

Suppuration

The formation of pus in tissues is called suppuration. Suppuration is usually caused by pyogenic bacteria like Streptococci, Staphylococci, Pseudomonas aeruginosa, Escherichia. coli, etc. Suppuration can also be caused by irritants like turpentine, calomel, croton oil, etc.

Pus *consists* of "Pus corpuscles" (cellular matter composed of especially polymorphs), and pus serum. Enzymes from leucocytes, bacteria and tissue debris are also present. Pus may be mixed with serum, mucous or blood when it is called seropus, mucopus or sanious pus, as the case may be. The *colour* of pus may vary from opaque, yellowish or greenish. The *consistency* of pus may be creamy, curdy, cheesy or ichorus (thin and acrid). Pus may be Living pus (Laudable pus), Sterile pus, Dead pus, and Septic pus (Infectious pus).

Living Pus (*Laudable Pus*): It contains living phagocytic cells and may be "*sterile*". It has phagocytic, bactericidal, bacteriostatic, bacteriolytic and antitoxic properties. The antiseptic property of living pus is decreased by dilution and use of strong antiseptics.

Dead Pus: Dead pus contains dead cells and do not possess bactericidal and phagocytic properties. It may also be infectious as it may contain the infective organisms.

Septic Pus: It contains living pathogenic organisms and bacterial toxins that the pus corpuscles could not destroy.

Empyema: It is collection of pus in a body cavity, e.g., empyema of frontal sinus, empyema of maxillary sinus, empyema of a joint (pyarthrosis), empyema of pericardium (pyopericardium), empyema of pleura (pyothorax, purulent pleurisy), etc.

Phlegmon (*Cellulitis*): It is an acute inflammation involving the connective tissues, in the form of a diffuse suppurative or serous lesion causing tissue necrosis, abscess formation and ulceration.

Abscess

An abscess is an abnormal cavity containing pus. The cavity is formed in tissues, due to local suppurative inflammation. Tissue reaction against the invading organism or foreign body as well as degenerative changes are evident in the zone of tissue surrounding the pus. This zone is called *'pyogenic membrane'* even though there is no membrane as such.

Classification

1. *Acute (hot) abscess*: In this the inflammatory symptoms are quite active.

2. *Chronic (cold) abscess*: In this the inflammatory symptoms are less active. In chronic abscess the pus may become partly inspissated or liquefied. (See also page 101).

3. *Superficial abscess*: It is situated superficially.

4. *Deep abscess*: An abscess that is deep-seated.

5. *Embolic abscess*: Developing from a septic embolus.

6. *Pyaemic or metastatic abscess*: A number of abscesses developing in different parts of the body.

SYMPTOMS

Acute abscesses developing superficially appear at first as a localised, painful, inflammatory swelling. The centre of the swelling gradually becomes soft and the skin at this point becomes thin when the abscess is said to be "pointing" or "maturing" or "ripening". Later, the abscess ruptures at this point and discharges pus. Febrile disturbances are usually absent in superficial abscesses. Deep abscesses developing under thick layers of tissue (like facia, muscle) give rise to pyrexia and pain on manipulation of the part. After such an abscess ruptures the pus migrates along the line of least resistance. Abscesses situated close to the rectum, pharynx, larynx and spinal cord create serious functional disturbances.

Termination of an Abscess

1. The pus inside an abscess tries to move along the direction of least resistance. When the pus reaches close to a surface, an

elevation is noticed at that point. The point becomes necrosed and appears yellowish or pale. This is called pointing of the abscess. The necrosed area at the point eventually sloughs discharging the pus. This is called rupturing of the abscess. A superficial abscess usually points and ruptures, discharging the pus and thereafter healing may follow. Hence the normal sequence that an abscess might follow are pointing or maturing, rupture, and draining. As already mentioned, the contents of an abscess may be sterile or septic. Draining may be followed by healing or the abscess may form again if the drainage is defective or if infection is not controlled. During the maturation stage, there is a varying degree of cellulitis of surrounding tissues, pain, rise of temperature, and functional disturbances of the affected part. There is more chance for spread of infection and septicaemia at this stage.

A pointed (matured or ripened) abscess may be helped to drain by incising at the "point", but incising an abscess before it points is likely to cause undue surgical trauma and create complications like spread of infection or cellulitis.

(2) If an abscess does not rupture the pus may be retained. The retained pus becomes thick (inspissated) because of absorption of its fluid content. The contents may appear curd-like. Retained pus may get encapsulated or calcified. It may sometimes get absorbed.

(3) When a deep-seated abscess ruptures, pus moves towards the surface through the surrounding tissues, following the line of least resistance.

Differential Diagnosis

An abscess should be differentiated from a cyst, a haematoma, a synovial distention or an abdominal hernia. A cyst develops slowly and fluctuates uniformly. A haematoma (which contains coagulated blood and serum) has a doughy consistency and may crepitate on palpation. It is not painful and does not point like an abscess. A distended synovial sheath is recognised by its location and by careful palpation. An abdominal hernia can be differentiated by the presence of the hernial ring. To confirm differential diagnosis, exploratory puncture may be made to find out the nature of contents.

TREATMENT

Fomentation and/or applications of blisters are advised to bring about early maturation of the abscess. The blister commonly used is Biniodide of mercury ointment (1 in 32 to 1 in 8). When the abscess is ripe the pus collects in a cavity. It is not ordinarily advisable to open an abscess which is not fully ripe as secondary abscess may form afterwards. However abscesses situated close to a joint or peritoneum may have to be opened before fully mature, to avoid the chance of rupture into the joint or peritoneal cavity.

The site where it is proposed to open and the surrounding areas should be cleaned and prepared as for a surgical operation: after shaving and washing the area with soap and water, drying and applying a suitable antiseptic like tincture iodire.

A sterilised "Syme's Abscess Knife" or scalpel may be used to open the abscess. The opening should be at the site where it "points". It should as far as possible be in a "dependant portion" to facilitate drainage. Dependant portion here means a lower area through which drainage by gravity is possible in the normal position of the patient. If the abscess is not pointing at a dependant portion it is sometimes necessary to make another opening in the dependant portion to provide drainage. This is called a "counter-opening". In order to make a counter-opening, a seton-needle may be passed through the first opening made and taken out through the dependant portion. Afterwards a "seton" (gauze dipped in antiseptic solution) may be passed through the eye of the seton-needle and carried through the openings and tied, in order to keep the openings patent. The seton is changed each day after cleaning the abscess cavity. However, many abscesses drain satisfactorily without a counter-opening and it is sufficient to make a single opening at the place where it "points".

After opening the abscess, the contents usually start draining. The abscess cavity should be irrigated with hypertonic saline. Afterwards it is stuffed with gauze dipped in Tincture iodine. This is intended to destroy any infection remaining therein and also to exert a mild irritant action to stimulate the healing process.

The gauze packs are removed after twenty-four hours (i.e., second day) and then the abscess cavity is irrigated with a mild antiseptic lotion. The conventional method was to irrigate with 1 in 500 solution of Acriflavin sulphate as it is a solution which retains its antiseptic properties even in the presence of pus. In modern times many patent antiseptic solutions like dettol, savlon, etc., are available.

The abscess cavity from the second day onwards is packed with sterile gauze dipped in Magnesium sulphate-Glycerine paste, which greatly favours drainage and absorption of fluid exudates. Topical application of antiseptics or antibiotics in the form of ointments or dusting powder is indicated if virulent infection is suspected, and systemic use of antibiotics may also be necessary in some cases.

Bismuth-iodoform-paraffin paste (BIPP) is a conventional antiseptic dressing used. It contains Bismuth submitras (1 part) and Iodoform (2 parts) mixed in Liquid paraffin to form a paste of desired consistency.

The normal time required for the healing of an opened out ·abscess is usually *three weeks.* (See also "Antibioma" page 101).

Acne

Acne is an abscess involving the sebacious gland. (See page 654)

INCIDENCE

The disease occurs in all domestic animals but is common in the horse and dog. In the dog it is more common in short haired breeds. The regions rich in sebacious glands (like nose, lips, sheath, etc.) are often affected.

ETIOLOGY

The infection is caused by Staphylococci. Local irritation from any cause (e.g., friction from saddle or collor) predisposes to the infection.

SYMPTOMS

The lesion may appear as single pustules or as furuncles (=a group of pustules). The pustule may have the size of a pea. When it ruptures greyish white pus is given out. A greyish white core of necrotic tissue comes out when the pustule is compressed between fingers.

TREATMENT

Wash thoroughly with soap and warm water. Apply an

antiseptic ointment like Carbolised vaseline (2% to 5%), Boro vaseline (2%), Salicylic acid ointment etc. In chronic cases with induration Unguntum Hydrargyri Oxidi Flavi is found to be effective. Some of the pustules may require to be incised to remove the necrotic core. They are afterwards touched with Tinct iodine. Penicillin topically and systemically is very effective. Other antibiotics also may be tried. (See also page 654)

Note: It is better to avoid preparations containing mercury and carbolic acid for the dog for fear of poisoning.

Furunculosis

Furunculosis is characterised by groups of boils in different parts of the body. A boil is an abscess involving the hair follicle caused by the infection by staphylococci.

TREATMENT

On the same lines as for Acne.

Alteratives and tonics and a liberal supply of nourishing foods. Administration of Vitamin B Complex or yeast has given good results in the dog. In obstinate cases use antibiotics.

Impetigo

Impetigo is a mildly contageous disease met with in human beings characterised by a number of vesiculo-pustular eruptions appearing on different parts of the body caused by Staphylococci.

TREATMENT

Penicillin is very effective.

Carbuncle

Carbuncle is a condition produced by small boils rupturing subcutaneously and draining inadequately through many tiny openings on the skin. The condition may start as a single boil which breaks into and extends along loose areolar and fatty subcutaneous tissue letting out pus through small openings here and there. Carbuncles are common in diabetic patients. They are usually caused by staphylococcal infections of the superficial facia. Penicillin is effective in most cases.

Antibioma

When an abscess has developed and pus has been formed in it proper healing will not take place if it is not drained. If treated with antibiotics, without proper drainage, there will be fibrosis around the abscess cavity and fluids in it may get absorbed making the pus inspissated. Such a clinical condition resulting from improper treatment of an abscess is called an "antibioma".

Questions

1. Describe the symptoms, differential diagnosis and treatment of an abscess.
2. Differentiate between hot abscess and cold abscess. Illustrate your answer with suitable examples giving their relative incidence.
3. Write short notes on:—a. Furunculosis   b. Sterile abscess c. Antibioma.

Addendum

The term 'cold abscess' is generally used in human medicine for a tuberculous abscess because the skin temperature is not raised as in ordinary developing abscess. The redness and pointing develop slowly or may not appear at all; sometimes the pus may get absorbed and resolution may occur.

Systemic treatment becomes necessary in treating a tuberculous abscess.

In veterinary practice, the term 'cold abscess' generally means a chronic abscess which need not necessarily be tuberculous.

CHAPTER 16

Necrosis and Gangrene

Necrosis is the death of a cell or group of cells in a living body, due to pathological reasons.

Examples of necrosis are:

1. Avascular necrosis (bland necrosis; simple necrosis; spontaneous necrosis; anaemic necrosis; or aseptic necrosis) wherein the necrosis is caused without infection and inflammation.

2. Coagulation necrosis is most frequently seen in infarction wherein the cell form and arrangement are not altered.

3. Liquefactive (colliquative) necrosis results in death of the cells involved:

4. Ischaemic necrosis is due to occlusion of an artery supplying the region.

5. Embolic necrosis is caused by embolism.

6. Diphtheretic necrosis is necrosis of a mucous membrane wherein a tough membranous layer called "diphtheritic membrane" is formed by the coagulated cells and fibrin.

Gangrene is the death of extensive area or mass of tissue due to failure of blood supply, disease, or injury.

ETIOLOGY

1. Due to certain bacterial infections like black quarter, malignant oedema, fusiformis necroforus, streptococci and staphylococci.

2. Burns and scalds, frost bite.

3. Caustic chemicals (strong acids and alkalies).

4. Traumatic injuries causing destruction of tissue or interfering with the nerve and blood supply to a part. Bed sore (dry gangrene caused by constant pressure on bony prominence of body) and "sit fast" also are included under this category.

5. Dimunition in the local resistance of tissue due to infiltration with urine, bile etc.

6. Due to the interference with the blood or nerve supply to a part.

7. Toxins.

CLASSIFICATION

1. *Dry Gangrene*: In dry gangrene the dead tissues become diy and reduced in volume.

2. *Moist gangrene*: It is seen in tissues having high fluid content. There is disintegration and liquefaction of tissue and a blood-stained, foul-smelling fluid is noticed. The absorption of this fluid containing toxic substances may also cause constitutional disturbances.

LOCAL SYMPTOMS

In *dry gangrene* contraction of tissue and the loss of normal appearance of the tissue becomes evident, e.g., the skin presents a wrinkled appearance with its hair dry and erect.

In *moist gangrene* the enlargement of the tissue with blood and serum causes an initial increase in the volume and change in the colour of tissue. At this stage there is severe pain. The tissues may present a blackish or purple or greenish appearance. When death of tissue takes place they appear cold and insensitive and pain disappears. A dark red, foul-smelling discharge is noticed.

TERMINATION

Local inflammation can be noticed around the dead tissues and a distinct line of demarkation gradually develops. In favourable cases the dead tissues are later cast off (sloughs) and the healing takes place of the resulting wound. The process of gangrene is marked by three stages, viz., (1) death of tissue, (2) separation of slough, and (3) healing (cicatrisation) of the resulting wound. Dead pieces of tissues like bone, cartilage, ligament and tendons are very slow to separate.

COMPLICATIONS

1. Death resulting from toxaemia or secondary bacterial infection.

2. Secondary haemorrhage if a vessel has been included in the slough.

3. If tendon sheath or joint cavities are opened by the sloughing, septic synovitis or arthritis may follow.

DIAGNOSIS

From the symptoms.

PROGNOSIS

Prognosis depends on the extent of the lesion, the resulting toxaemia and the virulence of the infecting organism, if any.

TREATMENT

The cause of gangrene should be removed and the spreading of the lesion to surrounding tissues should be prevented. Sloughing of the dead tissues should be facilitated.

2. Application of an irritant to the area to induce hyperaemia and separation of the slough.

3. Scarification of the tissue is sometimes advised to allow the discharges to escape from the dead tissue and to make possible penetration of antiseptics into the tissues but it may provide chances for fresh bacterial invasion.

4. Excision of the dead tissue is comparatively safe in the case of dry gangrene but may at times give rise to septic complications.

Questions

1. Give the causes, symptoms and treatment of gangrene.
2. Write short notes on
   (i) Dry gangrene, (ii) Necrosis.

CHAPTER 17

Ulcer

An ulcer is an inflammatory lesion of the skin or mucous membrane with loss of surface epithelium. The healing process in an ulcer is slow and it may show a tendency to persist or extend to surrounding areas.

CLASSIFICATION

1. *Traumatic ulcer*: It is an ulcer resulting from trauma.

2. *Decubitus ulcer*: Resulting from continued pressure (decubitus). The pressure interferes with the local nutrition of tissues and therefore called trophic ulcers (trophic = relating to nutrition) or pressure sores or bed sores.

3. *Pyogenic ulcer*: Also known as septic ulcer, streptococcic ulcer, tuberculous ulcer, actinobacillosis ulcer, etc., it is caused by bacterial and fungal infections.

4. Ulcers resulting from burns.

5. Irradiation ulcers resulting from exposure to X-rays, UV rays, IR rays, etc.

6. Varicose ulcer resulting from vascular disease.

7. Ulcers resulting from lymphatic obstruction.

8. Specific ulcers due to ulcerative lymphangitis, glanders, tuberculosis, etc.

9. *Healing ulcer*: The edges of a healing ulcer are sloping, and the floor is covered by firm granulation tissue. The exudate is very little and is serous and non-irritating. A bluish-white peripheral layer of growing epithelium may be evident.

10. *Spreading ulcer*: The edges and surrounding tissues of a spreading ulcer are inflammed or necrotic and there is usually a purulent and foul smelling discharge.

11. *Phagedenic ulcers*: An ulcer infected with pathogenic organisms and is spreading.

12. *Weak ulcer*: An ulcer in which there is abundance of soft granulation tissue (proud flesh) and in which epithelisation is delayed.

13. *Indurated ulcer*: An ulcer in which the edges are indurated or thickened.

14. *Indolent ulcer*: A chronic ulcer that does not show any tendency to heal, is rather inactive and painless.

15. *Callous ulcers*: Ulcers having a thick, callous (hardened) lining and edges.

16. *Malignant ulcer*: Ulcer resulting from a malignant lesion.

17. *Ulcers due to specific diseases*: Examples are ulcerative lymphangitis, glanders, tuberculosis, etc.

TREATMENT

1. *Removal of the cause*: The causes might be want of immobilisation of the part, rubbing by the patient, etc.

2. *Warm antiseptic irrigations*: Keeping the affected part in warm antiseptic baths, or irrigating with warm antiseptic solutions.

3. Antiseptic dressings like for example, BIPP.

4. Application of caustics is indicated when there is infection, when there is plenty of necrosed tissue or when there is excess of granulation tissue. For example, a septic ulcer may be touched with carbolic acid. Removal of necrotic tissue is favoured by repeated applications of 0.5% hydrochloric acid or urea. The excess granulation tissue can be suppressed by application of caustics like copper sulphate, powdered potassium permanganate etc.

5. *Exposure to ultraviolet rays*: These rays have bactericidal properties and are of special value in infected ulcers.

6. *Use of thermocautery*: Touching the ulcer with red-hot iron will help check infection.

7. *Excision of the ulcer* (*debridement*): This is described in the chapter on wounds.

8. *Bier's hyperaemia*: (This is described in chapter 19).

9. *Treatment of weak ulcers*: In these ulcers there is usually redundant or exuberant granulation (proud flesh). Moist dressings, ointments and septic exudates favour deyelopment of such flabby and oedematous granulations which are deficient in blood supply. These granulations project above the level of the surrounding skin and delay epithelisation. In treating these ulcers, caustics like copper sulphate, potassium permanganate, zinc chloride etc., are used for suppressing the excess granula-

tions. If an oily dressing has been used previously, clean the ulcer with turpentine followed by alcohol. Then apply either powdered copper sulphate or powdered potassium permanganate and put on a pressure bandage. Repeat this daily or on alternate days until healthy granulations appear. Afterwards Dry Dressing Powder may be applied (e.g., zinc oxide plus boric acid plus iodoform).

10. *Treatment of callous ulcers*: The thick callous lining is scraped or excised (under local anaesthesia). The necrotic tissue is cauterised with 10% solution of silver nitrate (or zinc chloride 5 to 10% solution, or zinc sulphate 5 to 10%) and is then treated on general principles.

11. Phagedenic ulcers are treated by first cauterising. Cauterisation may be done by red-hot iron or by chemicals. Chemicals used for the purpose are, phenol followed by tincture iodine; or application of copper sulphate crystals.

12. Irritable ulcers are touched with phenol followed by tincture iodine and are dressed daily with BIPP.

13. It is not advisable to treat tuberculous ulcers in animals for fear of communication of the infection to humans. If they are to be treated, the treatment mentioned for phagedenic ulcers is combined with systemic treatment for TB. In some cases, healing of the ulcer is favoured by producing a strong reaction by injecting a mixture of bovine and human tuberculin.

Questions

1. Define the term ulcer. State the causes and symptoms of non-specific ulcers and the general principles of their treatment.

2. Write short notes on: (i) Serpigenous ulcer, (ii) Indolent ulcer.

Addendum

A 'rodent ulcer' is a malignant ulcer caused by basal-celled carcinoma. Generally it occurs on the upper part of the face close to the eyes. In untreated cases, it erodes the bones of the skull and the patient ultimately dies of septic meningitis.

CHAPTER 18

Sinuses and Fistulae

Sinus

A *sinus* is a tubular, inflammatory tract leading from a deeper inflammatory area, with one or more external openings upon a mucous or cutaneous surface.

The interior of a sinus is lined by granulation tissue. There might be partial ingrowth of surface epithelium. In chronic cases there is thickening around the sinus tract due to fibroconnective tissue.

ETIOLOGY

1. Presence of foreign substance or dead tissue, e.g., metal or glass pieces, infected suture material, necrotic bone, parasites, etc.

2. Infections like actinomycosis, botryomycosis, or specific lesions like carcinoma.

3. A sinus persists when there is inadequate drainage especially when it has a tortuous course. Constant movement of the walls of the sinus interferes with healing process. When it develops thick connective tissue walls and callous or epithelial lining, healing of the sinus is further delayed.

DIAGNOSIS

Fluids injected into the sinus may show its capacity and a probe passed through the sinus may indicate its depth and direction.

TREATMENT

1. Remove the foreign body, if any, causing the condition.

2. The sinus tract is cleaned with 5% to 10% Zinc chloride lotion or is swabbed with Phenol followed by Tincture iodine. The use of solid or liquid caustics is specially indicated when there is thick callous lining. It also helps separation of necrotic tissue.

3. Drainage can be facilitated by injecting and filling the sinus with a 50% solution of Bismuth subiodide in white petrolatum. This is better than filling the cavity with gauze which will obstruct drainage. When there is lot of necrotic tissue, this treatment may not be effective.

4. Drainage can be provided by making a counteropening and passing a seton dipped in antiseptic solution. The seton is changed daily.

5. Opening out the sinus. Before opening a sinus it is better to inject into it a coloured antiseptic solution like methylene blue (1%) so that it will be easier to identify the tract.

6. Use of antibiotics.

7. Bier's hyperaemia.

8. Inoculations of autogenous vaccine.

Fistula

A *fistula* is a tubular inflammatory tract open at both ends connecting two surfaces covered by epithelium or at times mesothelium. It may be caused by injury, a destructive inflammatory or neoplastic process, or may be a congenital defect.

Note: A fistula always leads to a natural cavity. A sinus may communicate with an abscess cavity in connective tissues, bone, or muscle.

CLASSIFICATION

1. Congenital fistula present at birth due to some developmental abnormality, e.g., lacrimal fistula connecting lacrimal duct with the skin surface, anal fistula, rectovaginal fistula, pervious urachus, etc.

2. Acquired fistula: Those that are not congenital.

3. Complete fistula, having more than one opening.

4. Incomplete or blind fistula, having only one opening (sinus).

5. Pathologic fistula.

6. Purulent fistula.

7. Excretory fistula.

8. Secretory fistula.

TREATMENT

Congenital fistulas, excretory and secretory fistulas may

require surgical correction, depending on its location and the organ involved. Other varieties are treated more or less on general principles of treatment as for sinus.

Questions

1. What are sinuses and fistulae? How are they caused? Describe their symptoms and treatment.
2. Write short notes on:
(i). Fistula, (ii) Costal fistula.

CHAPTER 19

Bier's Hyperaemia

Bier's hyperaemia is a method of treatment recommended for septic inflammatory lesions. The *object* of treatment is to bring about passive hyperaemia by venous congestion in the affected region. This causes more extravasation of serum and leucocytes; and the leucocytes and the antibodies contained in the serum will bring about destruction of bacteria and their toxins.

Method

Bier's hyperaemia can be brought about in extremities like limbs and tail. A moderately tight elastic ligature is applied proximal to the lesion. After a few minutes the region below the ligature becomes slightly swollen and just warm. The bandage is removed after four to six hours and may be reapplied, if necessary.

A piece of elastic band 2½ inches wide may be used for ligation. The ligature should not be very tight; it may be as tight as to allow only one finger to pass through under the ligature with difficulty. (If the ligature is very tight, the animal exhibits pain, becomes restless, and the region appears greatly swollen and cold. When this happens, the ligature should be immediately loosened.)

The ligature when properly placed, restricts the venous flow from the region without much interference to the arterial blood supply to the part. This results in congestion in capillaries and induces extravasation of blood plasma and leucocytes.

CHAPTER 20

Yoke Gall; Saddle Gall; Bed Sore; and Sit Fast

Gall

A *gall* is a localised *acute inflammation* of the skin and subcutis due to constant irritation resulting from friction. A gall is characterised by a swelling due to the accumulation of inflammatory exudate collected subcutaneously or between the layers of the skin, e.g., yoke gall in cattle, saddle gall in horses.

Yoke Gall

A yoke gall is a localised acute inflammation of the skin and subcutis on the neck of cattle due to constant friction caused by the yoke.

A yoke gall may involve either the skin alone or the subcutaneous tissue also. Rarely is the subfacial tissue also involved. The condition is caused by the uneven pressure on the skin at certain points. The pressure of the yoke combined with its movement induces friction, causing separation of the layers of the skin and subcutaneous tissue. This is followed by infiltration of serum and inflammatory exudate and a more or less circular diffused swelling results. The size of the swelling may be small or as large as a foot-ball. The moist condition of the skin due to rain or sweat favours formation of a gall.

ETIOLOGY

Young animals with tender skin are prone to yoke gall. Putting animals to prolonged work is an exciting factor. A yoke with a rough surface is more likely to cause the injury. Undue and irregular pressure of the yoke may be caused either due to improper adjustment of weight or due to improper selection of the pair of animals.

CLINICAL SYMPTOMS

A yoke gall is an acute inflammatory swelling. The swelling appears warm and painful in the initial stages. The occurrence of the swelling is sudden and may not be noticed during the course of work but may develop suddenly after the yoke is removed. So long as the yoke is in position the capillaries underneath are compressed and because of the constant pressure the normal tone of capillary walls may be impaired. Therefore when the yoke is removed, there is an overdistension of these capillaries. The damaged capillary walls favour exudation of serum into the tissues and swelling results.

A yoke gall may become infected and form an abscess. The abscess may be an *acute (hot) abscess* or a *chronic (cold) abscess*.

DIAGNOSIS

Diagnosis is easy from the symptoms mentioned and the history. Confirmation of abscess formation can be made by exploratory puncture.

TERMINATION

1. *Resolution*: The exudate may get re-absorbed within about eight to ten days.

2. *Suppuration*: It may ensue if pyogenic organisms have gained entry, and an abscess results.

3. *Gangrene* and sloughing may take place if the injury is severe.

4. The swelling *may persist*, become fibrous and in the course of time appear like a fibrous tumour. This is commonly referred to as *tumour neck*. There may also be suppurating areas within the fibrous mass. These are actually chronic (cold) abscesses surrounded by fibrous tissue.

TREATMENT

1. In the initial stages (one or two days after onset) fomentations and application of freshly prepared acetic acid-chalk paste, Kaolin paste, or Mag Sulph-Glycerin paste, is helpful to reduce the swelling. Iodine ointment may be rubbed over the swelling to facilitate re-absorption of the exudate.

2. If an abscess has developed, it is better to open it surgically. Otherwise spontaneous rupture may leave an irregular

wound which would require more time for healing. Opening of the abscess should be done only after it matures; otherwise cellulitis may develop. (Cellulitis is an infection of subcutaneous tissue with pyogenic bacteria. Common causes of cellulitis are streptococcal and staphylococcal infection.) If the abscess has not matured fully, a blistering ointment may be applied to make it mature.

For opening the abscess a Syme's abscess knife may be used. The knife is thrust through the "point" of the abscess or, sometimes, through the dependant part. The dependant part is the lower-most part of the abscess cavity and by opening through this maximum drainage can be obtained. After opening the abscess drain the pus and flush the cavity with hypertonic saline (2 to 5%) followed by iodine solution 1 in 1000. Pack the cavity with moist antiseptic gauze dipped in Tincture iodine. On subsequent days do not use any irritant antiseptics like Tincture iodine because it will injure the newly formed granulation tissue; a non-irritant antiseptic like Acriflavine is preferable.

Acriflavine lotion (1 in 500) may be used for irrigation and a gauze dipped in 1% Acriflavine may be introduced into the wound.

3. If the swelling is well-developed and hard in the form of a fibrous mass called *"tumour neck"* enucleation (extirpation) may be done. Local infiltration anaesthesia may be used around the base of the tumour. Make an elliptical skin incision across the swelling. The incision should extend at either end a little beyond the swelling and should enclose necrosed areas of skin, if any, to be removed. If the incision is not long enough there might be pouch formation while suturing the skin edges after the operation. The incision should be *slightly oblique* rather than longitudinal or vertical, to avoid tendency to gape when the animal lowers its head. After cutting through the skin, dissect outwards subcutaneously, reach the base of the fibrous mass and enucleate it completely. Stop haemorrhage and suture the wound and allow it to heal by first intention. (See also page 478)

Complications of this operation are:

(i) Failure of healing by first intention due to: infection, improper apposition of the cut ends, failure of arrest of haemorrhage, use of irritant antiseptics, excessive trauma during operation and/or interference by the animal after operation.

(ii) Formation of an abnormally large scar, which interferes with the usefulness of the animal for work.

Saddle Gall

Saddle galls are seen on the back of horses due to the constant pressure and friction of the saddle. The lesion is somewhat similar to yoke gall in cattle. When a saddle gall develops into an abscess there is chance of suppuration extending to the underlying rib. This may cause necrosis of portion of the bone and thus delay healing.

Bed Sore

This is a local necrosis (dry gangrene) of the skin and subcutaneous tissue due to constant pressure on bony prominences. Animals that are forced to lie down in the recumbent state for a long time by disease or debility are likely to suffer from bed sores. Development of bed sores can be prevented to a certain extent by providing good bedding.

Sit Fast

It is a dry gangrene caused by the pressure of the collar on the top of the neck of the horse. The necrosed tissue is cone-shaped with the base of the cone above. The apex of the cone may have firm attachments to the ligamentum nuchae, so that separation of the dead tissue takes a long time.

PROGNOSIS

When properly treated, sloughing of dead tissue and healing of the resulting wound takes place in about two to four weeks.

COMPLICATIONS

(1) Secondary infections like tetanus and malignant oedema, (2) Maggot infestation.

TREATMENT

Discontinue use of the collar. Give a prophylatic dose of antitetanic serum. The hair is closely clipped. The superficial part of the dead tissue is cut and removed and Salicylic acid powder is packed into the lesion to favour early sloughing of its deeper part. This dressing is repeated daily until sloughing is complete, and afterwards ordinary wound dressings will be sufficient to bring about healing. Dry dressing is preferable. A fly-repellant like neem oil may be applied in the surrounding region.

Questions

1. Describe the surgical technique including anaesthesia in the treatment of yoke tumour.
2. Write short notes on:
(i) Yoke gall, (ii) Sit fast.
3. Write a short essay on inflammatory changes manifested in yoke-galls of working cattle and explain the reparative process accompanying such tissue reaction.
4. What is a cold abscess? Describe the etiology and diagnostic features with special reference to working cattle.
5. What is "tumour neck"? Describe the etiology and treatment of acute and chronic yoke galls in cattle.
6. What is a "tumour neck"? How does it differ from a simple yoke-gall? Outline the differential diagnosis and the treatment of either of these conditions.

CHAPTER 21

General Inflammatory Conditions Affecting Bones

Structure of Bone

Bone is composed of three types of osseous tissue, viz., the outer layer of compact bone or cortex; the middle layer of cancellous bone; and the medullary bone. The medullary bone is the connective tissue found in the interspaces of cancellous bone as well as in the marrow cavity. The medullary bone gives support to the bone marrow and the blood vessels.

The *bone marrow* in the growing stage is completely red and fills the entire marrow cavity. In the adult animal most of the marrow becomes fatty and yellowish and is seen only in the sternum, ribs, vertebrae, skull, pelvis, in the proximal epiphyses of long bones like femur and humerus, etc. (Bone marrow for diagnostic purpose is usually taken from sternum or crest of ilium.)

The *compact bone* (*cortex*) contains longitudinal channels called Haversian canals. Surrounding each Haversian canal are thin ring-like bones called lamellae. Between these rings are spaces called lacunae containing osteocytes. The lacunae are interconnected by microscopic channels called canaliculi. Haversian canals are occupied by small arterioles derived from the periosteal and medullary arteries. (Since hard bone is incapable of expansion, the collection of inflammatory exudates in these canals cause obliteration of the vessels due to pressure, and causes necrosis of the area of bone involved.)

The *cancellous bone* is composed of bony tissue arranged in the form of trabaculae. Cancellous bone does not contain any Haversian system. (Inflammation of the cancellous tissue and marrow differs from that of compact bone. In cancellous bone the blood vessels are not so readily occluded and thus necrosis is less likely to result.)

The proportion of cortical bone and cancellous bone varies

greatly. In flat bones the outer compact layers form two plates, between which lies a small amount of cancellous tissue. In the short bones a thin layer of compact bone is found covering a disproportionately large amount of cancellous tissue. The long bones are made up of a shaft, which is composed of a tube of compact bone known as *diphysis* joined to either end by cartilage known as the epiphyseal cartilage.

Bone Formation

Two types of bone formation takes place in the embryo: (1) by intramembranous ossification of connective tissue cells, e.g., most bones of the skull; and (2) by endochondral bone formation from a hyaline mould—e.g., long bones of the body.

In the development of a long bone there is first the formation of a hyaline cartilage model containing three centres of ossification, one located at the centre of the diphysis and the other two at the epiphyses. Longitudinal growth of bone progresses from the epiphyseal centres throughout the growing period and the longitudinal growth of bone ceases when the epiphyseal plates (*metaphyses*) get ossified.

Blood supply to the bone is from the periosteum lining the outer surface of bone and from the endosteum lining the inner surface. In the case of long bones there is in addition, the nutrient artery which enters the bone through the shaft. The nutrient artery breaks up into small branches in the endosteum and also enter Haversian systems to anastomose with branches from periosteal vessels.

Nerve supply to bone: The periosteum and endosteum are supplied with sensory nerve endings.

Cartilage

There are three types of cartilages in the body: elastic cartilage, fibrocartilage and hyaline cartilage.

Elastic cartilage contains elastic fibres and is therefore flexible, e.g., external ear, epiglottis.

Fibrocartilage: It contains collagen fibres arranged in lines parallel to the line of stress, and therefore has great tensile strength, e.g., Annular fibrosus of intervertebral disc; Menisci of the stifle, Ligamentum teres of femur, Insertions of tendons.

Hyaline cartilage: It consists of cartilage cells surrounded by a homogenous mass of collagen fibres, e.g., Trachea, costal cartilage, articular cartilage, cartilage of the nose. Hyaline cartilage is the precursor of bone and is widely distributed in the body.

Ostitis

Ostitis or inflammation of bone is usually due to concussion, or sprain of ligaments at their points of insertion. The inflammation may be of periosteum (periostitis), or periosteum and bone (osteoperiostitis). Osteomyelitis is inflammation involving chiefly the bone marrow.

Ostitis may be acute, chronic or suppurative. Suppurative (purulent) osteomyelitis is due to entrance of infection into the bone either through open wounds or through the blood stream. Purulent osteomyelitis affecting the maxilla and mandible is seen in cattle and horses as a complication of alveolar periostitis. Ostitis causes rarefaction of bone due to increased vascularity which predisposes it to fracture, e.g., rarefying ostitis of ospedis. A familiar example of osteoperiostitis resulting from concussion is splints. Rarefaction or depletion of mineral matter in the bone (de-calcification) seen in initial stages of inflammation is followed by increased mineral deposition when the vascularity decreases. This mineralisation may proceed beyond the replacement of loss from initial decalcification, resulting in exostosis or condensation of bone filling up the cancellous bone and Haversian canals, as is seen in chronic ostitis.

SYMPTOMS

General symptoms are of acute or chronic inflammation as the case may be. If there is infection the symptoms are much aggravated. In chronic cases the chief symptom noticed is the presence of osseous deposits (exostoses). Lameness is not marked unless the exostosis interferes with the movements of joints or tendons.

Purulent osteomyelitis is characterised by multiple abscess formation in the bone.

PROGNOSIS

Aseptic inflammations usually terminate in resolution. Prognosis in septic inflammations is guarded as it depends on the severity of infection and the virulence of the organism.

TREATMENT

On general principles. In suppurative ostitis proper drainage should be provided and any dead piece of bone (sequestrum) should be removed.

Necrosis and Caries of Bone

Necrosis of bone is death of bone due to interference in its blood supply. Caries is a progressive, molecular destruction of bone due to infection by *pyogenic* organisms. Febrile disturbances due to toxaemia and septicaemia may be present in caries.

TREATMENT

1. The dead portions of bone (called sequestrum) will have to separate for healing to take place. The sequestrum may be removed by curetting or excision, taking care not to injure the surrounding bone tissue. It may be possible in some cases to decalcify the sequestrum by injecting 2% to 3% solution of hydrochloric acid. A mixture of hydrochloric acid 16 minims plus pepsin ½ drachm plus distilled water 8 ounce may be used to digest the sequestrum and the liquefied matter is removed by irrigations of hypertonic saline.

2. Dressings containing antiseptics like iodoform, or antibiotics may be used to check infection.

Questions

1. Write short notes on: (i) Caries, (ii) Ostitis.

2. Discuss the special features of inflammatory reaction and repair in osseous tissue as against soft tissue with reference to histo-pathological changes and clinical findings.

CHAPTER 22

General Inflammatory Conditions Affecting Joints

Anatomical Considerations

A joint is a closed cavity between the ends of bones forming the articulation. The articulating surfaces of the bones are covered with a layer of hyaline cartilage known as the articular cartilage. In some joints there are additional structures such as the round ligament of the hip, semilunar cartilage of stifle, etc.

The joint is enclosed in the joint capsule. The joint capsule consists of an inner lining of synovial membrane and an outer fibrous layer. It is supported outside by ligaments, tendons and muscles which are attached to the bones of either side. The synovial membrane secretes a fluid called the synovia which normally is sufficient only to lubricate the articulating surfaces. But during inflammation of the joint there is an excess secretion of synovia which distends the joint capsule. The movements of a joint are controlled by muscles which originate from, or are inserted on to, the bones forming the joint.

1. Arthritis

Inflammation of a joint.

CLASSIFICATION

(1) Acute arthritis. (2) Chronic arthritis. (3) Serous arthritis: characterised by increased secretion of synovia and distension of joint capsule due to the trauma. (4) Suppurative (infectious) arthritis: characterised by pus inside the joint due to infection. (5) Osteoarthritis (which may be hypertrophic and/or degenerative): characterised by degeneration and hypertrophy of bone and cartilage. (6) Adhesive arthritis (anchylosis): characterised by ulceration and erosion of joint surfaces and osseous proliferation

characterised by finger like growths from the synovial layer. (8) Specific arthritis: e.g.,"Joint ill" in calves. (9) Arthritis due to metabolic diseases: e.g., rickets. (10) Neoplastic arthritis: due to neoplastic growths in or around the joint. (11) Traumatic arthritis: due to trauma or injury to the joint.

SYMPTOMS

Physical symptoms like enlargement of the joint. Pain and functional disturbances like lameness.

DIFFERENTIAL DIAGNOSIS

Based on laboratory examination of synovial fluids, the differentiation of traumatic arthritis from infective arthritis is possible because:

		Traumatic arthritis	*Infective arthritis*
1.	Physical appearance of synovial fluid	Clear	Clear to turbid, usually coagulates
2.	Leucocytes per cubic mm.	up to 1000	Higher, up to 3000
3.	Neutrophils	up to 500	Higher, up to 1000
4.	Protein	4 gm %	4 to 9 gm %
5.	These above findings should be correlated in the light of complete history, physical examination and other clinical findings.		

PROGNOSIS

Guarded to unfavourable.

TREATMENT

In the acute stage use local anaesthetics and sedatives to reduce pain. Supporting bandages are used. Excess synovia may be withdrawn, if necessary. Hydrocortisone 50 mg to 100 mg may be injected into the joint and corticosteroids may also be given systemically.

In chronic cases, use of corticosteroids, blistering, firing, Infra-red irradiation, etc. can be tried.

In suppurative arthritis, the pus is drained and the synovial cavity is cleaned with normal saline. The pus may be examined to identify the causal organism. A suitable antibiotic is injected into the joint with hydrocortisone. The antibiotics commonly used are Penicillin G. Sodium (3 to 12 lakhs units in the dilution of 3 lakhs per cc), Dihydrostreptomycin (0.5 to 3.0 g in the dilution of 0.5 g. per cc), and Neomycin (200 to 800 mg in the dilution of 200 mg per cc).

When arthritis is due to systemic diseases like rickets, specific treatment for the disease concerned becomes necessary. Pantothenic acid deficiency is a primary cause of arthritis and rheumatism. (Barton-Wright, 1978).

2. Sprain of Joints

Sprain of a joint may be complete tear of some of the supporting structures of the joint produced usually by a temporary dislocation. The causes of sprain are mechanical injuries (like movement beyond the physiological limits in the direction of extension, flexion, abduction or adduction) which may result from slipping, falling, false stepping, etc. Any one or more of the following injuries may result: the joint capsule is torn, the ligaments are ruptured partially or completely, the articular cartilages are bruised, the tendons passing over the joint are overstretched or ruptured. There may be haemorrhages within the joint (haemarthosis) and into periarticular tissues. (See also page 654)

SYMPTOMS

Acute local inflammation and lameness. Pain is evident on pressing over the affected portion and also on passive movement of the joint, especially in the direction in which the sprain was caused. Swelling due to extravasation of blood and inflammatory exudate is noticed around the joint.

PROGNOSIS

If the sprain is slight recovery may take place. If there is complete rupture of ligaments, or if articular cartilages are crushed permanent deformity results.

TREATMENT

(a) Provide rest for the affected joint. (b) Cold and astringent applications in the initial stages. (c) Application of moist .heat. (d) The application of Iodine ointment or Reducine to help reabsorption of exudates. (e) Chronic cases blistering or firing. (f) Regulated and mild exercise in necessary during the period of recovery to prevent adhesions forming in and around the joint.

3. Open Joint

Open joint is a condition caused by open wounds penetrating into the joint. The wounds are caused by sharp objects like nails, stones, broken glass, etc. In the horse the common joint affected in this way is the knee joint as a result of stumbing and falling on the knee. Wounds caused in front of the knee due to "falling on the knee" is referred to popularly as *broken knee*. These wounds, if deep, may also cause open joint of the knee.

Open joint is characterised by the escape of synovia. Infection is likely to enter into the joint and may cause septic arthritis. The wound if large may be sutured, leaving space for drainage.

TREATMENT

On general principles as for open wounds and septic arthritis.

Questions

1. Write short notes on:—
   (i) Open joint
   (ii) Anchylosis
   (iii) Broken knee.
2. Explain in detail the symptoms and treatment in a case of open knee joint and state the possible complications.
3. Write an essay on arthritis, its classifications, causes, symptoms and sequelae with reference to working cattle and illustrate your answers with suitable examples.

CHAPTER 23

Counter-irritation; Physiotherapy; and Actinotherapy

Counter-irritants are agents applied over the surface of skin to bring about beneficial effects on deep-seated lesions. They are indicated in subacute and chronic inflammatory conditions so as to induce acute inflammation under controlled conditions and thus stimulate the reparative processes. Methods of counter-irritation in a broad sense include: (1) Application of linaments, (2) Blistering, (3) Fomentation, (4) Massage, (5) Firing, (6) Chemical cauterisation, (7) Diathermy, and (8) Use of Infra-red and Ultraviolet rays.

The liniments used are Linimentum Saponis, Lint. Terebinth, Lint. Camphor, etc. The commonly used blister is Biniodide of mercury ointment (Unguntum Hydrargyri Iodidi Rubrum). A strength of 1 in 32 is used for horses. For cattle strengths up to 1 in 8 can be used. The skin should be shaved and dried before applying the blister. The surrounding areas should be protected with vaseline. The animal should be prevented from licking the blister.

Fomentation

Fomentation may be done with *moist heat* (using cloth dipped in boiling water and squeezed) or *dry heat* (using heated rice bran or sand bundled in a cloth). The evaporation of moisture left on the skin in moist fomentation causes quicker cooling than in dry fomentation. But moist heat is generally preferred because it has a soothening effect.

Massage

Massage improves local circulation of blood and lymph, reabsorption of exudates and prevents to a certain extent muscular atrophy.

METHODS

(i)   Massage causing *slight friction* is performed by rubbing the skin with the tips of the fingers or the hand in a circular manner.

(ii)   Massage by methodical pressure consists of applying firm pressure on the tissues with the fingers or the palm of the hand or with a closed fist.

(iii)   Massage by individual compression of muscles. Portions of the muscle are seized and compressed between the fingers and thump and is massaged from its insertion towards its origin.

(iv)   Massage by percussion consists of superficial or deep percussion of the tissues by striking the part perpendicularly with the fingers or with the closed fist.

Massage is done towards the direction of venous and lymphatic flow after vaseline or a mild liniment is smeared over the part. Massage is continued for five to ten minutes at a time.

Firing (Thermo-Cautery)

Firing is done under regional or local infiltration anaesthesia. General anaesthesia may be necessary when there is difficulty in controlling the patient. The animal is cast and secured in a convenient position depending on the region to be operated upon. The skin in the area should be prepared as for an aseptic surgical operation after clipping the hair.

The piece of iron (usually provided with a wooden handle) used for firing is called a *firing iron*. The iron is heated in the fire until it is made dull red-hot. (If the iron is heated further it becomes *white hot* which is not suitable for the operation.) Three types of firing irons are in common use, viz., Line-firing iron, Bud-point firing iron, and Pin-point or Needle-point firing iron.

Superficial line firing: Superficial line firing is usually done on the hip, shoulder, back tendons, etc. Lines are drawn on the prepared skin using the heated line firing iron. The lines should neither be too close nor too far apart. They should not unite with each other. The optimum distance between lines is $\frac{1}{2}''$ to $\frac{1}{4}''$. It is convenient to mark the lines on skin beforehand with a grease pencil or some coloured solution.

The heated iron is drawn over the lines only lightly but may be repeatedly used on the same line until the desired depth is obtained. The degree of firing is classified into the following three types of which it is desirable to obtain the *second degree* firing. In *first degree firing* the lines appear shallow having a yellowish brown base and containing a few drops of serous exudate. In *second degree firing* the lines are deeper with their base golden yellow and with more pronounced exudations. In *third degree firing* the lines cut almost through the entire thickness of skin, have straw coloured bases and contain profuse serous discharge.

Bud-point firing: For this the bud-point firing iron is used and instead of drawing lines the heated point is pressed on the skin over a number of points. The points are chosen $\frac{1}{2}''$ to $\frac{3}{4}''$ apart. Point firing can be more effective than line firing because deeper penetration is possible.

Needle-point firing: Needle-point firing penetrates very deep and therefore is indicated in spavin, ring bone, synovitis, etc.

Mixed firing: To increase the efficacy of line firing, point firing is sometimes done between the lines. This is called mixed firing.

A blister is sometimes applied after firing to make it more intensive.

After firing an acute inflammation develops within one or two days. Local swelling and exudation are noticed. Lameness is increased. Within about fourteen to twenty days the inflammation gradually subsides, the exudate dries up to form scabs and the scabs later fall off giving pink cicatrices on the skin. The swelling in the region may persist for a few more days. Complete rest to the affected region should be provided during the first two weeks after firing. Mild exercises may be given after the first two weeks. Some authorities, however, believe that firing is a crude method of treatment and that most of the good results claimed for it are only due to the prolonged rest given afterwards.

Firing in cattle will have to be done more deeply since the bovine skin is thicker than of the horse. In the dog firing is only very rarely used and is limited to certain types of ostitis and arthritis. Needle-point firing is most suitable in such cases.

Chemical Cauterisation

Chemical cauterisation is done by touching the area of skin at different points ($\frac{1}{2}''$ to $\frac{1}{4}''$ apart) with a cork dipped in strong sulphuric acid. The effect is almost similar to bud point firing.

Diathermy

Diathermy is a method of heating the tissues in depth by passing through them modified high frequency electric current. To avoid danger and discomfort due to excitation of nerve and muscle tissues, and to produce electrolytic effects, the alternating current (*sinusoidal current*) having 500,000 cycles per second is used. Special apparatus and appliances are available for the purpose. The current is modified in such a way that muscular contractions are not produced. Diathermy has been used with success in arthritis, certain skin diseases, neuralgia, muscular atrophy, paralysis, etc.

Infra-red Rays and Ultra-violet Rays

Infra-red and Ultra-violet rays are commonly used for therapeutic purpose. The infra-red rays have wave lengths between 7700 to 8800 Angstrom units. . The wave lengths of ultra-violet rays fall within a range of 2000 to 4000 AU. The ordinary (coloured) rays, *vibgyor*, are within the range of 4000 to 7700 AU.

The infra-red rays are hot rays. They can heat up deep-seated tissues. Marked dilatation of vessel, warmth and analgesic effect are produced by exposure to infra-red rays. Prolonged exposure may cause reactions due to overheating.

Ultra-violet rays have very little penetrating power but have powerful bactericidal action. Over-exposure causes erythema and burning of the skin. These reactions are not noticed immediately after exposure but only after a period of two to eight hours.

Electric lamps emitting I-R and U-V rays are available for therapeutic use.

Indications for use of I-R rays: Sprains, arthritis, neuralgia, rheumatic conditions, paralysis. Certain skin diseases also respond favourably even though the rays have no bactericidal effect.

Indications for use of U-V rays: Eczema, acne, chronic ulcers, pruritis.

Technique for I-R irradiation: The duration of exposure is fifteen minutes to one hour. The distance from the lamp can be as close as one foot depending on physical comfort. The eyes should be protected. Inflammable articles like celluloid should not be exposed.

Technique for U-V irradiation: Before use the lamp should be allowed to burn for two to three minutes. The eyes should be well-protected with coloured glasses. Initial exposure of one to two minutes may be given on the first day keeping a distance of thirty inches from the lamp. The reaction if any, will be noticed after two to eight hours after irradiation. If there is no reaction, increase the time by half a minute on subsequent days. If there is any reaction, suspend treatment for at least two days.

Physiotherapy (Physical Therapy)

Physiotherapy is the treatment of diseases using physical agents like fresh air, water, heat, cold, electric current, sound waves, etc. (e.g. Fomentation, firing, diathermy, ultrasonic massage.)

Actinotherapy

Actinotherapy is the treatment of diseases using rays of light, especially ultra-violet or 'actinic' rays.

Ultrasonic Therapy

Ultrasonic therapy is treatment of diseases using sound waves which have frequencies higher than what the human ear can hear. (Ultra=higher; Sonus=sound)

Use of Laser

LASER (Light Amplification by Stimulated Emission of Radiation) is used to perform delicate surgery in deep-seated organs. The types of lasser are: Carbon dioxide laser, Argon laser, Neodynium-treated Yttrium Aluminium laser (YAG laser), Dye laser, Gold Vapour laser, Electron Beam laser, Excimer laser, etc.

YAG laser is generally used for removal of tumours, to stop bleeding in gastric ulcers, haemorrhoidectomy, tonsillectomy, anastomoses of minute vessels and nerves, treatment of dental caries, etc.

The major advantages of laser surgery are: (1) the need of only short-duration anaesthesia, (2) precision, (3) sterile conditions, (4) minimum damage to adjoining normal tissues, (5) minimum loss of blood and clear operative field, (6) minimum post-operative pain, and (7) quicker convalescence.

Ionisation*

It is believed that ions contained in certain electrolyte solutions can be made to pass through tissues with the help of electric current by a process of ionisation. This ionisation has been found to be beneficial in the treatment of conditions like ulcers, neuritis and rheumatism.

Principle

The molecules of some drugs in solution are split up into ions when electric current is passed through the solution. The positively charged ions (example: zinc) go towards the negative electrode and the negatively charged ones flow in the opposite direction. So it is presumed that when the current is made to pass through the body with the electrodes properly placed over the body and soaked in the solution, the ions infiltrate into the tissues. The galvanic current (DC) is employed. One of the electrodes is placed in close contact with the affected region and covered with a thick layer of cotton wool well-soaked in the solution. An elastic bandage may be applied to keep them in position. The other electrode is placed over a suitable area so as to enable current to flow through the required part. The choice of the electrode that is to be placed over the affected region depends on the ion that is to be made use of.

For example, if a negatively charged ion is to be infiltrated into the affected parts of a hind limb, the negative electrode will be placed over it alongwith cotton wool soaked in the electrolyte solution. The other electrode (positive) located in the lumbar region will attract these ions when the current flow starts, and this will cause migration of the ions through the tissues.

* Iontophoreiss; Iontherapy; or Galvano-ionisation.

Examples

Drug in solution	Ion and charge	Electrode to be placed over hind limb	Electrode to be placed over lumbar region
1. Zinc sulphate	Zinc (+)	+	—
2. Perchloride of mercury	Mercury (+)	+	—
3. Cocaine hydrochloride	Cocaine (+)	+	—
4. Potassium iodide	Iodide (—)	—	+
5. Sodium salicylate	Salicyl (—)	—	+

The current is only gradually increased to a tolerable degree. It is applied for ten to thirty minutes and then gradually reduced and switched off. The treatment is repeated on alternate days.

CHAPTER 25

Fundamentals of Radiology

Radiology (*Roentgenology*) is a science which deals with the use of x-rays for therapeutic and diagnostic purposes. Roentgen (1843-1923) discovered x-rays in 1895; hence it is called *Roentgenology*.

X-Rays for Therapeutic Purpose

X-rays are harmful to living cells especially to gonadal cells and immature embryonal cells. They cause biological changes, somatic as well as genetic. In higher doses they are capable of bringing about actual destruction of cells and they have a selective affinity for malignant tissues. These properties are taken advantage of in the use of x-rays for thereapeutic purpose and the treatment of malignant lesions. A device called *r-meter* or *Roentgen-meter* placed in the x-ray beam can be used to determine the quantity of x-rays produced by a given x-ray machine used for treating tumours and other diseases. The unit of measurement, regardless of the quality of radiation is designated by a small "r". The unit of absorbed dose of x-ray is called *rad.* Certain element, like radium, emit x-rays and these elements can also be used for x-ray therapy, e.g., Radium needles.

X-Rays for Diagnostic Purpose

(Since x-rays are able to penetrate most substances including certain metals like aluminium and are capable of producing chemical changes on a photographic film, they are useful in *Radiography*.

A *Radiograph* ("x-ray picture") is a photographic record produced by the passing of x-rays through an object or body and recorded on a special film.

Fluoroscopy (Radioscopy; Screening): Though x-rays cannot be seen directly they can cause certain chemicals (Calcium tungstate, Barium lead sulphate, Zinc sulphide, Zinc cadmium sulphide, Barium platinocyanide, etc.) to fluoresce or emit visible rays. A fluorescent screen used for this purpose usually consists of a board smeared over with *calcium tungstate*. The x-rays coming through the patient falls on this screen and the image becomes visible on it. The advantage of fluoroscopy is that actual *movement* of an internal organ or part can be observed whereas in radiography only a photograph of the same is obtained. Fluoroscopy is therefore more helpful in dislocations, etc. But the disadvantages are that it does not give a permanent record like a radiograph, and involves additional risk of irradiation to the patient and the observer due to the increased duration of exposure to x-rays. However, fluoroscopy is sometimes necessary for diagnosing conditions like pulmonary emphysema and pericardial effusions in which a radiograph may not be of much diagnostic value. Fluoroscopy in pulmonary emphysema reveals a flattened diaphragm which does not show normal inspiratory and expiratory movements (but only "pulsates"). The image of the heart in pericardial effusions does not show the normal systolic and diastolyic movements but only vibrates.

X-rays

X-rays are included in the category of electro-magnetic ray. The wavelength of x-rays, is expressed in Angstrom Units (AU). One AU. is $1/100,000,000$ cm. or $1/10,000,000$ mm. Like all other light rays, x-rays travel at the rate of about 186,000 miles per second. A comparative note on the approximate wavelengths of various electro-magnetic rays are given below.

APPROXIMATE WAVELENGTHS OF SOME OF THE RAYS

(a) *Measured in Angstrom Units*

Less than about 1/10	: X-rays used for industrial radiology
1/10 to 1/2	: Medical radiology
1/2 to 25	: Very soft x-rays
25 to 4,000	: UV rays
4,000 to 7,700	: Visible rays (Vibgyor)
7,700 to 10,000,000 AU or 7,700 to 1/1,000 M	: Infrared rays.

(b) *Measured in Metres*

Close to 1/100 M   :   Micro-wave (Radar)
,,   ,,   1 M   :   Television
,,   ,,   100 M to 1,000 M :   Communications
,,   ,,   10,000,000 M   :   60 cycles AC

X-rays used for industrial radiography and for therapeutic purpose have wavelength less than 1/2 AU; Very soft x-rays have ½ to 25 AU. X-rays can pass through most substances. The shorter the wavelength, the greater is the penetrating power. X-rays can pass through aluminium. Other metals are practically opaque. Substances through which x-rays can pass through are called *Radio transparent*. Others are called *radiopaque*.

X-ray Tube

X-rays are produced by using electric currents of very high voltage. Over 10 kilovolts are required to produce even soft x-rays. 30 to 100 KVP (kilovolt peak), or more are required in the x-ray machines used for radiography and fluoroscopy. For x-ray machines used for therapeutic irradiation, still higher voltages are required. [1 kilovolt = 1000 volts]

The x-ray tube consists of a vacuum glass bulb containing an anode and a cathode kept apart by a small distance. The anode (+) is called the target and the cathode (—) is called the filament. When current is made to flow, electrons travel from the filament and strike the target with great force. The energy thus released is mostly converted into heat and only partly (about 1%) into light rays including x-rays.

The x-ray tube is enclosed in a lead-protected box which has a small opening on one side covered by an aluminium plate. Since x-rays can pass through aluminium, they come through the aluminium while the ordinary rays are retained. The quantity of the x-rays coming out can be regulated by an adjustable lead diaphragm.

Radiography

For taking the radiograph, the film is first loaded into a cassette or an x-ray Film Holder, in the dark room. *Intensifying screens*, may be used with the film, according to requirement.

The part to be exposed is kept closest to the loaded cassette and the x-rays are permitted to flow through the tissue and fall on the film for the specified duration. The cassette is again taken to the dark room and unloaded. The film is processed to make the *radiograph* or *roentgenogram*, popularly called an "*X-ray picture*". A printed x-ray picture is called a *skiagram*.

A *cassette* is a flat, light-proof, metal box made of aluminium used for keeping the film for exposure. Its bottom and sides are protected with lead. The x-rays enter the cassette through the surface not protected with lead, fall on the film and are subsequently absorbed by the lead plates. The cassette can also accommodate intensifying screens whenever necessary. The film is kept between two intensifying screens.

An X-ray Film Holder is a light proof, cardboard folder with lead protection at the bottom. It can be used instead of a cassette.

An *intensifying screen* is a thin sheet containing fluorescent substance like Calcium tungstate or Barium lead sulphate. When x-rays fall on the intensifying screen ordinary coloured rays are also produced because of the fluorescent effect of the screen and therefore the photographic effect of the x-rays is intensified. So when the special film which is sensitive to both x-rays and coloured rays is used, exposure time can be shortened. While loading the cassette the film is placed between two intensifying screens. Three types of intensifying screens are available. (1) Hi-speed screens provide high intensification, (2) Slow speed screens produce better image sharpness. (3) Par speed screens provide medium speed and medium sharpness.

Use of Grid

The x-rays coming directly from the focal spot are called primary rays When these rays get reflected after falling on some object the reflected rays are called *secondary rays* or *scattered radiation*.

(It may be mentioned that while taking a radiograph all the primary rays falling on the tissue exposed do not pass through it. Some of the rays pass through, some others get reflected at various levels in the thickness of the tissue, and the remaining are absorbed by the tissue.) The reflected rays cause scattered radiation. The scattered radiations falling on the film alongwith the primary rays produce blurring of the image obtained on the film. To avoid scattered radiations, an additional equipment called *grid* is sometimes used in radiography. Use of grid is advisable whenever the thickness of tissue exposed exceeds 11 centimetres. The grid is placed between the part exposed and the cassette. There are *stationary* grids and *movable grids*. A grid is composed of alternating strips of lead and radiotransparent material such as wood or aluminium arranged in such a way that when the focal spot is centred over the grid the plane of each lead strip is in line with the primary beam. A familiar example of the device containing a movable grid is the Potter-Bucky Diaphragm (or, "Bucky"). This grid is kept moving during the period of exposure. When a stationary grid is used, fine lines representing the image of lead strips can be noticed in the radiograph. These lines are avoided by using a movable grid.

STEPS IN THE PROCESSING OF THE FILM

The processing is done in the dark room. The optimum temperature of the solutions used is 60 to 75°F.

The steps in processing consist of: Developing, Rinsing in running water, Fixing, Rinsing in running water again and Drying.

QUALITIES OF A RADIOGRAPH

1. *Density* (Radiographic density): The "blackness" in a radiograph is defined as density. Greater densities represent areas where more x-rays had fallen on the film and had chemically reacted with the silver salt on the film and had converted it into black, metalic silver.

2. *Contrast* (Radiographic contrast): The difference in density in the various part of the radiograph is called contrast. The factors influencing contrast are: (1) the relative transparency to x-rays of the various structures that are radiographed, (2) the type of film used, (3) the processing of the film after exposure, (4) the intensifying screens, (5) kilovoltage, and (6) scattered radiation.

Lower kilovoltages produce *high contrast* and higher kilovoltages produce *low contrast*.

3. *Sharpness* (Definition): The sharpness or *definition* in a radiograph is indicated by the well-defined demarcation between various structures that are recorded in it.

4. *Detail*: Detail is a quality of the radiograph based on the sharpness (definition) of the outlines and contrast between

various structures recorded in it. When the outlines are well defined and clear the detail is said to be good.

Factors to be Considered in Taking Radiograph

(EXPOSURE FACTORS)

1. *KVP:* When the KVP or kilovoltage is increased, x-rays with more penetrating power are produced. When the penetrating power of rays increases, the contrast of the image that is obtained in the radiograph *decreases.* So an optimum has to be set.

2. *ma:* When the milliamperage is increased, the quantity of rays produced increases and therefore better definition (sharpness) is obtained in the radiograph.

3. *Time of exposure (seconds):* Either over exposure or under-exposure may affect the radiograph adversely. It is better to reduce the exposure time to the minimum to avoid movement by the patient during exposure.

4. *Focal spot-Film distance.* (Focus-Film distance): When the distance is made short the intensity increases, but there is tendency for magnification. Therefore an optimum distance is to be chosen. Usually this distance ("D") is kept constant as 36 inches.

5. *Part film distance:* The distance between the part exposed and the film should be the minimum possible in order to get good definition and avoid magnification. This distance is made zero by keeping the part in contact with the cassette.

6. *The thickness of tissue:* When the thickness of tissue increases the KVP may have to be increased to obtain rays having more penetrating power.

7. *The type of film used:* Different films, with or without intensifying screens, are to be chosen according to need.

Of the seven factors mentioned above, two factors (viz, the focal-film distance and the part-film distance) are usually made constant.

If three more factors are kept constant, a readymade chart can be prepared for changes in the remaining two variable factors. Since the KVP decides the penetrating power of x-rays, it is related to thickness of tissue more than any other factor. Therefore, KVP and thickness of tissue are taken as variable factors. A chart prepared on the above lines is given below.

Example of a Chart for Radiography

[Ref: Banks, W. C., J. A. V. M. A., Nov. 1, 1959]

Keep the following 5 factors constant:

1. Milliamperes $=10$
2. Exposure time $=\frac{1}{4}$ second
3. Distance $=36$ inches. (90 cm.)
4. Film with "Hi-Speed" screens.
5. Part-Film distance at zero.

Thickness of tissue in cm	KVP.	Thickness of tissue in cm	KVP.
1	40	13	64
2	42	14	66
3	44	15	68
4	46	16	70
5	48	17	72
6	50	18	74
7	52	19	76
8	54	20	78
9	56	21	80
10	58	22	82
11	60	23	84
12	62		

Positioning the Animal for Radiography

In describing position, the term first mentioned denotes the aspect through which x-rays entered the tissue exposed and the term last mentioned denotes the aspect that has been closer to the film.

The common positions in which radiographs of various regions are taken are listed below:

(i) *Skull*: ( ) Ventro-dorsal, (2) Lateral, (3) Antero-posterior.

(ii) *Cervical region*: (1) Ventro-dorsal, (2) Dorso-ventral, (3) Lateral.

(iii) *Thorax*: (1) Dorso-ventral, (2) Lateral, (3) Standing lateral.

(iv) *Thoracic spines*: (1) Ventro-dorsal, (2) Lateral.

(v) *Abdomen*: (1) Dorso-ventral, (2) Lateral, (3) Standing lateral.

(vi) *Lumbar spine:* (1) Ventro-dorsal, (2) Lateral.

(vii) *Pelvis:* (1) Ventro-dorsal, (2) Ventro-dorsal frog position, (3) Lateral.

(viii) *Pelvic limbs:*

(1) Femur: (a) Antero-posterior*, (b) Postero-anterior, (c) Lateral.

(2) Stifle: (a) Postero-anterior, (b) Lateral.

(3) Tibia: (a) Postero-anterior, (b) Lateral.

(4) Hock joint and foot: (a) Antero-posterior, (b) Lateral.

(ix) *Pectoral limbs:*

(1) Scapula: (a) Postero-anterior, (b) Lateral.

(2) Shoulder joint: (a) Postero-anterior, (b) Lateral. (Details given later in this chapter.)

(3) Humerus: (a) Antero-posterior, (b) Postero-anterior, (c) Lateral.

(4) Elbow joint: (a) Antero-posterior, (b) Lateral.

(5) Radius and Ulna: (a) Antero-posterior, (b) Lateral.

(6) Carpal joint and foot: (a) Antero-posterior, (b) Lateral.

POSITIONING FOR RADIOGRAPHY OF THE HIP AND SHOULDER IN SMALL ANIMALS

1. *Ventro-dorsal Pelvis Position:* Place the animal in dorsal recumbency with its pelvis centred on the film. The hind limbs are drawn backwards and parallel to each other by holding one hock in each hand so as to obtain both hips symmetrical in the radiograph. The hocks are slightly rotated outwards so that the stifle joints will get rotated inwards. This is necessary to get a good view of both the femoral necks, heads and trochanter majors. The V-D pelvis position is ideal for diagnosing dislocations, fractures, and other irregularities of the hip.

2. *Ventro-dorsal Frog Position of Pelvis:* This is similar to the V-D position described already, except for the difference that the femora are held forwards (symmetrically) slightly anterior to the acetabulae that each femur forms an angle of 45° with the film. This position is sometimes chosen for diagnosing hip dysplasia.

3. *Postero-anterior Position of Shoulder:* Place the animal

*In the case of a limb an Antero-posterior view can also be called a Dorso-ventral view.

in the dorsal recumbency. The affected limb is pulled forward and the shoulder is kept in contact with and centred on the cassette. The animal may be slightly tilted to the opposite side away from the scapula, to an angle of about 60° to the table.

4. *Lateral Position of Shoulder*: The animal is placed in lateral recumbency with the affected shoulder in contact with and centred on the cassette. The other forelimb is pulled forward or backward to avoid overlapping.

Lateral Position of Pelvis

The animal is placed in lateral recumbency with the affected side closest to the film. The upper limb is raised and held horizontally, parallel to the other. The two hip joints should exactly coincide with each other in the radiograph and for this the central beam of x-ray should pass through both joints. At the same time overlapping of the two hind limbs should be avoided by keeping one of them forward.

The Central Beam

The central ray that is emanating from the focal spot of the target in the x-ray tube is called the central beam or the central ray. While taking radiograph the x-ray tube and positioning should be so adjusted that the central beam falls perpendicular to the film surface.

METHOD OF PLACING A RADIOGRAPH ON THE ILLUMINATOR

A radiograph can be seen clearly by placing it on a viewing lamp (or, illuminator). It is customary to follow a standard pattern for placing the radiograph on the illuminator

Examples: 1. *Dorso-ventral or ventro-dorsal position of abdomen, thorax or skull*: The right and left sides and the anterior and posterior aspects of the radiograph will appear on the illuminator as follows:

Anterior

Right   Left

Posterior

(While looking at the radiograph on the illuminator we will have the left side of it on our right side).

2. *Lateral position of abdomen, thorax and skull*:

Dorsal

Caudal   Cranial

Ventral

3. *Antero-posterior or postero-anterior position of a right limb*: (Fore or hind limb).

Proximal

Lateral   Medial

Distal

4. *Antero-posterior or postero-anterior position of a left fore or hind limb*:

Proximal

Medial   Lateral

Distal

5. *Lateral position of a right or left limb*: (Fore or hind limb).

Proximal

Posterior   Anterior

Distal

Some Terminologies, Synonyms and Abbreviations Used in Radiographic Positioning

Position (View)	Synonym	Abbreviations
Antero-posterior	. . . .	A—P
Postero-anterior	. . . .	P—A
Dorso-ventral	. . . .	D—V
Ventro-dorsal	. . . .	V—D
Antero-posterior of a limb	Dorso-ventral of the limb	A—P or D—V
Postero-anterior of a limb	Ventro-dorsal of the limb	P—A or V—D

Contrast Media

Some of the x-rays falling on a tissue get reflected, some others get absorbed by the tissue and only the remaining ones pass through the tissue. Bone absorbs most of the x-rays falling on it; soft tissues very little; and air (contained in lungs, gastrointestinal tract etc.) practically nil. This difference in the absorption capacity between different tissues is responsible for the "contrast" obtained in a radiograph. If the difference between the absorption capacity of adjacent tissues, is remarkable, good contrast is obtained. On the other hand, if the difference is negligible the contrast is poor and the picture may not be of any diagnostic value. For example, in a radiograph, the contrasts of the various soft tissues like kidney, liver, intestines, bladder, etc., are not very distinct. In such instances, good contrast can be obtained with the use of some radiopaque substance in the organ to be outlined. Such substances are called *contrast media*. The most commonly used contrast media are Barium sulphate and iodine containing fluids. Air is sometimes used as a contrast medium. Since air is not radiopaque like other contrast media, it is referred to as a *negative contrast medium*. Air distributes itself between tissues and provides demarcation between the tissues in the radiograph by virtue of its being more *radiolucent* (=permitting passage of x-rays) than any tissue.

1. *Contrast medium for digestive tract*: Barium sulphate is very commonly used. The powder is mixed with water to make a thick paste and is administered orally. For rectum and colon radiography, the substance may be given as an enema. For giving enema a *bardex catheter* may be used because it will help retain the substance.

For taking radiograph of the oesophagus about 5 to 20 cc of the paste is sufficient for a dog weighing 25 to 30 lb. For radiography of duodenum or intestines an additional 30 cc may be given about two to four hours before the exposure.

2. *Contrast media for urinary tract*: Iodine-containing fluids are usually used. For example, "Pyelectan" (Glaxo). Some of these preparations can be given intravenously. Others are injected through the urethra. A radiograph of the renal pelvis and ureters is called *pyelogram*. Air is used as a contrast medium for radiograpy of the urinary bladder. The radiograph is called *pueumocystogram*. The technique is that urine is removed by passing a catheter and using a three-way adapter and syringe; then air is injected through the catheter. About 50 cc is sufficient for a 30 lb dog. Have the radiograph taken and then withdraw the air.

3. *Contrast medium for abdominal viscera*: General outline of different abdominal viscera can be obtained by using air as contrast medium. Air is injected into the peritoneal cavity with proper aseptic precautions. After radiography air is withdrawn.

4. *For spinal canal*: Iodine-containing fluid (e.g., "Myodil" —(Glaxo)) is injected into the sub-arachnoid space. The radiograph is called **myelogram**. Up to about 3 cc can be injected in

a dog, withdrawing an equal quantity of cerebrospinal fluid, if necessary.

5. *For blood vessels, heart, etc.*: (Angiography; Angio-cardiography). The contrast medium (e.g., "Pyelosil" —(Glaxo)) is injected intravenously and the picture is taken immediately. The radiograph of the heart is called *angiocardiogram*.

Stereoscopic Radiography

The radiographs of the same part are taken from two different angles, without moving the part but by changing the position of the cassette and x-ray tube. These two radiographs are viewed in special "Stereoscopic Viewers" so as to get a three-dimension view of the part radiographed. This technique is most helpful for diagnosing conditions affecting the skull. (See also page 655)

Questions

1. How will you judge the quality of a radiograph? How will an increase in KVP affect "Contrast"?

2. What is the principle underlying the use of contrast media? Name the different types of contrast media commonly used for different organs and tissues.

3. Write short notes on:
   (i) Ventro-dorsal frog position.
   (ii) Radiograph in dislocation of shoulder.

4. Describe the radiological diagnosis of intussuception in a dog.

5. Briefly describe the principles involved in modern diagnostic imaging procedures. Mention the advantages and disadvantages of each of them, and uses.

Part II

Regional Surgery

Regional Surgery

CHAPTER 26

Surgical Conditions Affecting Bursae

Bursae are cavities lined by synovial membrane. Bursae are of two types:

1) Typical or deep bursae, present at birth, and
2) Atypical or superficial or acquired bursae, acquired after birth.

Synovial sheaths of tendons and joint capsules are also sometimes called bursae.

Examples of *typical bursae* are *navicular bursa* situated between the tendon of the deep digital flexor and the os-navicularis; *bicipital bursa* situated between the bicipital groove of the humerus and the tendon of biceps brachii muscle; *bursa* between the common digital extensor and the fetlock joint, etc.

Acquired bursae or atypical bursae are seen to develop over bony prominences (between the bone and overlying skin, or, between the bone and an overlying tendon) where there is constant friction or mild and repeated trauma.

Examples of *atypical* bursae are *subcutaneous bursae* lying between the skin and bony prominences at the point of the elbow and point of the hock; *atlantal bursa* lying between the ligamentum nuchae and the dorsal arch of the atlas; *supraspinous bursae* between the spines of thoracic vertebrae and the ligamentum nuchae; the *subcutaneous bursa* in front of the knee, etc.

Some bursae may be destroyed or excised without causing much disability. When excised it often replaces itself by regeneration from neighbouring connective tissue.

Bursitis

Bursitis (inflammation of a bursa) causes synovial effusions into the bursal cavity. The resulting swelling may be painful.

The common cause of bursitis is direct trauma. Severe trauma gives rise to acute bursitis while mild and repeated trauma results in chronic bursitis. Bacterial infection, toxaemia, etc., are other causes.

Acute Bursitis

ETIOLOGY

1) Direct violence, 2) An extension of inflammation from local tendinitis in the case of bursitis involving the tendon sheaths, 3) Open wounds involving the bursa, 4) Bacterial infection, 5) Toxaemia of bacterial diseases like influenza and stangles, and 6) Due to rheumatism.

SYMPTOMS

In the initial stages there is not much swelling or exudation but there is pain especially during extension or flexion of the joints in the affected region. This type of bursitis wherein the exudation is more or less absent is called *dry bursitis*. Dry bursitis may be followed by serous bursitis. In serous bursitis there is pronounced exudation and swelling. When bursitis is caused or complicated by infection by pyogenic organisms, it is called *purulent bursitis* or *suppurative bursitis*.

TREATMENT

Acute bursitis is treated on general principles as for acute inflammation. Hydrocortisone acetate (0.5 cc of a 25 mg per cc solution) injected into the bursa helps to suppress the inflammation. When bursitis is due to infection antibiotics may be injected into the bursa. Penicillin G Sodium (3 to 12 lakh units in the dilution of 3 lakh per cc); Dihydrostreptomycin (0.5 to 3g, in the dilution of 0.5g. per cc); and Neomycin (200 to 800 mg in the dilution of 200 mg per cc) are the antibiotics commonly used.

Purulent bursitis is treated like an abscess, by aspirating the contents or incising the bursa and providing drainage. Local and parenteral administration of antibiotics might he helpful.

In rheumatoid bursitis, use of Soda salicylas is indicated.

Chronic Bursitis

Chronic bursitis results from mild and repeated trauma or it may follow acute bursitis. There is swelling, but pain may not be marked so much, unlike in acute bursitis. Chronic bursitis affecting the point of the elbow ("capped elbow"), the anterior aspect of the knee ("capped knee"), and the point of the hock ("capped hock") are frequently encountered.

The following are some of the common forms of chronic bursitis.

1. *Cystic form*: In this type the bursal sac contains a variable quantity of a viscid opalescent fluid. The wall of the bursa becomes thickened with fibrous tissue. In longstanding cases the bursa may contain cartilaginous or calcareous material.

2. *Proliferative form*: The interior of the bursal sac contains vegetative growths which might be infiltrated with cartilageous material.

3. *Fibrous form*: In this type there is extensive fibrous thickening of the bursa and it appears like a fibroma containing a small quantity of fluid in its centre.

4. *Haemorrhagic form*: This is characterised by the presence of extravasated blood in the bursa. This is evidently the result of trauma. (The haemorrhagic form of bursitis is sometimes classified under acute bursitis.)

SYMPTOMS

There is distension of the bursa. When situated close to a joint, it may be mistaken for arthritis. When the inflammation of a subcutaneous bursa has been in existence for a long time the skin overlying it may develop horny or wart-like thickenings (as is sometimes seen on "capped knee"). Usually there is not much of functional disability, but the distension of bursa may cause mechanical interference and may look unsightly.

Chronic bursitis may become acute as a result of more severe injury. Infection may gain entrance and suppurative bursitis may result.

TREATMENT

1. Remove the cause.
2. Local application of absorbant topics like Iodine ointment or reducine, "antiphlogistics." (Reducine contains: Iodine 4 parts plus Potassium iodide 16 parts plus Glycerine 80 parts.)
3. Application of a counter-irritant like Biniodide of mercury ointment (1 in 32 to 1 in 8).

4. Needle-point firing.

5. Exposure to infra-red rays.

6. Aspiration of contents by using a syringe and inoculation needle followed by injection of an irritant solution like Tincture iodine, Carbolic acid 3 to 5%, etc. Afterwards a pressure bandage is applied. The irritant destroys the lining of the bursa which is followed by granulation, cicatrisation and obliteration of the cavity.

7. Passing a seton through the bursa. This facilitates drainage and quicker healing. During the healing process the cavity of the bursa gets obliterated.

8. Lancing and drainage (Incision) of the bursa at a dependant part to evacuate its contents followed by application of an irritant to its interior. This method is better than those previously described. Vegetative growths and semi-solid materials are to be removed from the bursa in proliferative bursitis.

9. *Excision:* (Extirpation) In longstanding cases when the enlarged bursa is composed mostly of fibrous tissue, fairly circumscribed, it may be dissected out and removed. It is sometimes possible to remove a bursa by ligation when it is well separated from surrounding tissues. e.g., some cases of "capped elbow".

Poll Evil*

Poll evil is a condition met with in horses, resulting from bursitis of the atlantal bursa.

(The atlantal bursa is an acquired bursa found between the dorsal arch of the atlas and the funicular part of the ligamentum nuchae.)

ETIOLOGY

1) Repeated trauma, 2) Bacterial infection, 3) Parasitic infection like Onchocercosis.

SYMPTOMS

A lobulated, fluctuating swelling behind the poll. The head is held high up, with the nose pointing upwards, to relieve tension on the bursa. When the horse is made to walk, it keeps the head steady and stiff, unwilling to move.

* Bursitis of the Atlanal Bursa.

The bursa may rupture and infection may spread, leading to formation of abscesses. The pus that is discharged moves along the line of least resistance and may open out through a number of sinus-like openings on the skin near the poll. The skin is thickened (indurated) around these sinus openings. The suppuration may spread on to ligamentum nuchae and cause necrosis of that structure.

PROGNOSIS

Poll evil can be cured if treated early. If neglected, the necrosis may spread causing arthritis of the intervertebral joints. The suppuration may extend to the spinal cord causing death.

TREATMENT

The bursa and surrounding dead tissues are removed. The operation is done under general anaesthesia. Make a 6 inch long incision commencing from the poll backwards, on the superior aspect of the neck. Sever through the funicular portion of the ligamentum nuchae behind the necrosed part. Dissect and reflect it forwards and detach from its insertion to the occipital crest. Remove the necrosed tissues adherent to the bone by scraping and curetting. The bone surface may then be touched with caustics if necessary. Bleeding is fairly severe during the operation and will have to be controlled. (The important vessels are the ascending branches of the occipital arteries.) After removal of dead tissues the wound cavity is packed with sterile gauze and the skin incision is sutured from behind leaving a small space *anteriorly* for drainage. The gauze packs are removed twenty-four to forty-eight hours later and the wound is subsequently treated in the usual manner. It may take six to eight weeks for healing.

For the first few days after the operation there may be a tendency for the head to drop down because of the severance of the ligamentum nuchae, but this deformity gets corrected in due course by the compensatory action of the cervical muscles.

Capped Elbow*

Capped elbow is a condition caused by subcutaneous bursitis at the point of the elbow. It may appear either as a simple

* Hygroma of the elbow: "Shoe-boil"; olecranon bursitis.

bursitis or may be associated with parabursitis and thickening of the surrounding tissues. The condition may occasionally develop into a purulent inflammation resulting in abscess formation. The abscess becomes painful and may rupture.

INCIDENCE

Capped elbow is common in horses and dogs. Heavy breeds like Great Danes are particularly pre-disposed. Rare in cattle.

ETIOLOGY

Usually due to repeated trauma. Sometimes as a complication of infectious diseases like influenza and strangles. The cause of repeated trauma may be any of the following.

1. The heel of the shoe repeatedly coming in contact with the point of the elbow when the horse is lying with folded knee. Cart horses shod with long-heeled shoes or calkins are more subject to this type of injury.

2. The elbow frequently coming in contact with rough, hard ground while getting up (in horses).

3. Bad conformation of the limb. Horses with prominent elbows are more pre-disposed to this condition.

4. The corresponding hind foot striking against the point of elbow during galloping.

SYMPTOMS

The symptoms may be in the form of an acute or chronic inflammation. The most common type is the chronic form. Occasionally it may appear in the form of cold abscess.

The chronic form appears in the form of a fluctuating fibrous mass because of the thickening of the walls of the bursa and surrounding tissue (bursitis and parabursitis). There is no pain or lameness. In the cystic form occasionally the fluid gets absorbed leaving an empty cutaneous sac. Chronic bursitis may become acute due to subsequent infection or more severe trauma. The pain and swelling are well marked in the acute form. If there is infection it develops into an abscess. The abscess may burst and communicate with the outside in the form of small istulous tracts.

PROGNOSIS

Prognosis is favourable when properly treated; but due to the difficulty in removing the causes, the condition is likely to recur.

TREATMENT

1. A soft litter (bedding) of straw may be provided.
2. When the case is acute cold and astringent applications are indicated.
3. Warm fomentations, Iodine ointment/Biniodide of mercury ointment, may be applied to reduce the swelling. When it is of a cystic nature, incise the bursa and touch the interior with irritant solution so as to bring about destruction and obliteration of the synovial sac. Needle-point firing also may be tried. When the lining is vegetative, it may be necessary to scrape it with a knife or cauterise it with hot iron.
4. Another method of treatment of the cystic form is by inserting a seton through the bursa.
5. If the condition is of a suppurative type, it is treated just like an abscess.
6. Extirpation of the bursa is the best method of treatment especially when there is fibrous thickening.

Removal of the bursa is done either by ligation or by dissection. For removal by ligation, an elastic ligature is applied at the base of the swelling. Sloughing takes place within about ten days leaving a small wound which soon heals up. During the period of sloughing an antiseptic dressing may be applied daily to prevent chances of infection.

Extirpation: An elliptical cutaneous incision is placed enclosing the bursa and it is removed by blunt dissection. The edges of the wound are sutured. Sufficient portion of the skin should be removed with the fibrous swelling as otherwise there will be pouch formation after suturing. On the other hand, if too much of skin is removed there will be gaping of the wound which will retard the healing process. The incision is placed slightly along the lateral aspect of the point of the elbow rather than behind it. The bursa should be removed completely; if a portion of the synovial sac is left behind, healing will be delayed. All dead portions of the skin should be removed with the incision. After operation, movement of the area should be restricted (immobilisation) to facilitate healing. For this purpose the animal may be put on slings if necessary.

Capped Hock (*Hygroma of the Hock*)

Capped hock is caused by the bursitis of the superficial bursa at the point of the hock.

INCIDENCE

It is a common condition in horses. Occasionally met with in cattle and dogs also.

ETIOLOGY

Trauma. The trauma may result from friction against hard ground while lying down and getting up, by kicking against the wall of the stable, etc.

SYMPTOMS

Similar to those seen in capped elbow, but lameness is not usually noticed.

TREATMENT

Soft litter to be provided to avoid friction. The sides of the stable may be padded, if possible. General principles of treatment similar to capped elbow but surgical removal is not done in the case of capped hock. Aspiration of contents and injection of Tincture iodine into the bursal sac may be done.

Deep Capped Hock

The distension of the small bursa situated between the gastrocnemius and superficial flexor tendons at the point of the hock is called *Deep Capped Hock*. In this case the swelling is observed slightly above the point of the hock and on either side of it. (Not so high as in thoroughpin.) Pain and lameness are usually absent.

TREATMENT

1. Needle-point firing and blistering. 2. Aspiration of contents and injection of an irritant solution.

Incising the bursa is not advised as this might cause infection and necrosis of the tendons.

Capped Knee (*Hygroma of the Knee*)
Distension of the subcutaneous bursa in front of the knee.

INCIDENCE
Hygroma of the knee is seen more commonly in cattle. It may also occur in the horse.

ETIOLOGY
The common cause is trauma. In cattle the constant rubbing with rough flooring while the animal lies down and gets up is a common cause. In the horse frequent falling during progression may cause it.

SYMPTOMS
A diffuse swelling is noticed on the anterior aspect of the knee due to bursitis and parabursitis. On palpation it may appear to contain fluid. Most of the fluid is not in the form of free fluid in the bursal cavity but intercellular. Hence the name hygroma. In chronic cases there may be thickening or induration of skin. If there is an external wound, it may get infected and suppurative bursitis may follow.

DIAGNOSIS
The swelling should be differentiated from distension of tendon sheaths in the region. Hygroma presents a diffuse extensive swelling whereas the distensions of tendon sheaths (e.g., extensor tendon sheath) conforms to the position of the synovial sheath involved. For example, the distension of the tendon sheath of common digital extensor presents a swelling on the anteroexternal aspect of the knee; and the distension of the extensor metacarpi obliqus sheath is seen on the anterointernal aspect of the knee.
In cattle hygroma may be in the form of chronic bursitis which is the most common form and is called a typical hygroma; a suppurating bursitis due to infection of the part; a diffuse fibrous enlargement; and rarely as an acute bursitis.

TREATMENT
See general treatment for bursitis and also page 165.

Capped Fetlock

Distension of the subcutaneous bursa in front of the fetlock. The condition is common in horses. The common cause is trauma due to rubbing or striking on rough, hard ground. Knuckling is a predisposing factor.

Treatment is on general principles.

Fistulous Withers (*Supraspinous bursitis*)

Fistulous withers results from inflammation of the bursae situated over the spines of the second to fifth thoracic vertebrae.

INCIDENCE

The condition is more common in the horse.

ETIOLOGY

Predisposing causes: (1) The withers of the horse (unlike that of cattle) does not have much muscular covering and therefore is more exposed to trauma, (2) Bad conformation.

Exciting causes: (1) The most common cause of supraspinous bursitis is trauma resulting from an ill-fitting saddle. A saddle which is too small or too big for the animal may cause trauma. In a narrow-chested animal the saddle may frequently slip forward and cause trauma. (2) Infections due to Brucella abortus, Actinomycosis, parasitic infection (Onchocerca reticulata, Vitamin E deficiency, etc. are also mentioned as causes for the condition (O'connor, 1950).

SYMPTOMS

There is local swelling due to distension of the bursa. In long standing cases the bursal enlargement may extend into the surrounding tissues in the form of pockets. The condition might become suppurative and the bursa may rupture like an abscess. The pus escapes through small sinus openings on the skin in the region of the withers. Hence the term fistulous withers.

The pus migrates downwards and spreads easily through the intermuscular spaces of the external thoracic and cervical muscles and thus may collect either in front of the shoulder or behind the shoulder. The collection of pus gives rise to a soft, abscess-like swelling.

Suppuration may also extend to neighbouring tissues like

ligamentum nuchae, supraspinous ligament, the cartilages of the dorsal spines, the cartilaginous portion of scapula, the ribs, etc. Very rarely, the pus may pass along the costo-vertebral groove and into the vertebral canal.

PROGNOSIS

Prognosis is guarded. Prolonged treatment is necessary. The condition is serious if it is extensive. It is very difficult to provide adequate drainage. Fistulous withers in horse with high withers responds more readily to treatment than when it affects animals with low withers.

TREATMENT

Discontinue the use of the saddle. Enlarge the sinus openings to provide drainage. Touch the interior with caustics. Remove the necrotic tissues. If pus has migrated downwards up to the level of the shoulder, it might be necessary to open at this point like an abscess to drain the pus. Antibiotics may be used locally and parenterally to check infection.

Bursitis Intertubercularis (*Bicipital Bursitis*)

The bicipital bursa or intertubercular bursa is situated between the bicipital groove of the humerous and the tendon of Biceps brachii *m*. (Coroco radialis *m*; Flexor brachi *m*.). This is a very extensive bursa. The inflammation of the bursa is a common cause for shoulder lameness. The inflammation may be acute or chronic.

ETIOLOGY

(1) Injury to the bursa resulting from pressure of the collor in draft horses.

(2) An extension of inflammation from local tendinitis. The sprain of the tendon of Biceps brachii muscle results from over-stretching of the muscle, slipping backwards or due to violent efforts to extricate the limb when fixed.

(3) Toxaemia resulting from infectious diseases.

SYMPTOMS

Local symptoms are not pronounced in many cases. Diffuse swelling may be noticed in the shoulder region on one or both sides of the tendon. In acute cases there is typical shoulder lameness. Weight is not borne on the affected limb during progression because of pain. The opposite limb is quickly taken forward in a "hopping" fashion in an effort to relieve the affected limb. During standing the shoulder joint is somewhat extended and the knee is flexed, the foot being placed behind the opposite limb and resting on the toe. There is marked local inflammation just below the point of the shoulder in some cases. Characteristic symptoms are shown when the animal is in progression. There is inability in advancing the limb. The affected limb is dragged on its toe while a short step is being taken by the opposite limb, in a hopping fashion. When both limbs are involved, the animal seems *"tied at the shoulder"*. However, when backed, the limb is used in an almost normal manner. In chronic cases the symptoms are not obvious at rest but are evident during progression. Atrophy of the shoulder muscles is seen in longstanding cases.

DIAGNOSIS

Diagnosis is made from the symptoms and the history of the case. Pain is evident when the limb is lifted and flexed backwards. (As this will stretch the biceps brachii muscle and cause pressure on the bursa.) Local pressure in the region of the shoulder may also reveal pain in some cases.

PROGNOSIS

Guarded. Usually, recovery takes place within six to eight weeks; but sometimes the condition may become chronic and incurable. Chronic cases are not very painful and the animal may continue to be used for work. Ulceration of the bicipital groove and formation of exostosis are possible sequelae.

TREATMENT

(1) During the acute stage the use of cold water over the area is advisable.

(2) Counter-irritation. Blistering ointments (Biniodide of mercury ointment alone or in combination with Iodine ointment) may be used.

Trochanteric Bursitis (*Trochanteric Lameness*)

Inflammation of the bursa situated between the tendon of the middle gluteus muscle and the great trochanter of the femur.

ETIOLOGY

1. Trauma (e.g., due to a blow or a strain of the tendon).
2. Consequent to equine influenza or strangles.

SYMPTOMS

In the acute case there is swelling and pain on pressure over the great trochanter. At rest the limb is kept relaxed. During progression there is difficulty in advancing the limb and the hind quarters of the affected side is raised. In chronic cases disuse atrophy of the gluteal muscles may be seen.

PROGNOSIS

Guarded. The inflammation usually subsides wihin four to six weeks when treated properly. Rarely, it may persist as a chronic bursitis.

TREATMENT

As for bursitis intertubercularis.

Surgical Conditions Affecting Synovial Sheaths of Tendons

The movement of tendon over bony prominences and joints is facilitated by the presence of tendon sheaths (thecae or vaginae). The sheaths of the flexor tendons are more extensive than those of extensor tendons so much so injuries and infection of the flexor sheaths are more serious.

Contusions and Open Wounds

Contusions and open wounds of the synovial sheaths are caused by various types of trauma. The characteristic feature of open wound of a synovial sheath is the discharge of synovia through the opening. The synovia is coloured straw-yellow and is thin in consistency. It coagulates when exposed to air for sometime and is recognised as a yellow coagulum in the wound resembling a pad of fat. Open wounds of synovial sheaths situated close to a joint may be confused with an open joint.

Treatment is the same as for wounds in general. Once infection is checked healing takes place quickly.

Acute Synovitis

Normally synovial fluid is secreted by the synovial membrane and is re-absorbed. When the lining membrane of a synovial sheath is irritated due to injury or infection there is likely to be an excessive secretion of synovial fluid not readily reabsorbed and a distension of the tendon sheath results.

CLASSIFICATION

(1) *Dry synovitis*: In this type the lining membrane becomes thickened and rough and when the tendon moves through it crepitation may be felt due to friction.

(2) *Plastic synovitis*: It is characterised by fibrinous deposits which may cause adhesion between the tendon and the tendon sheath.

(3) *Serous synovitis*: It is the commonest type. There is an increased formation of synovia, causing distension of the sheath.

ETIOLOGY

1. Trauma. Traumatic injury of the sheaths may occur from striking against the wall or other hard objects, small foreign bodies like thorns penetrating into the sheath, etc.

2. In most cases synovitis occurs from overwork or from sprain of the tendon.

SYMPTOMS

In the acute stage there appears sudden and pronounced distension of the affected sheath, and sensitiveness on palpation. If the inflammation is very acute lameness may be shown. Synovitis of the flexor tendon sheath is a rather serious condition and produces well-marked lameness.

PROGNOSIS

Favourable, if properly treated in the early stages. However, in some old animals and in neglected cases fibrous thickening may develop and lameness persists.

TREATMENT
1. Rest.
2. During the stage of acute inflammation applications of cold water and astringent lotions are advisable. A thick layer of cotton pad dipped in white lotion or in magnesium sulphate-glycerine paste, is placed and a bandage is applied.
3. In subacute and chronic cases a blister ointment may be applied.

Infectious Synovitis

Infectious synovitis may be seen during the course of infections diseases like equine influenza, strangles and pneumonia.

SYMPTOMS
The pain and lameness are pronounced. The horse in many cases refuses to bear weight-on the limb.

TREATMENT
1. Immerse the affected portion of the limb in warm antiseptic solution.
2. Administration of antibiotics or sulphonamides parenterally.
3. Injection of antibiotics and corticosteroids into the synovial sheath.
4. Injection of polyvalent antiserum is advantageous.

Purulent Synovitis (Purulent Tenovaginitis)

This is synovitis characterised by accumulation of pus.

ETIOLOGY
1. Open wound of the synovial sheath and its consequent infection.
2. An extension of infection due to rupture of a neighbouring abscess.

SYMPTOMS
The symptoms are those of acute septic inflammation and of a synovial fistula discharging synovia mixed with pus and having foetid odour. The tendon sheath is tensely distended, causing a prominent swelling in the region. Pain is intense and the animal

refuses to put any weight on the limb. Febrile symptoms may also be present.

DIAGNOSIS

From the symptoms. The following points might help in differentiating tendinous synovitis from articular synovitis when the lesion appears in the viscinity of a joint. In a joint the inflammation is around the joint whereas in a tendon sheath it roughly conforms to the course of the tendon. The inflammatory symptoms and lameness are more marked in articular synovitis than in tendinous synovitis.

PROGNOSIS

Guarded. Purulent synovitis affecting the great sesamoidean, carpal or tarsal sheaths is a serious condition because the infection is likely to cause necrosis of the tendon and render the case hopeless. In some cases of suppurative synovitis, the spread of infection is checked by adhesions developing around it. In these cases recovery is likely to ensue.

Sequela

Adhesions may develop between the tendon and its sheath, as a result of suppurative tenovaginitis causing permanent lameness.

TREATMENT

1. Warm antiseptic irrigations using perchloride of mercury 1 in 1000 or formalin 1% is given for at least two hours a day for a few days. The area is covered with a thick pad of cotton dipped in the antiseptic lotion and is bandaged.

2. The tendon sheath may be incised (synoviotomy) to drain the pus. The cavity is then irrigated with warm normal saline. Hydrogen peroxide is used to clean it further. Afterwards any one of the following antiseptic solutions may be injected into it: (1) Perchloride of mercury in glycerine 1 in 1000. In addition to the antiseptic property this solution has good penetrating power because of the affinity of glycerine for moisture. (2) Carbolic acid in glycerine (3%). (3) Ether. (4) Irrigating with lactoserum (see treatment of "wounds"). (5) Injecting antibiotics into the tendon sheath. (6) Bier's hyperaemia treatment. (7) When the suppuration has been controlled and tendency towards healing

is evident, light exercise should be given to prevent formation of adhesions.

Chronic Synovitis (*Dropsy of Synovial Sheath*)

Chronic synovitis is marked by distension of the synovial sheath with accumulation of synovia.

CAUSES

1. Constant hardwork is the common cause of chronic synovitis.
2. It may sometimes follow acute synovitis.

SYMPTOMS

Pain is usually absent. Distension of the synovial sheath may be the only prominent symptom. Lameness may or may not be present. The interior of the synovial sheath sometimes contains fibrinous and riziform (rice-like) bodies in addition to synovial fluid.

TREATMENT

1. Needle-point firing and blister ointments. The synovia drains through the perforations caused by the firing. The synovial discharge ceases within a few days and the swelling gradually disappears.

2. Thecocentesis and injection of irritants: The synovial sheath (theca) is punctured with a needle and the contents are aspirated with a syringe. An irritant solution is then injected into the sheath. [Any one of the following solutions may be used: Tincture iodine; carbolic acid 3-5%; perchloride of mercury 1 in 1000; iodoform in glycerine 1 in 10; tannin in 96% alcohol 1 in 100.] After the injection local symptoms of acute inflammation are noticed. Febrile reaction (temperature up to 105°F) may be noticed for one or two days. Adhesions should be prevented by mild exercise. Recovery may take two to three months.

3. In some cases the synovial sheath bursts automatically. Then it must be treated as an open wound of the synovial sheath.

4. Synoviotomy (opening of the synovial sheath) is required especially when there are solid contents (riziform bodies). The operation must be done with all aseptic precautions and is not

usually recommended for fear of septic complications. Synoviotomy is specially risky in the case of large flexor tendons.

Note: A mild type of chronic synovitis is seen in young
animals freshly put to hard work. This usually subsides when
the animal is given proper rest.

Wind Galls

Distension of the great sesamoidean sheath is called *wind
galls*. It is characterised by a soft swelling above the level of the
proximal sesamoid bones. Wind galls may be due to chronic
synovitis or may be of a non-inflammatory nature.

INCIDENCE
More common in older horses.

SYMPTOMS
Besides the swelling no other abnormality may be noticed.
Lameness is usually absent.

TREATMENT
Not usually attempted because there is no lameness. General
treatment for bursitis (tenosynovitis) like aspiration, needle-point
firing, etc., may be tried.

Articular Wind Galls

The distension of the synovial capsule of the fetlock joint is
called articular windgalls. The distension is seen immediately
above the fetlock on either side, between the edge of the suspensory ligament and the metatarsal (or, metacarpal) bone.

Thoroughpin

Distension of the tarsal sheath due to chronic synovitis. The
swelling is noticed at the hollow of the hock on either side of
tendoachilis. Lameness may or may not be present.

TREATMENT
On general principles.

Extirpation of Hygroma of Knee

In long-standing cases of hygroma of knee in cattle, with welldefined fibrous thickening, it is better to extirpate the bursa including its fibrous thickening. Under local infiltration anaesthesia, put an elliptical incision vertically enclosing the required area of skin. By blunt dissection extirpate the mass. Control haemorrhage. Suture skin edges (after trimming excess skin) by interrupted apposition sutures or preferably by vertical mattress sutures. Trimming of excess skin was necessary to prevent "pocket formation"; but if too much skin is removed there will be difficulty in flexion of knee and the sutures may consequently cut through.

Questions

1. Write an account of fistulous withers in horse.
2. Describe the causes, symptoms and treatment of capped elbow in the dog.
3. Write short notes on:—a. Synovitis b. Bursae c. Bursitis intertubercularis d. Capped knee e. Wind galls f. Saddle galls g. Perforating wound into tendon sheath h. General principles for treating bursitis.
4. What are bursae? What are their functions? Name the different forms of bursitis and describe the symptoms and treatment of one such form commonly met with in cattle.

CHAPTER 27

Fractures

A *fracture* is a break in the continuity of hard tissues like bone, cartilage, etc.

ETIOLOGY
1. *Predisposing or Indirect Causes*
1. Fractures are common in certain bones because of their superficial position, shape, osseous structure or their function as levers during muscular movements.
2. Smooth roads and slippery floors of stables and sheds.
3. Diseased condition of bones like: osteomalacia, osteoporosis, ostitis, necrosis of bone, caries of bone etc.
4. Old age.

2. *Exciting (Direct) Causes*
1. External violence e.g., blows, kicks, etc.
2. Internal violence, excessive or incoordinate muscular action, e.g., fractures occurring in horses during galloping or jumping or due to struggling when cast for operations.

CLASSIFICATION
Fractures may be broadly classified into three types, viz. simple, compound, and complicated fractures.

(i) *Simple fracture* (closed fracture): A fracture which does not communicate with the outside, i.e., there is no wound on the skin leading to the fracture site.

(ii) *Compound fracture* (open fracture): A fracture which is communicating with an open wound on the skin.

A fracture in which the wound is caused at the time of fracture either from external trauma or by protrusion of a bone fragment through the skin, is called a primary compound fracture.

When a simple fracture has later been rendered compound,

it is called a secondary compound fracture.

(iii) *Complicated fracture*: A closed fracture in which there is considerable injury to important neighbouring vessels or nerves or is accompanied by the opening of a joint or visceral cavity, e.g., complicated fracture of rib.

A fracture may be incomplete or complete.

1. *An incomplete fracture*
   It is a fracture which does not extend through complete thickness of the bone, e.g., Greenstick fracture, fissured fracture, deferred fracture, etc.

   Greenstick fract re: Fracture in which the bone is partly broken like a bent green stick. Greenstick fracture occurs in young animals.

   Partial or splintered fracture: When splinters of bone are separated from the main bone as a result of direct violence as may be caused by firearms.

   Fissured fracture: In a fissured fracture there is a fissure (crack) extending through the bone without causing any displacement of the fragments. The fissures in the bone may be longitudinal, transverse or oblique. Fissured fractures are seen in the tibia, radius, metacarpus and os-suffraginis.

   Sub-periosteal (Intra-periosteal) fracture: A fracture of the cortical bone without rupture of the periosteum.

   Deferred fracture is an incomplete fracture in which separation of fragments occur only after a varying period after the incident due to subsequent violence, strain, or concussion, e.g., some cases of "broken back" in the horse.

2. *A complete fracture*
   It is a fracture in which the bone is broken completely through its thickness. The following are examples of complete fractures:

   Single fracture: When the bone is broken in one place only it is called a single fracture.

   Double fracture: When there are two fractures in the same bone.

   Multiple fracture (Comminuted fracture): When the bone is broken into more than two pieces.

3. *Avulsion fracture*

The tearing of bony prominences (like tuberosity) by forcible pull of its tendinous or muscular attachments.

Based on the portion of the bone involved, fractures may be classified as:

(a) *Diphysary fracture*: A fracture involving the diphysis (shaft) of a long bone.

(b) *Epiphysary fracture* (*Epiphysary separation*): Fracture at the junction of the epiphysis and shaft of bone. This type of fracture is common in young animals in whom the calcification of epiphysis is incomplete, e.g., epiphysary fracture of the proximal end of tibia in calves; epiphysary fracture of distal end of femur in dogs.

(c) *Supracondylar fracture*: A fracture above the condyle, e.g., supracondylar fracture of humerus.

(d) *Condyloid fracture* (*condylar fracture*): A fracture in which small fragments including the condyle is separated from the bone, e.g., condyloid fractures of humerous, femur, etc.

(e) *Transcondylar fracture*: A fracture of the humerus of femur in which the line of fracture is at the level of the condyles.

(f) *Intercondylar fracture*: A fracture between the condyles of the humerus.

An intercondylar fracture and a transcondylar fracture may coexist, making a T-shaped fracture.

(g) *Pertrochanteric fracture:* Fracture of the femur passing through the great trochanter.

(h) *Transcervical fracture:* Fracture through the neck of the femur.

Note: The "anatomical neck" of femur is that portion of the femur which is closest to its head; the portion of the neck of femur where fractures usually take place is referred to as the "surgical neck" of femur.

(i) *Periarticular fracture:* When a bone is fractured close to its articulating extremity without extending into the joint, a periarticular fracture results.

(j) *Articular fracture (joint fracture):* Fracture involving the articular surface of a bone.

(k) *Extracapsular fracture:* A fracture near a joint but not entering within the joint capsule.

(l) *Intercapsular fracture*: A fracture within the joint capsule.

Depending on the direction of the fracture, a fracture may be:

1. *Transverse fracture*: A fracture at right angles to the axis of the bone.

2. *Longitudinal fracture*: A fracture extending in a longitudinal direction, e.g., "split pastern" in the horse, wherein there is a longitudinal fracture of the os-suffragins.

3. *Oblique fracture*: A break in a bone extending in an oblique direction.

4. *Spiral fracture*: A fracture which is in a spiral direction.

Depending on relationship between the fragments in the fracture:

1. *Torsion fracture*: A fracture in which one of the fragments has been twisted and separated.

2. *Impacted fracture*: Fracture in which one fragment is firmly driven into another or one bone is driven into the fracture site of another, e.g., head of femur being driven into a fractured acetabulum.

3. *Dentate fracture*: A fracture in which the ends of the fragments are toothed and interlocked.

4. *Riding fracture* (over-riding fracture): A fracture in which the fragments lie side by side, causing shortening of the limb.

5. *Distracted fracture*: A fracture in which the fragments are separated by muscular pull, e.g., Fracture of olecranon.

A fracture could be:

1. *Compression fracture*: A fracture produced by compression, causing apparent reduction in the size of the bone due to pressure, e.g., some fractures occurring in cancellous bones like vertebrae.

2. *Depressed fracture*: A fracture of the skull in which a fragment is depressed below the surface.

3. *Colle's fracture*: Fracture of the distal end of radius. Abduction of paw is noticed in Colle's fracture.

4. *Pathological fracture* (*Spontaneous fracture; secondary fracture*): A fracture occurring due to a weakening of bone by disease and not due to trauma.

5. *Congenital (Intra-uterine) fracture*: Fracture of the bone of a foetus in the uterus.

INCIDENCE

The bones commonly fractured in the dog are the femur and pelvis. Less frequently fractures of the tibia, radius, ulna, humerus and mandible are encountered. Fracture of other bones are comparatively rare.

In the *bovine* fractures of tibia, humerus, metatarsus and pelvis are relatively common. Radius, ulna, femur, scapula, carpus and tarsus are but rarely fractured. Fracture of the patella is unusual in cattle. Fracture through the epiphyseal cartilage between the head and neck of femur is of frequent occurrence in the bovine below three years.

In the *horse* the frequency of occurrence of fractures is as follows: pelvis (especially of the external angle of ilium), *tibia*, humerus, ulna, metacarpus, metatarsus, phalanges ("split pastern") proximal sesamoids, radius, vertebrae, os-pedis and os-navicularis. Fractures of femur, patella, carpus, tarsus, os-calcis, scapula and astragalus occur very rarely.

It may be mentioned that fracture of femur is very common in the dog but rare in large animals and that vertebral fractures may occasionally occur in the horse and dog but are very rare in cattle.

HEALING OF FRACTURE

The healing of a fracture may be described in four stages, viz., (1) formation of haematoma, (2) formation of soft callus, (3) formation of primary bone callus, and (4) formation of secondary bone callus.

1. *Formation of haematoma*: Fracture causes injury to blood vessels in the bone and surrounding soft tissues causing haemorrhage. This blood collects around the seat of fracture forming a haematoma which later coagulates. The haematoma is well-formed within about twenty four hours.

2. *Formation of soft callus* (*fibrous callus or temporary callus*): Within about twenty four hours the ingrowth of fibroblasts and capillaries into the clot starts, the growth of capillaries takes place from periosteum, Haversian canals, endosteum and bone marrow. Macrophages (wandering phagocytic cells) make their

way into the blood clot to remove the extravasated RBC and debris. The clot at this stage contains fibrin, fibroblasts and newly formed blood vessels and resembles granulation tissue. This fibrovascular tissue thus formed between the broken ends is called *soft callus* or *fibrous callus* or temporary callus.

The callus fills the space between the broken ends. The size of the callus is large when the bleeding and haemotoma at the fracture site is extensive. The soft callus is formed within *one* or *two weeks*.

The vascularity of the granulation tissue is diminished when it is converted into fibrous callus.

3. *Formation of primary bone callus*: During the early stages of fracture the reaction of the clot is acidic. The presence of cellular debris consisting of damaged tissue and haemorrhage is responsible for this lowering of the ph. The acidity favours mobilisation of calcium from the bone fragments (as calcium phosphate) and from the blood. The enzyme phosphatase released by osteoclasts also facilitates release of calcium phosphate from plasma so as to cause a supersaturation of calcium in the haematoma surrounding the fracture, even though there is no appreciable variation in the general blood level of calcium. The calcium mobilised from bone fragments and plasma is held in solution so long as the ph is on the acidic side. Later, it becomes deposited when the reaction slowly turns alkaline, and forms the primary bone callus. The reaction is now changing towards alkalinity which is favourable for the deposition of calcium in the area. Osteoblasts derived from the bone fragments invade the callus and calcium is deposited in the intercellular space. [Osteoblasts are most numerous in periosteum and the endosteum and extremely few in the compact bone. Therefore mineralisation is more at the peripheral and central zones of the callus while it is meagre in the intermediary zone. The mineralisation formed at the peripheral and central zones affords a temporary union and immobilises the fragments until normal bony tissue is formed later.] The primary callus now presents a granular appearance and feels like an irregular hard mass of cartilage and bone. Calcification commences on the *tenth day* and by about the *third week* it becomes radiographically visible. Clinically it can be felt as a firm round mass around the seat of fracture. Within about four to eight weeks,

depending upon the size of bone and the age of the patient, the primary callus becomes sufficiently firm to prevent any movement and *clinical union* is said to have taken place; but radiographically the union may not appear complete. (When there is clinical union there is presence of a palpable callus. No pain is evinced on movement.)

It is to be emphasised that an alkaline reaction is essential for a proper deposition of calcium. Lack of proper immobilisation of a fracture and consequent tissue injury at the site will cause an acidic reaction and cause interference in the mineralisation of the callus and delay the healing of fracture.

4. *Formation of secondary bone callus and functional reconstruction of the healing bone* (*Formation of mature bone*): The secondary bone callus develops from four to eight weeks. During this period the primary callus is organised by a process of consolidation or ossification. The excess connective tissue cells and debris are removed by osteoclasts. Simultaneously deposition of new bone is brought about by osteoblasts. Contraction and organisation of the callus takes place and the excess thickening over the periphery disappears (resorption). The union at this stage is complete radiographically. Radiographic evidence of complete union of a fracture is characterised by uniform calcification of the callus approaching the density of mature bone and the new bone uniting the fragments appears like normal bone except that it does not have the Haversian systems.

SYMPTOMS

The symptoms that are likely to be noticed in a fracture are: (1) Deformity, (2) Loss of function, (3) Abnormal mobility, (4) Pain, and (5) Crepitus.

1. *Deformity*: Deformity is due to the displacement of fragments and may be manifested by deviation from the normal posture or position, viz. shortening, angulation, rotation, adduction, abduction, etc. The local swelling at the seat of fracture may also cause some deformity. In certain types of fractures, deformity is characteristic, e.g., abduction of the paw in Colle's fracture of radius (fracture of distal end of radius); supination (=turning outward) of palm in fracture of the lateral condyle of humerus in man.

FRACTURES 173

2. *Loss of function*: In the case of a limb, the loss of function is manifested by its inability to bear weight. In incomplete fractures loss of function is sometimes relatively less.

3. *Abnormal mobility*: It is exhibited by the ability to move the affected part at a point or in a direction in which movement is not normally possible. The movement of one extremity of the fractured bone is not transmitted to the other end of it.

4. *Pain* is evinced especially when the fragments are moved. In man, the initial pain exhibited at the time of fracture vanishes after a few minutes and there is a short period (lasting ten to twenty minutes) when no pain is felt at the seat of fracture. During this period of "numbness" there is also muscular relaxation and therefore reduction of fracture is easy. This period of numbness is, however, again followed by pain and muscular contraction. Pain is less in impacted fractures and may be absent in pathological fractures. Pain disappears within twenty-four hours after reduction and immobilisation.

5. *Crepitus (Crepitation)*: Crepitus can be produced by manipulation making the fractured ends rub against one another. Crepitation can be heard or felt. Crepitus obviously is not possible when there is interposition of soft tissue between the fragments and in the case of distracted fractures, etc. In fractures involving vertebral column crepitus can be appreciated only very rarely. The coarse grating sound in fracture should be differentiated from the soft crepitus feft in arthritis, tenosynovitis and emphysema.

Other symptoms noticed in fracture: In some cases of fracture there is rise of temperature to about 2 to 3 degrees F and albuminurea and lipuria may be detected.

DIAGNOSIS

From the symptoms. If a radiograph is taken it will help confirmation.

TREATMENT

The treatment of a fracture includes : (1) reduction of the fracture and (2) Retension and Immobilization.

1. *Reduction of a Fracture*

The correction of the displacement of the fractured ends of

the bone so as to bring the fragments into normal alignment and apposition, is called "reduction of the fracture". If the displacement is slight, reduction can be effected by holding rigidly the upper segment of the bone and then moving the lower segment into the correct position. When the displacement is well marked as in the case of an over-riding fracture, it may be necessary to administer general or epidural anaesthesia or a muscle relaxant. The over-riding can be usually corrected by "extension" and "counter-extension" combined with local manipulation. Exerting traction on the distal fragment is called traction or extension. In the case of a limb this can be effected by tying a rope round the pastern. The traction should be exerted along the normal direction of the limb. Counter-extension is the procedure adopted for pulling the proximal fragment in the opposite direction. This can be effected by fixing the upper part of the limb, while the lower part of it is being pulled.

2. *Retention and Immobilisation of a Fracture*

Application of a "charge" is one of the methods employed for immobilisation. A "charge" is an immobilising dressing prepared by smearing melted pitch and cut pieces of tow over a region. It is very useful for immobilising fractures of shoulder and hip regions. "Coaptation splints" and "casts" are very commonly used for immobilising fractures. They consist of materials like cloth bandages, plaster of paris, wooden pieces, metal strips, metal sheets, etc., which are applied around the affected part as mentioned below:

(a) *Gum bandage*: Ordinary gauze bandage soaked in gum is good for immobilising fractures in birds and small animals.

(b) *Starch bandage*: Powdered starch made into a paste with water and incorporated in gauze bandage can be used for immobilising fractures in small animals.

(c) *Splints and bandages*: Splints made out of light metal or wooden sticks may be used for immobilising a fracture. A good padding of cotton wool or tow is given to prevent injury to the skin and underlying soft tissues and over this the splints are placed and bandaged. For proper immobilisation, it is necessary to include within the splint the two joints involving either end of the fractured bone. It is difficult to retain splints for fractures above the knee and hock. Plaster of Paris bandages are better and more convenient than splints.

(d) *Plaster of Paris*: Gauze bandages impregnated with Plaster of Paris are available (e.g. "Gypsona Plaster of Paris bandages"). The bandage is immersed in water until bubbling of air stops and is immediately used for bandaging. The Plaster of Paris solidifies in a few minutes and then the whole bandage becomes a stiff cast over the region facilitating immobilisation. This is called a *plaster cast*. Before putting the plaster cast it is necessary to spread a uniform layer of cotton wool over the area to prevent injury due to friction or compression. It is also advisable to apply Tincture Benzoin or collodion over the skin before spreading the cotton wool so that it will stick to the skin. This will to some extent prevent slipping of the plaster cast. For proper immobilisation, the joints immediately above and below the fracture site should be included in the plaster cast.

(e) *Plaster of Paris splints and gutters*: Plaster of Paris splints are prepared by impregnating gauze pieces with Plaster of Paris made into a paste with water. Pieces of gauze containing Plaster of Paris are then placed one over the other or are folded into layers of varying thickness conforming to the shape required. About 2 to 4 splints are used for immobilising a part. The splints are placed over the part and are kept in position by bandages or cords. The advantage of these splints is that they can be loosened or tightened at will.

A *"plaster gutter splint"* is a plaster splint which is bent longitudinally into an angular shape resembling the shape of gutter. The length and breadth of these gutters are so adjusted as to adapt to the shape of the part to which they are applied.

(f) *Poroplastic felt*: Poroplastic felt is a porous piece of felt which has been impregnated with a resinous substance. This is dipped in boiling water or exposed to heat immediately before being used as a bandage. When heated it becomes soft and facilitates bandaging. After sometime it becomes stiff by cooling and thus acts like an immobilising cast. Because of its being porous, it permits transpiration and thereby prevents retention of perspiration and consequent necrosis of skin.

(g) *Thomas splints*: Modified Thomas splints are useful both for correction and immobilisation of fractures of small animals. They are made out of light metal rods (duraluminium rods). These rods are available in sizes of $\frac{8}{16}''$, $\frac{1}{4}''$, $\frac{3}{8}''$ etc., and 6 to 12 feet long.   These rods are bent to the required shape and are properly padded before application.

(h) *Mason meta-splints.*   These are flat metal splints made of aluminum, conforming to the shape of the metacarpal region including the carpal and fetlock joints (or, the metatarsal region including tarsal and fetlock joints).   They are usually used in small animals.

(i) *Suturing bone fragments*: The fractured ends are exposed surgically and after reducing the fracture the ends are united by stainless steel wire sutures.   Holes are made in the bone by using a bone drill and through these holes the wires are passed and tied. In oblique fractures the holes should be drilled at right angles to the fractured surfaces in order to prevent displacement.

(j) *Applying bone plates*:   Vitellium bone plates and screws are used to unite the broken ends.   The plates are kept in position by means of screws.   At least two screws should be fixed to each fragment to prevent displacement.   It is necessary to drill holes into the bone for fixing the screws. (See also page 581)

(k) *By using bone pins*: Stainless steel bone pins are used. There are two methods of pinning: (A) External pinning, and (B) Intramedullary pinning.

(A) *External pinning* (cortical pinning; external fixation): Examples are Kirschner Splints, Stader splints, etc.

Two pins are driven into each fragment at an angle of about 40° to each other by using a chuck. (The pins penetrate through the overlying skin and soft tissues before they get into the bone. They must be firmly landed in the cortex by going through almost the entire thickness of the bone.)   The two pins fixed to each fragment are then connected outside by a short assembling pin, using specially designed screws and nuts (clamps).   The short assemblies on each fragment are next connected by a long assembling pin after adjusting the fragments into correct alignment and apposition. External pinning is done on the side of the bone where the bone is most superficial, e.g., for femur: posterolateral aspect; for humerus: anterolateral aspect; for tibia: medial aspect; for radius: medial aspect.

(B) *Intramedullary pinning* (*Internal fixation*): In this the pin is driven through the medullary cavity of the bone.   There are two methods for doing this: viz., the open method (open-reduction) and the closed method (closed reduction).

In the open method a pin pointed at both ends is required. The seat of fracture is opened by a surgical incision and by the use of a chuck the pin is first driven from there into the proximal fragment until the upper end of the pin comes out through the skin. The chuck is then disconnected and is fixed on to the upper exposed end of the pin in order to drive the pin through the distal fragment also until it properly lands into the epiphysis. The excess portion of the pin at the upper end is cut and removed. After healing of the fracture the pin may either be retained or removed.

In the closed method the fracture site is not opened surgically. The pin is driven from one end of the bone to the other by following certain landmarks.

Examples: For fracture of the shaft of femur the pin is driven through the trochanteric fossa which is ·located by feeling the trochanter major and then directing the pin along its medial aspect. For fracture of the shaft of humerus the pin is introduced through a point ¼ inch below the ridge on the lateral tuberosity. For tibia the pin is driven ¼ inch below the medial meniscus and between the anterior and medial tuberosities. (See also page 580).

COMPLICATIONS OF FRACTURE

1. Injury to a nerve causing paralysis of the muscles supplied by it.

2. Injury to important vessels causing impairment in blood supply to a dependent region. Injury to the main vessels supplying an important muscle may cause degeneration and atrophy of the muscle.

3. Non-union and delayed union may result from defective reduction or lack of proper immobilisation.

Non-union: Non-union of a fracture might result if the gap between the fracture ends are very wide; interposition of soft tissue between the fragments; incomplete reduction; lack of immobilisation; and presence of infection at the fracture site causing autolysis of the fibrin clot, thus interfering with the formation of a callus. The commonest cause of non-union in compound fractures is the presence of infection.

Delayed union: Delayed union of a fracture is caused by repeated movements interfering with the mineralisation of the callus. This can usually be rectified by proper and continued immobilisation.

Some Fractures Met with in Domestic Animals

Fractures of the skull: These are usually depression fractures. Fractures involving cranial bones may cause injury to the brain.

Fractures of the scapula: Fractures of the scapula occur only rarely. The fracture may involve any of the following regions viz., the acromion process, superior angles, body, neck, articular cavity etc. Fracture of the lower portions of the scapula are more serious. Immobilisation can be tried by applying a "charge". (A "charge" is an immobilisation dressing made out by spreading alternate layers of warm melted pitch and chopped tow. The charge hardens on cooling.) But in horses treatment is not likely to be successful. Euthanasia of the horse is therefore advisable. In cattle recovery is possible. In small animals (dog, cat) recovery is the rule except when articular surfaces are involved. In the case of compound fractures, infection may set in.

Fracture of humerus: Fractures of the humerus may happen due to direct violence or by falling or jumping from a height. In dogs and cats the fracture usually involves condyles. Immobilisation can be effected by the use of a charge. When displacement is slight recovery is possible. Dogs and cats usually recover as a rule. Lameness may disappear gradually after the fracture has healed.

Fracture of ulna: Usually happens at the olecranon process. In dogs, cats and pigs the shaft of ulna may fracture with fracture of radius.

When there is fracture of olecranon, the fragment is pulled upwards by triceps muscle and the fore-arm has an oblique position but the *metacarpus is in a vertical position*. Crepitation may be felt.

Treatment is on general principles. In large animals cure is difficult. In cattle not used for work, a fibrous union may be obtained so as to enable use of the limb. In small animals (dogs, cats) good healing usually takes place.

Fracture of first phalanx: The fracture of os-suffraginis or first phalanx is usually met with in horses doing fast work. The condition is called *split pastern*. The horse stops suddenly, keeping the limb resting on the toe. If there is no displacement recovery usually takes place, provided sufficient rest is given. When there is displacement, healing is slow and too much exostoses develops causing lameness.

In dogs fracture of phalangeal bones usually responds to treatment favourably, even when it is a compound fracture provided the necrosed pieces of bone, if any, are removed.

Fracture of pelvis: The bones involved in pelvic fracture may be the ilium, pubis or ischeum. The fracture may also happen through the cotyloid cavity. (See also page 180).

Fracture of ilium: Fracture of the external angle of ilium is frequently met with in the horse. The fractured fragment is pulled downward and forward by the muscle Tensor facia lata. The deformity can be easily recognised by looking from behind and comparing the two hips. The condition is called *down in the hip*. The horse is said to be *"hipped"*. There is lameness in the beginning but it disappears when the local inflammation subsides.

Fracture of internal angle of ilium: This is rare. When there is fracture crepitation may be palpated on external manipulation.

Fracture of shaft of ilium: The affected quarter appears to be not symmetrical to the opposite quarter. Crepitation can be palpated externally or per rectum. Severe lameness is present. Prognosis is guarded. Deformity and lameness may persist even when union takes place. Displacement of fragments may sometimes injure important vessels in the pelvis causing fatal haemorrhage.

Fracture through the cotyloid cavity. Usually happens by falling on the great trochanter of femur. Sometimes the head of femur may also get fractured simultaneously. Crepitation may be felt on passive movement of the limb. There is severe lameness. The case is incurable.

Fracture of femur: Common in the dog. The fracture may be through the head, neck, shaft or condyles of femur. Bone pinning, use of Thomas splints, etc., can be tried for successful treatment of the condition.

Fracture of tibia: In the horse fracture of tibia is very common (next only to fracture of pelvis). In large sized horses prognosis is grave. In ponies, foals, etc., recovery may take place if treated properly. In dogs and cats the condition is usually treated successfully. An immobilising bandage from the foot to stifle (including stifle) is necessary.

Fracture of patella: There is inability to bear weight on the limb. Causes severe lameness. Prognosis is grave. Lameness persists even if healing takes place. In dogs the fragments can be removed surgically to relieve lameness.

Fracture of pelvis in dog: Some cases can be treated by bone-pinning, depending on the part of bone involved. The best conservative treatment is "cage rest", which is followed by recovery in a few cases. But generally prognosis in pelvic fracture is guarded.

Questions

1. Classify fractures. Describe the modern methods of surgical immobilisation.

2. Write short notes on: (1) False joint, (2) Split pastern, (3) Deferred fracture.

3. Define a fracture. What are the complications arising in the healing of fracture of bones? How will you treat them?

4. Define a compound fracture. Describe the principles of treatment of such a fracture involving the shaft of a long bone.

5. Describe the essential features of reparative processes taking place in compound and complicated fractures.

6. Describe the principles and practice of immobilisation of simple fractures in dogs and specify the precautions taken to promote bone repair.

7. Discuss the incidence of fractures of the fore-arm in cattle and dogs and describe the diagnostic procedure and therapeutic measures advised.

8. What is a false joint? Describe the steps to be taken for preventing the formation of false joints or for favouring such a termination in bone repair.

9. Discuss the incidence of fractures of long bones in dogs and cats. Describe the procedure for reduction and retention of simple fractures as well as the post-operative care required. State how you would confirm that re-union is complete.

10. Describe briefly the healing process in a bone fracture. Mention the conditions under which healing is retarded.

CHAPTER 28

Dislocations (Luxations)

Dislocation (luxation) is the separation of articular surfaces of bones. When there is only a slight change in the relationship of the articular surfaces of bones it is called a partial dislocation or subluxation. (The Latin word *Locare* means *to place*. Dislocation means displacement. The word *luare* in Latin means *to dislocate* and hence luxation means dislocation.)

CLASSIFICATION

1. *Complete dislocation*: A dislocation in which the articular surfaces are completely separated.

2. *Partial dislocation* (*Incomplete luxation*; or *subluxation*): When some parts of the articular surfaces are still in contact.

3. *Acute* (*recent*) *luxation*: When it is of recent occurrence.

4. *Chronic luxation*: A dislocation that has been in existence for a long time.

5. *Recurrent luxation*: Showing recurrence after corrrection of an earlier occurrence.

6. *Simple* (*closed*) *luxation*: When there is no open wound communicating with the joint.

7. *Compound luxation*: When the joint communicates with the external air through a penetrating wound.

8. *Complicated luxation*: When luxation is associated with other important injuries like fracture.

9. *Fracture dislocation*: Dislocation combined with fracture of the related bones close to their articular surfaces.

Examples: Luxations of the vertebral joints are usually combined with fracture of one or more articular processes. Dislocation of hip slmultaneously with fracture of head of femur.

10. *Pathological dislocation*: A dislocation resulting from

paralysis or some other local pathological lesion.

(*Note*: Luxations of immovable joints (synarthrosis) like the symphysis pelvis are commonly referred to as fractures.)

INCIDENCE

Dislocations are not so common when compared to fractures. Diarthroidal joints like hip, shoulder, elbow etc. are more commonly affected. Rare in vertebral joints. The frequency of occurrence of common dislocations in different species are:

Bovine: (1) Femoropatellar articulation, (2) hip, (3) rarely shoulder, and (4) other joints.

Equine: (1) Fetlock, (2) stifle, (3) hip, (4) rarely, elbow, hock or knee, and (5) very rarely, shoulder and other joints.

Canine: (1) Hip, (2) shoulder, (3) rarely, phalangeal joints, (4) very rarely, the cervical vertebrae, and (5) other joints.

ETIOLOGY

1. Direct violence as may be caused during jumping, accidental slipping, etc. (Traumatic dislocation).

2. Due to some pathological condition affecting the joint, articular ligaments or paralysis of certain muscles (Pathological dislocation).

3. Dislocations sometimes occur congenitally (Congenital dislocations).

PROGNOSIS

In congenital and pathological dislocations the prognosis is unfavourable. In traumatic dislocations the prognosis is guarded.

SYMPTOMS

1 In a dislocation there is usually rupture of the joint capsule and sprain of the articular ligaments. Some of the muscles concerned with the movement of the joint may also be sprained. When the violence is severe, the displaced articular extremity may be forced through the skin causing a compound dislocation. *Pain* is present in a dislocation.

2. There is either *immobility* or *restricted mobility* of the affected joint in the normal directions because free movement is prevented by the displaced articular ends. At the same time

increased movement might be possible in abnormal directions. Sometimes increased mobility of a dislocated bone can be produced if all the articular ligaments and the joint capsule are ruptured.

3. *Functional interference.* There is inability to use the joint or the limb (or part) properly.

4. *Deformity* is the most important symptom of dislocation. A prominence may occur in an abnormal situation and corresponding depression may occur elsewhere because of the displacement of the articular ends. Besides this there is also deformity of the limb as a whole. The limb is often placed in a characteristic position depending on the joint involved and the direction of displacement. Deformity may be in the form of deviation in direction of the limb, shortening or lengthening of the limb, or variation in the normal angularity of the surface of the joint or the difference in the position of certain landmarks over the surface of the articulation (e.g., disappearance of the prominence of great trochanter in obturator dislocation of the hip).

5. Inflammatory swelling may be noticed around the joint.

Differential Diagnosis

Differential diagnosis between fracture and dislocation is generally easy. Some of the differentiating signs are: the pain due to dislocation is constant; there is no period of numbness as in fracture. The tenderness present in dislocation is less intense and more diffuse than it is in a fracture. In fracture, when the concerned extremities are moved there is crepitation, whereas in dislocation there is rather a rocking noise. In dislocation crepitation is absent unless there is associated fracture also. (Sometimes, however, a fracture and dislocation may occur together involving the same bones.)

4. A fracture when reduced recurs immediately unless properly supported. A dislocation once reduced has very little tendency to re-occur provided rest is given.

5. A rather constant muscle spasm and rigidity about the injured part is maintained in dislocation. Abnormal mobility is present in the case of a complete fracture.

6. The local symptoms of dislocation are noticed in the viscinity of a joint. In fractures it need not be so, unless it is close to the joint.

7. The normal appearance of the joint is altered in dislocation. For example, in the posterior dislocation of the elbow joint when the olecranon is displaced from the corresponding fossa of the humerus the usual triangular relationship between the olecranon and the condyles of the humerus is altered.

8. In dislocation the limb is often fixed in a particular posture and movement is generally restricted; abnormal and free mobility is characteristic of fracture.

9. The abnormal posture of the limb is fairly suggestive of the type of dislocation.

10. Radiography or fluoroscopy may be necessary to confirm the diagnosis in certain cases.

PROGNOSIS

The prognosis varies according to the nature of dislocation and the extent of injury to the articular ligaments and other soft tissues. If correction of displacement is delayed, the articular cavity may be filled with blood-tinged inflammatory exudate. This exudate may cogulate and form a *chicken-fat clot*. The presence of this clot makes correction of the dislocation very difficult. In large animals reduction of a dislocation becomes very difficult or impossible at times. Sometimes even after reduction the case may not progress well because of cicatrical contraction of ruptured ligaments and ankylosis of the joint may follow.

When a dislocation is not corrected, a "false joint" (pseudo-arthorsis) may form because of certain changes in the soft tissues accommodating the displaced articular end of the bone. The *false joint* will have also a synovial membrane formed resembling an ordinary joint. After the false joint is formed the animal will be able to use the limb in an almost normal manner though with some degree of lameness.

When there is an open wound communicating with the joint, it sometimes leads to septic arthritis and the prognosis in these cases is generally unfavourable. A fracture dislocation usually results in a stiff joint after healing.

GENERAL PRINCIPLES OF TREATMENT

Treatment of a dislocation consists of reduction and retension.

Reduction: Traction is applied on the two displaced bones in opposite directions until the articulating surfaces come to the same level and afterwards they are pushed to their normal position. Most of the simple dislocations get corrected automatically with a characteristic "clicking" noise when the articulating surfaces are brought to the same level by traction. Excessive manipulation of a dislocation should be avoided since this will cause unnecessary trauma. For this it is necessary to have a clear idea about the relationship of articulating surfaces. Radiography or fluoroscopy of the affected joint will be helpful in this regard. If a dislocation has been in existence for a long time there might be adhesions. Some of these adhesions can be separated by careful manipulations. The muscle spasm present in dislocation is generally not much as in fractures. Gradual traction may cause fatigue in these muscles and may thus help overcome muscle spasm. A muscle relaxant or general anaesthetic is advisable if the muscle spasm is too much, if the manipulations are painful or if there is difficulty in controlling the patient. Manipulations are generally easy in small animals. But in large animals the assistance of two or more persons may be required. Traction in large animals is usually done by means of two ropes; one applied to the proximal and the other to the distal parts of the limb. In small animals *open reduction* of the dislocation may be tried if the joint cavitis are damaged or if there is interposition of soft tissues. If reduction is impossible resection of the articular head of the bones may be considered so as to enable formation of a false joint.

Retention: After reduction proper rest should be given to the affected joint for a few days. Complete immobilisation is advisable during this period, if practicable. A tranquiliser may be used, if necessary. Slings may be used in the horse. Mild exercise is advisable later to improve blood circulation and to prevent anchylosis and muscular atrophy.

Repair of Dislocations: The dislocation might have caused extravasation of blood and tear of ligaments, joint capsule muscles, etc. When it is reduced without much trauma and is immobilised, the extravasated blood may get reabsorbed and the damaged tissues may heal by the formation of scar tissue.

Hip Dislocation (*Coxo-femoral dislocation*)

Dislocation of the hip is common in the dog and ox; less common in sheep and goat; and is rare in the horse. In the hip joint of the horse an accessory ligament (pubo-femoral ligament) is present unlike in other species. This may be one of the reasons for the relatively few incidence of hip dislocation in the species. In the bovine peculiarities like shallowness of the acetabulum and the small radius of curvature of the femoral head probably predisposes to the occurrence of dislocation. Hip dislocation in the cow occurs during oestrum or during parturition.

Hip Dislocation in Large Animals

ETIOLOGY

Movement beyond physiological limits caused by slipping outwards, falling from a height, etc.

CLASSIFICATION

The dislocation may affact one or both hind limbs (i.e., may be unilateral or bilateral.) Bilateral dislocation sometimes occurs in the cow due to both hind limbs slipping outwards. The common types of hip dislocation in Large Animals are of two types:

(1) Upward and forward (antero-dorsal) dislocation wherein the head of femur is displaced anteriorly and upwards towards the shaft of ilium; and

(2) The head of femur is displaced into the obturator foramen.

SYMPTOMS

In all types of hip dislocations stiffness of the affected limb and circumduction are noticed during progression. The affected limb is turned slightly outward and the stifle and hock joints are extended. The foot of the affected limb is placed in front of the opposite hind foot.

In upward and forward dislocation there is shortening of the limb: only the toe may touch the ground. Adduction of the limb is easy but abduction is limited. The great trochanter of the femur appears very prominent and is displaced upward and forward.

In obturator dislocation the limb appears longer. The great trochanter of the femur appears less prominent as compared to the normal side. On rectal palpation the head of the femur can be felt in the obturator foramen. When the animal walks a "rocking noise" can be heard sometimes due to the friction çaused by the movement of the femoral head in the obturator foramen and the trochanteric ridge striking against the ischium.

Note: When a heifer below three years shows the symptoms of hip dislocation, suspect first an epiphyseal fracture through the junction of head and neck of femur than a dislocation.

PROGNOSIS

Guarded. Reduction of the dislocation is at times difficult or impossible. Immobilisation to prevent re-occurrence is also difficult. Some cows affected with dislocation may show inability to get up for about one month or more. They may subsequently get up but may continue to show lameness.

TREATMENT

The animal is put under general or epidural anaesthesia and is cast and secured in lateral recumbency with the affected limb above. Only three limbs are secured together leaving the affected limb free. A rope is tied to this free limb above the fetlock for traction. Counter-extension can be provided by passing a rope or a smooth wooden bar through the groins and securing the same to a fixed object (like a nearby tree). During traction the *foot should be as close to the ground as possible*. Pull the limb in this manner downward and forward to reduce an "upward and forward dislocation". For dislocation into the obturator foramen the direction of traction is straight or slightly backward. A clicking noise is heard when dislocation is corrected. Treatment is successful in dislocations of recent occurrence.

Hip Dislocation in Small Animals

INCIDENCE

The most common dislocation in the dog and cat is hip dislocation and of this the anterior dislocation is commonest (Leonard, 1960).

ETIOLOGY

Jumping from a height, automobile accidents, etc.

CLASSIFICATION

According to the direction of displacement of the femoral head, hip dislocations are classified into four types.

1. *Anterior* (Precotyloid or Pre acetabular) dislocation in which the head of femur is displaced antero-dorsal and lateral to the acetabulum.

2. *Dorsal* (Supracotyloid or Supra-acetabular or outward) luxation in which the femur head is shifted dorsolaterally over the acetabular rim.

3. *Posterior* (Postcotyloid or Postacetabular or Ischiatic) luxation in which the femur head is seen displaced postero-laterally along the body of ischium.

4. *Intrapelvic* (Internal pubic or Obturatorial) luxation which in small animals occurs only when there is fracture of acetabulum.

PATHOLOGY

During dislocation, injuries may be caused to surrounding soft tissues which may also cause haemorrhage. For example, in anterior dislocation the iliopsoas and rectus femoris muscles; in dorsal dislocation the gluteal muscles; and in posterior dislocation the quadratus femoris muscles, may be damaged. The sciatic nerve may be paralysed in cases of posterior dislocation. Blood collecting in the acetabular cavity organises within a few days making reduction difficult. If the luxation is not reduced, the torn joint capsule may heal across the acetabulum and cover the organised blood clot. Anchylosis of the joint do not generally occur unless the damage to the articular surfaces are very extensive. Necrosis of the head of femur also does not happen in hip dislocation except in very rare instances in which there is also fracture of the femoral neck.

SYMPTOMS

1. Abduction of the limb is noticed in all types of hip luxations *except* in posterior luxation. (This is also a symptom in fracture of the neck of femur in which case the abduction is still more pronounced). In posterior luxation there is pronounced inward rotation of the limb; in anterior luxation rotation of the limb is outwards; in dorsal and intrapelvic luxations rotation of the limb may not be significant.

2. Make a careful examination by palpation of the great

trochanter of femur. If necessary the animal may be put under short-acting general anaesthesia for this purpose. The trochanter may seem to be elevated, depressed, rotated outwards or rotated inwards depending on the type of dislocation. The position of trochanter can be ascertained in relation to an imaginary line connecting the external angle of ilium and tuber ischii. Outward rotation is indicated by the trochanter being drawn towards the external angle of ilium and inward rotation by its being drawn away from it. The trochanter is elevated in anterior, dorsal and posterior luxations, fractures of the head and neck of femur, etc. In posterior luxation the trochanter is rotated inward and in anterior luxation there is outward rotation of it.

3. Press the thumb firmly between the trochanter major and the tuber ischii and palpate here while rotating the femur outwards on its long axis. If the joint is normal the trochanter can be made to "pinch" the thumb when moved in this manner; but if there is either luxation of the joint or fracture of the femoral neck the trochanter will only slide away without the so called pinching.

4. Place the animal in dorsal recumbency. Grasp the hocks and keep both hind limbs extended upwards and compare their lengths. A dorsal luxation makes the affected limb appear shorter *in this position*. Then extend the limbs backwards horizontally in a similar manner. In the latter position an anterior luxation will cause the affected limb appear shorter and a posterior luxation will make it appear longer than the opposite normal limb.

DIAGNOSIS

Diagnosis can be made from the symptoms. A ventro-dorsal radiograph with hind limbs extended symmetrically backwards, is of value in confirming the diagnosis.

PROGNOSIS

In intrapelvic luxations and in chronic recurrent luxations prognosis is guarded. In other types prognosis is generally favourable if reduction is effected within forty eight hours. A false joint may form in unreduced cases and there may be functional recovery though with slight deformity. If the sciatic nerve is injured, temporary or permanent paralysis may result depending on the severity of injury.

TREATMENT

Treatment consists of reduction and retention. *Reduction* of dislocation can be attempted as follows. The animal is anaesthetised and kept in lateral recumbency with the affected limb above. The pelvis may be supported either with the use of bandage passed through the groins or with the use of a Thomas splint. Traction is applied by holding the limb below the stifle keeping the joint flexed and the femur rotated inwards or outwards depending on the type of dislocation. In anterior and dorsal luxations femur is to be rotated inwards and in posterior luxation outwards.

During this procedure the other hand is used to palpate and guide the upper extremity of femur so as to guide the replacement of femoral head into the acetabulum. This is done by gripping the thigh from behind with the fingers over the trochanter and thumb in the acetabular region. If reduction is not possible by the above methods open reduction may have to be tried.

In recurrent luxations, the limb must be kept *immobilised* for about five to ten days by any of the methods listed below. (Details may be obtained from Leonard, 1960, p. 200.)

1. The limb is flexed and abducted and is bandaged with the body keeping the thigh rotated inward in anterior luxation and rotated outward in posterior luxation. An effective bandage of this type including both the hind limbs can be put against a properly paded wooden board placed across the rump above. Such a bandage has been described as a "butterfly cast" or "spread cast" or an "air plane cast", because of its shape.

2. Keeping the limb in a fixed degree of flexion and rotation by using the Thomas splint combined with bone tongs applied to the distal end of femur.

3. By using Stader an d Kirschner pins anchored to the ilium and ischium.

4. By the De Vita's method using a long intramedullary pin passed through the facia ventral to the tuber ischii and above the femoral neck and fixed to the wing of ilium.

5. By the Yarborough method using two pins crossing over

the femoral neck and landing respectively into the body of ilium and the body of ischium.

In cases where open reduction is attempted, it is better to suture the joint-capsule with a non-absorbable suture material like stainless steel wire to prevent re-occurrence before healing is complete. Reconstructing the ligamentum teres with facia or plastic has been suggested to make the replacement more secure. Another method proposed for firm retention of the femoral head in the acetabulum is by the use of "toggle" threaded with facia or plastic threads. The toggle is passed through holes drilled through the trochanter major and the acetabulum.

Hip Dysplasia

Hip Dysplasia is a general term used to denote a badly formed hip joint due to development abnormalities. It causes unequal wear and tear of the different components of the hip joint and predisposes to various deformities and arthritis of the joint. The condition has been met with more commonly in the canine and is supposed to be hereditory.

Examples of hip dysplasia are *Coxa magna* in which condition the head and neck of femur are unusually broad. *Coxa plana* in which the articular surface is flattend in the longitudinal direction due to osteochondrosis of the capitular epiphysis. This condition is called *Legg-Perthes' disease. Coxa valga* in which the normal angulation of the neck of femur with its shaft is modified in such a way that the neck is in an almost straight line along the shaft. In other words, the angle formed by the axis of the shaft and the axis of the head and neck is increased. *Coxa vara* in which the angle mentioned above is decreased i.e., the opposite of coxa valga.

SYMPTOMS

Symptoms are usually noticed when the pup is three to nine months old. Abnormal gait, limping, wincing on pressure over the hips, and sitting in abnormal positions are the usual symptoms. Outward rotation of the stifle, prominent trochanters are other symptoms. Some cases exhibit pain; some others have difficulty in climbing stairs. The hind limbs are used in a "hopping" or "rabbit-like" fashion while running. In chronic cases there is atrophy of the thigh muscles. When viewed from behind the hips are wide and flat. In coxa plana there is symptomatic relief when the dog reaches maturity (ten to twelve months old) possibly due to the compensatory effect of the related muscles.

DIAGNOSIS

From the symptoms. A ventro-dorsal radiograph with hind limbs extended backwards parallel to midline is helpful for confirmation.

PROGNOSIS

Guarded. In some cases where the acetabulum is very flat, prognosis is very poor. Frequent luxations occur in these types. In coxa plana prognosis is fair because the symptoms disappear with age. Using the animal for breeding purpose should be discouraged.

TREATMENT

No satisfactory treatment. Use of corticosteroids etc. may be helpful in some cases to relieve inflammation and pain.

Shoulder Dislocation (*Scapulo-humeral dislocation*)

Dislocation of the shoulder joint is a rare condition in animals. It is extremely rare in the dog.

SHOULDER DISLOCATION IN LARGE ANIMALS

The luxation of shoulder generally happens when there is excessive flexion of the joint with simultaneous flexion of the elbow joint during jumping or due to falling down. With the flexion of the above joints there is relaxation of the biceps muscle and this facilitate *upward and forward* displacement of the articular surface of humerus. Complications like the fracture of scapula and humerus, rupture of vessels and nerves in the axilla etc., may happen.

Types: 1. Upward and forward displacement of the humerus is the most common.

2. Very rarely an inward luxation is met with as a result of excessive abduction of the limb.

SYMPTOMS

General symptoms of shoulder lameness. No weight-bearing on the affected limb. Shortening of the limb. Pain on palpation. On manipulation adduction and abduction are easy while flexion and extension are difficult and cause pain.

PROGNOSIS

If the dislocation is reduced cure is usually effected within about two to three weeks. Reduction may be impossible in some cases.

TREATMENT

Cast the animal with the affected limb above. General anaesthesia is advisable. Counter-extension is provided by a rope passed around the neck and thorax through the axilla and tied to a fixed object. The pastern of the limb is secured by another rope and steady traction is exerted by an assistant. The operator palpates the shoulder joint to supervise the direction of traction. A clicking sound is heard when the dislocation is corrected.

Shoulder Dislocation in Small Animals

In Small Animals the displacement is usually lateral with the humeral head resting on the acromion.

SYMPTOMS

The limb is abducted and extended. Slight outward rotation of the limb and elevation of the point of the shoulder is also evident.

DIAGNOSIS

From the symptoms. Deep digital palpation of the glenoid cavity of scapula may be possible. Confirmation can be done by radiography (Postero-anterior view of shoulder).

PROGNOSIS

Favourable except in recurrent cases. Guarded in chronic or recurrent cases.

TREATMENT

Extend the limb and draw it medially while the head of the humerus is being pressed with the palm of the other hand. The dislocation is easily corrected and immobilisation is not necessary in a simple case. In chronic and recurrent cases and when there is appreciable damage to the joint capsule and ligaments, immobilisation for about two weeks is necessary. This can be provided by a "sling cast" around the body or by keeping the limb in the normal flexed position in a Thomas splint.

Elbow Dislocation (*Humero-radio-ulnar Dislocation*)

This is a rare condition. In the dog i tmay sometimes occur congenitally. In large animals treatment is rather impossible.

Elbow Dislocation in the Dog

ETIOLOGY

The dislocation may happen during excessive flexion of the joint with weight-bearing on the foot. Forceful twisting of the limb in the adducted or abducted position may also cause it.

PATHOLOGY

The radius and ulna gets displaced laterally. The joint capsule and medial and lateral articular ligaments may be sprained or ruptured. A temporary paralysis of the flexor muscles of the limb indicates possible injury to the ulnar nerve where it passes behind the medial epicondyle of humerus.

Rarely when combined with fracture of ulna, a forward and upward luxation of radius is also possible. But lateral displacement is common even in this instance.

SYMPTOMS

No weight-bearing on the limb, abduction of elbow, inward rotation of forearm, and impossibility for full extension of the elbow joint. The joints of the limb may be in a semi-flexed state provided there is no injury to the ulnar nerve. It may be possible to palpate the trochlear surface on the medial epicondyle of humerus.

Pain is severe when the luxation is combined with fracture of ulna and the symptoms also vary slightly. The luxated radial extremity can be easily palpated and flexion of the joint beyond 90 degrees becomes impossible.

DIAGNOSIS

From the symptoms. Confirmation can be made by radiography. An anteroposterior view of the elbow joint is taken as follows. Place the animal in ventral recumbency with the affected limb pulled forwards and the elbow centred over the cassette. During exposure the cassette is placed slightly tilted from behind and the x-ray tube adjusted in such a way that the beam falls perpendicular to the film.

PROGNOSIS

Favourable, unless complicated by fracture. Prognosis is guarded in fracture dislocations.

TREATMENT

The patient is anaesthetised and placed in lateral recumbency with the affected limb above. All the joints of the limb are flexed. The elbow joint especially should be flexed to less than 45 degrees so that the anconeal process of the ulna will not get obstructed by the lateral condyle of the humerus during reduction. The semilumar notch of ulna should face medially and this is made possible by having the foot rotated medially. Keeping the limb in this position, downward traction is applied on the fore arm so as to bring the radio-ulnar articular surfaces downwards; and simultaneously the proximal ends of the radio-ulna are pushed medially. The traction downwards of the radio-ulna can be made easier with a bone pin driven through the olecranon. (The pin is removed after accomplishing reduction.)

In some (chronic) cases a rocking motion is more effective for reduction than simple traction. The rocking motion can be produced by alternate pressure on the olecranon and the foot (Leonard, 1960).

Open reduction. Site: posterolateral aspect of elbow vertical incision extending from about 3 inches above the point of the elbow to 3 inches below it.

Patellar Dislocation

Dislocation of the patella may be caused by direct violence or

powerful muscular contractions. In dogs it is mostly congenital.

1. *Inward luxation*, the patella being displaced on the inner lip of the trochlea of femur.

2. *Outward luxation*, in which the patella is displaced on the outer trochlear lip.

INCIDENCE

In the dog inward luxation is more common. In the ox and horse luxation is rare but subluxation is common.

SYMPTOMS

In *inward luxation* flexion and extension of stifle becomes difficult or impossible; and the patellar ligaments and the quadriceps muscle are pulled inwards. The trochlea of femur becomes palpable.

In *outward luxation* the stifle is directed outwards and is semiflexed. Only the toe of the foot may touch the ground. Stiffness of the limb, shortened stride, and outward deviation of the quadriceps muscle. The abnormal situation of patella can be palpated.

TREATMENT

The limb is pulled forwards by an assistant with a rope applied to the pastern. The patella is manipulated simultaneously to effect reduction. Retention may be difficult. A blister applied over the area may induce swelling and thereby assist retention. In the dog reinforcement of the lateral patellar ligament or removal of patella is stated to be beneficial to prevent recurrent luxations.

Sub-luxation of Patella (*Fixation of Patella above the Trochlea*)

The upward luxation of patella by which the patella gets fixed above the trochlea of the femur is called subluxation of patella. The condition is common in the ox and horse.

PATHOLOGY

The patella gets fixed in the depression on the upper part of the trochlea. In this position the medial straight ligament of patella gets overstretched and slips above the medial trochlear ridge of femur. Since the ligament in this position gets applied against the prominent trochlear ridge its easy return downwards when the joint is flexed becomes difficult and therefore the patella gets locked up.

SYMPTOMS

When the animal starts to walk, the affected limb is kept rigidly extended backwards because the stifle and hock cannot be flexed. When the animal walks the toe is dragged. After a few steps the patella may, however, slip down and at this moment flexion of the stifle and hock joints also happen with a *jerk* or spasm. For each few more steps the joints are flexed in a jerky fashion but subsequently the limb may be used in an almost normal manner. The symptoms are very much pronounced when the animal is walked after a period of long rest (say, in the early morning). In other words it may be stated that the lameness *improves with exercise* and is exaggerented after a period of rest.

ETIOLOGY

The etiology is not well-understood. Rigid overextension of the limb may possibly be an exciting factor. General debility and weakness of muscles acting on the stifle have a predisposing effect.

TREATMENT

Using high-heeled shoes and providing saw-dust bedding are stated to exert some beneficial effect in subluxation of patella in the horse.

In the ox injection of Lugol's iodine solution or Tincture iodine (5 to 10 C.C.) into the femoro-patellar joint is stated to be effective in many cases. A swelling of the joint develops after the injection which gradually subsides within one to two weeks. The animal should be given rest for two to three weeks.

Patellar desmotomy or cutting the inner straight ligament of patella provides immediate symptomatic relief in most cases. For details see Operative Surgery.

Dislocation of the Fetlock

The following types of luxation of the fetlock joint have been reported: Anterior, Posterior, and Lateral.

The dislocation may be simple or compound. In compound dislocations the meta carpus (or meta tarsus, as the case may be) protrudes through the skin.

PROGNOSIS
Usually unfavourable, but complete recovery has been reported in some cases.

TREATMENT
Reduction and retention on general principles. For retention, a special immobilisation cast or apparatus conforming to the shape of pastern and fetlock may have to be devised.

Dislocation of the Hock
The dislocation may occur at the tibio-tarsal joint or at any of the internal joints. It may be complicated with fracture. General symptoms of dislocation and local inflammation are noticed. A radiograph may help confirm diagnosis. Prognosis is grave since perfect cure and correction of the deformity are difficult to achieve. In the horse and ox (work animals) euthanasia may have to be advised. In small animals treatment may be considered successful even though some deformity persists. When reduction is difficult by other means tenotomy of the tendoachilis may be tried in the dog (Dollar 1957; p. 929).

Dislocation of the Knee (*Carpal Dislocation*)
The dislocation may be complete or incomplete. It may be combined with fracture or complicated with fracture or with open joint.

SYMPTOMS
Inflammation of the knee joint. In complete dislocation no weight is borne on the limb and the animal virtually goes on three legs. The limb is abnormally mobile below the knee. In incomplete luxations the limb is deviated inwards or outwards at the knee.

PROGNOSIS
Unfavourable in complete and complicated dislocations. Guarded in simple incomplete dislocations.

TREATMENT

Reduction and retention, on general principles.

Dislocation of Phalangeal Joints

This is extremely rare in Large Animals. It is common in sporting dogs. Correction and treatment of the dislocation is easy but the condition often recur. Therefore excision of the affected phalanx is preferable. When the terminal phalanx is dislocated, the affected claw is seen lifted prominently. This is called "knocked up toe". Amputation of the terminal phalanx is indicated. Details of the above operations may be obtained from Operative Surgery.

Dislocation of the Jaw*

INCIDENCE

The dislocation of jaw cannot occur in Large Animals unless there is fracture of the coronoid process of the mandible. In the dog the dislocation can occur though very rarely. It may be unilateral or bilateral.

SYMPTOMS

Inability to close the mouth. Exophthalmos may be present. Tongue protrudes out. If luxation is unilateral, the lower jaw of the affected side appears depressed and pushed to the sound side.

DIAGNOSIS

Should be differentiated from rabies. The *"dropped jaw"* seen in rabies is not stiff as in temporo-mandibular dislocation and therefore can be passively lifted upwards. This may help differential diagnosis.

TREATMENT

To facilitate easy correction general anaesthesia is preferable. For correction of the dislocation a strong piece of stick is kept across the mouth as far behind as possible between the upper

---

*Dislocation of the mandible, Dislocation of the Temporo mandibular articulation; or Dislocation of Temporo-maxillary articulation.

and lower molars; and then using this as a fulcrum the upper and lower jaws are brought together by closing the mouth. When the mouth is being closed in this manner the vertical ramus moves downwards and if it is simultaneously pushed backwards the dislocation gets reduced.

Questions

1. What are the common dislocations met with in work bullocks? Describe in detail any one of them.

2. Discuss the causes, symptoms, diagnosis, prognosis and line of treatment of hip dislocation in the dog.

3. What is dislocation of joint? Describe its surgical pathology, symptoms, prognosis and treatment.

4. What is a dislocation? What are the symptoms which differentiate it from a fracture?

5. Define and differentiate a fracture from a dislocation giving suitable examples in illustration. State the main principles of treatment in fracture immobilisation and describe the cause for delayed union in uncomplicated simple fractures.

6. Write a short essay on the different methods and materials used for immobilisation of fractures/dislocations.

7. What are the common forms of dislocations of the hip met with in cattle? What is the prognosis and line of treatment if detected immediately?

8. Classify hip dislocations in the dog. Describe in detail the procedure you will adopt for reducing a hip dislocation in the dog.

9. Describe the condition described as subluxation of patella in cattle and its surgical treatment.

10. Write short notes on (i) Patellar desmotomy and (ii) Luxation of patella.

11. Describe the symptoms and treatment for dislocation in general.

CHAPTER 29

Paralysis

Paralysis or *akinesis* is the loss of function of muscles (i.e., their inability to contract in response to normal stimuli). A partial loss of function is called *palsy* or *paresis*. Loss of sensation in a particular area or part of the body is called sensory paralysis. Motor and sensory paralysis may co-exist. When the cause of paralysis is in the muscle it is called *myopathic paralysis*. When in the nerve supplying the muscle it is referred to as *neuropathic paralysis*. Paralysis may be due to lesions in the brain, spinal cord, nerves or in the muscle.

CLASSIFICATION
1. *Local paralysis* when only a single muscle or a group of muscles in a particular part is affected.
2. *Hemiplegia* affecting one side of body.
3. *Paraplegia*, affecting the hind quarters.
4. *Quadruplegia*, affecting all the four limbs.

SYMPTOMS
The affected muscle/muscles remain either in a relaxed state or in spasmodic contraction.
When main nerves like radial nerve, facial nerve, etc. are involved characteristic symptoms are noticed.

DIAGNOSIS
The degree of sensitivity, tendinous reflexes (e.g. patellar reflex) and electrical contractility of the affected muscles may be tested. The dimunition in *sensitivity* is tested by pricking with a needle or pin. Paralysed areas usually show diminished sensitivity though rarely there may be hypersensitivity. *Tendinous reflexes* (Patellar reflex, Tendo-achilis reflex, etc.) may be normal or diminished/suppressed. *Electrical contractility* may be present,

diminished, or absent depending on the degeneration undergone by the muscle. The lack of response to electrical stimulation indicates an unfavourable prognosis.

Electro-diagnosis

To stimulate contraction in muscles of the fore-limb, one of the electrodes (usually the positive) is placed on the skin, anterior to the dorsal vertebra. In case of the hind limb the same is placed in the lumbar region. The other electrode is placed distally and close to the concerned muscle. The following observations are made: (1) whether there is hyper excitability or hypoexcitability; (2) whether contractions are produced with both faradic (AC) and galvanic (DC) currents, or only with galvanic (DC) current; and (3) whether any difference in the contractions (excitability) is noticed by stimulation with galvanic current after interchanging the electrodes.

(1) *Hypoexcitability and Hyperexcitability*: Hypoexcitability is present when a stronger current than normal is required to induce contraction. In hyperexcitability contraction is obtained with a relatively weak current.

(2) *Response to AC/DC currents*: In a normal muscle contractions can be produced either with faradic current (AC) or with galvanic current (DC). But faradic current may not induce any contraction of a muscle with partial degeneration though galvanic current may still be able to produce mild contractions of it. When the muscle is completely degenerated neither faradic nor galvanic current produce any effect.

(3) *Response to interchange of electrodes*: On galvanic (DC) stimulation of a *normal muscle* maximum response is obtained when the current is made to flow with the cathode placed distally rather than with the anode distally. That is, the Cathode closing Contractions are greater than Anode closing Contractions (KCC is greater than ACC). On galvanic stimulation of a *partially degenerated muscle* maximum response is obtained when the current is made to flow with the anode placed distally. That is, ACC is greater than KCC. This reaction of partial degeneration (RPD) is known as the *Inversion formula* of muscular contraction under galvanic current.

Condition of muscle	A.C. (Faradic) current	D.C. (Galvanic) current	Remarks
Normal muscle	Normal contraction	Normal contraction KCC>ACC	
Muscle partially degenerated	No contraction	Slight contraction ACC>KCC	Reaction of partial degenera-tion(RPD)
Degenerated muscle	No contraction	No contraction	Reaction of complete degenera-tion(RCD)

ETIOLOGY

1. Injury to the nerve like open wounds, contusions, over-stretching of the nerve, fractures in the viscinity, etc., (2) Neurits, (3) Haemorrhage around the nerve causing pressure on it, (4) Neoplasms, (5) Toxins, (6) Some lesion in the muscle itself causing destruction of muscle fibres, i.e., myopathic paralysis, (7) Rheumatism.

Paralysis occurring suddenly is usually of traumatic or toxic origin. Paralysis slow in onset is generally the result of chronic neuritis or the development of a neoplasm close to the nerve. The cause is obscure in some cases.

PROGNOSIS

Prognosis varies according to the cause of the condition, the seriousness of the lesion in the muscle or nerve, the duration and the degree of degeneration undergone by the muscle. If there is muscular atrophy prognosis is generally unfavourable. If the trauma is slight the paralysis may last only for a few days. The longer the duration of paralysis the more pronounced is the atrophy of the muscles and lesser the chances of recovery.

TREATMENT

1. If the paralysis is due to a callus or tumour pressing on the nerve, it is desirable to remove the same.

2. When the paralysis is due to a minor injury and is of a temporary nature, application of counter-irritants locally may accelerate recovery. Pot. Iod may be given internally to promote absorption of inflammatory exudate pressing on the nerve.

3. Nerve tonics like Vitamin-B.1. (Thiamin or Anurin), Phospholecithin etc. are advisable. B.1. is capable of improving the blood supply to the nerves and thereby promote regeneration of the nerve.

4. Administration of calcium.

5. Nervine stimulents such as strychnine may also be useful. Liq. Strych. Hydrochlor may be given S/c in small and repeated doses. Arsenical preparations also have a beneficial effect.

6. To prevent muscular atrophy, mild exercises, massage and application of liniments or blisters are indicated. Manual movements of the joints will induce activity of the paralysed muscles and thereby prevent atrophy.

7. Electro-therapy accelerates recovery and prevents muscular atrophy. The negative electrode is applied on the region corresponding to the nerve trunk at a point where it is superficial and the positive electrode is placed over the muscles where the nerve ramifies. The voltage recommended in 50 to 60 volts. 3 to 20 milliamperes of the current is permitted to flow for about 5 to 20 minutes, the actual amperage and time depending on the area involved and the individual tolerance of the patient. To begin with, treatment may be done for about 5 minutes daily or for 10 minutes on alternate days. Electrical stimulation is very effective for preventing muscular atrophy.

8. Infra-red rays can penetrate into deeper tissues and being hot rays they stimulate regenerative processes largely by favouring hyperaemia.

9. If paralysis is due to rheumatism, Sod. salicylas is indicated.

10. Corticosteroid preparations may be effective in some cases to quicken the recovery.

Paralysis of the Facial Nerve (*Paralysis of the Seventh Cranial Nerve*)

[The facial nerve is the chief motor nerve of the face. It is, therefore, called the *nerve of expression*. The nerve passes through the facial canal of the petrous temporal bone and comes out through the stylo mastoid foramen. Afterwards the nerve travels close to the parotid salivary gland and crosses over to the lateral aspect of the mandible about 1 to 1½ inch below the temporomandibular articulation. It then divides into superior and inferior buccal nerves supplying the lips and muzzle. The facial nerve also supplies motor branches to the eye lids, ear and cheeks.]

INCIDENCE
     Paralysis of the facial nerve is more commonly seen in horses than in other animals. It is rare in cattle.

ETIOLOGY
     1. Injury to the nerve: Injury is common at the point where the nerve crosses over to the lateral aspect of the mandible, about 1 to 1½ inch below the temporomandibular articulation.
     2. Inflammation in the surrounding areas may exert pressure on the nerve, e.g., inflammation of petrous temporal bone, inflammation of the middle ear.
     3. Tumour within the facial canal or in the parotid region pressing on the nerve.
     4. Toxins produced in infectious diseases like strangles and equine influenza.
     5. Exposure to severe cold.
     6. Rheumatism.

SYMPTOMS
     The paralysis may be unilateral or bilateral. When paralysis affects only the superficial portion of the nerve after it crosses over the mandible it is called peripheral paralysis of the facial nerve. When paralysis involves the portion higher up at the intra-temporal portion of the nerve, it is called central paralysis of the facial nerve.
     In the latter case the branch supplying the ear and eye lids are also involved. In unilateral paralysis the lips are drawn towards the opposite (sound) side. Accumulation of feed between the teeth and cheek and quidding may also be noticed. When paralysis is bilateral the lips are paralysed and the lower lip appears pendulous. The nostrils appear constricted and the muzzle region of the horse presents an appearance similar to that of a camel (stupid look). The animal is unable to use the lips for prehension. For drinking water the animal has to dip the muzzle beyond the level of the angles of the mouth. The collapsed nostrils interfere with respirations and during exercise the respirations become noisy. The animal may evince difficulty in

breathing during trotting or galloping.

In central paralysis of the facial nerve the branches supplying the eyelids and ear also are affected. The animal is not able to close the eyelids completely because of paralysis of orbicularis oculi muscle. There is also ptosis or dropping of the upper eyelid. There is also dropping of the ear and loss of sensation in the inner surface of concha.

PROGNOSIS

Guarded. Peripheral paralysis usually gets cured in 5 to 6 weeks. Central paralysis may take a longer time even in favourable cases.

TREATMENT

(1) General treatment for paralysis. (2) If both sides are paralysed care should be taken to see that the animal is able to take food and water properly. (3) To relieve difficulty in breathing the nostrils may be kept dilated by means of clips or by a minor surgical operation consisting of putting two or three mattress sutures on the skin between two nostrils.

Trigeminal Paralysis*

[The trigeminal nerve is a mixed nerve consisting of three main branches as noted below: (1) the ophthalmic nerve (sensory) emerging through the foramen orbital later branching in to lacrimal, frontal and nasociliary nerves; (2) the superior maxillary nerve (sensory) emerging through the foramen rotundum and subsequently branch into zygomatic, sphenopalatine and infraobital nerves; (3) the inferior maxillary or mandibular nerve (mixed) passing through the oval notch of foramen lacerum and finally terminating as masseteric, deep temporal, buccinator, pterygoid, superficial temporal, temporal, mandibular, alveolar and lingual nerves.]

Paralysis of the fifth cranial nerve is seen rather commonly in the dog but is rare in horse and cattle.

ETIOLOGY

Rabies is one of the causes of trigeminal paralysis. But it may also occur due to any of the other causes for paralysis mentioned already.

* Trifacial paralysis; Paralysis of the fifth cranial nerve.

SYMPTOMS

The paralysis may be unilateral or bilateral, partial or complete, peripheral or central. Paralysis of the ophthalmic branch brings about loss of sensation in the cornea, conjunctiva and sclera. Paralysis of the superior maxillary nerve (which subsequently becomes the infraorbital nerve) causes loss of sensation in the nose, cheek, teeth and gums of upper jaw, upper lip, etc. When the mandibular branch which is a mixed nerve is affected, the muscles of mastication (masseter, buccinator and pterygoid muscles) are paralysed and then the typical symptoms of trigeminal paralysis are noticed. When paralysis is unilateral the lower jaw is deviated towards the sound side. Movement of tongue is possible normally but mastication is not possible in the affected side. During mastication the head is lowered and is turned towards the unaffected side. When there is complete bilateral paralysis the lower jaw is dropped ("dropped jaw") but the dog is able to lap liquids with its tongue. Swallowing is not affected.

PROGNOSIS

A temporary form of trigeminal paralysis is seen in dogs in which recovery takes place within five to ten days. In other cases where paralysis is permanent the muscles of mastication undergo atrophy and recovery may not take place. If due to rabies, the animal dies within ten days after the onset of the symptoms.

DIAGNOSIS

Diagnosis is made from the symptoms. The condition is to be differentiated from dislocation of the lower jaw and from rabies. In dislocation, the lower jaw appears dropped but is stiff and cannot be raised with the hand.

TREATMENT

General treatment for paralysis. The animal should be handled carefully and should be kept under observation for ten days to rule out the possibility of rabies.

Supra-scapular Paralysis*

[Supra scapular nerve arises from the brachial plexes, passes between the supraspinatus and subscapularis muscles and turns around the anterior border of the distal fourth of scapula. It then supplies the supraspinatus and infraspinatus muscles.] Suprascapular paralysis is frequently seen in young horses.

Etiology

(1) Direct injury to the nerve, e.g., due to a fall, pressure of the collor in draft horses, etc., (2) Overstretching/compression of the nerve.

Symptoms

(1) Difficulty in extending the shoulder joint. (2) Marked bulging outwards of the shoulder joint when weight is borne on the limb. The shoulder joint appears to slip outwards at each step and therefore the condition is called *shoulder slip*. (3) Atrophy of the supraspinatus and infraspinatus muscles.

Prognosis

Guarded. Recovery may take place in four to six weeks. If the muscular atrophy is rapid prognosis is unfavourable.

Treatment

General treatment for paralysis. Blistering over the shoulder region and over the affected muscles is often done.

Radial Paralysis**

Radial nerve is the largest nerve from the bracheal plexus. It passes downwards and outward along the musculospiral groove of the humerus. It supplies the triceps brachii, extensors of the carpus and digits. (i.e., Triceps brachii, Anconeus, Extensor carpi radialis, common extensor of the digit, Ulnaris lateralis, Lateral extensor of the digit, Extensor carpi obliqus, etc.)

Radial paralysis is more commonly seen in the horse and rarely in cattle and dog.

Etiology

Compression of the nerve between the shoulder and thorax

---

* Atrophy of Shoulder, Sweeny, "Shoulder slip."
** Paralysis of the musculo-spiral nerve; "Dropped elbow".

while casting the horse on a hard ground. Over-stretching of the nerve. Injury to the nerve accompanying fracture of the first rib.

SYMPTOMS

In complete paralysis of the radial nerve all its branches are affected. Partial paralysis involving either the branch supplying the triceps muscle, or the branches supplying the extensors of the digit and carpus may be noted. In complete paralysis affecting the entire nerve, all joints below the elbow are in a flexed state, and the point of the elbow is dropped (*dropped elbow*) because of the paralysis of the triceps muscle. The limb appears longer and the toe of the foot rests on the ground. When made to move forward, the toe is dragged. While standing the limb can be made to bear weight by supporting the knee from front with a hand.

If the *branches supplying the extensors* of the digit only are affected, the animal will be able to use the limb almost normally when walking on level ground but on uneven ground it stumbles and the foot is dragged.

If the branch to the triceps muscle only is affected, there is inability to bear weight on the limb, because it is not possible to extend the elbow. The limb presents an abnormal appearance since the point of the elbow is dropped and the knee is semi-flexed, but the planter surface of the foot touches the ground almost normally.

PROGNOSIS

In most cases prognosis is favourable. Recovery usually takes place in ten days to six weeks but some cases may require many months.

TREATMENT

General treatment for paralysis.

Sciatic Paralysis (*Paralysis of the Sciatic Nerve*)

All muscles of the hind limb *except* the Quadriceps extensor cruris muscle (Quadriceps femoris muscle) are supplied by the sciatic nerve.

Sciatic paralysis is occasionally seen in the horse, ox and dog.

ETIOLOGY
(1) Over-stretching of the nerve. (2) Injury to the nerve by falling on the corresponding quarter. (3) Toxaemia—e.g., in diseases like strangles, pneumonia, purpura haemorrhagica, distemper, etc. (4) Compression by tumour.

SYMPTOMS
Since all the muscles of the hind limb, except the Quadriceps extensor cruris (Quadriceps femoris) are supplied by the sciatic nerve, the hind limb hangs loosely in sciatic paralysis. When forced to move the limb is dragged with the toe of the foot and fetlock dragged along the ground, but simultaneously because of the action of the Quadriceps muscle the stifle is lifted forward and upward at each step. (Compare the symptoms with those of crural paralysis.)

TREATMENT
General treatment for paralysis.

Crural Paralysis*
The crural nerve supplies the Quadriceps extensor cruris muscle situated in front of the femur. This muscle, also known as the Quadriceps femoris muscle, actually consists of four muscles, viz., vastus medialis, rectus femoris and vastus internus muscles. *Origin*: Ilium, Proximal and anterior part of femur. *Insertion*: Patella. *Action*: To extend the stifle.

When there is paralysis of the crural nerve the Quadriceps extensor cruris muscle becomes functionless and the stifle remains "dropped". When the animal tries to put weight on the limb there is sudden flexion of stifle and then automatically of the hock and therefore no weight can be borne on the limb. The loose powerless appearance of the limb may resemble some fracture.

TREATMENT
General treatment for paralysis.

*Femoral paralysis. Paralysis of the crural nerve.

External Poplitial Paralysis*

The external poplitial nerve supplies the extensor muscles of the digit and flexor metatarsi (tibialis anterior) muscles.

[Flexor metatarsi (Tibialis anterior) muscle: *Origin*—crural facia, lateral condyle and tuberosity ·of tibia. *Insertion*: One branch to proximal end of large metatarsal bone and the other branch to the first tarsal (cuneiform parvum) bone. *Action*: To flex hock.]

When the animal is made to walk or trot, the hock is extended and the fetlock and digital joints are flexed. Therefore the limb is rigidly extended backwards with the front of the foot and fetlock dragging during progression.

Internal Poplitial Paralysis**

The flexors of the digit and extensors of the hock which are situated behind the tibia are affected. (Superficial and deep flexor muscles, Gastrocnemius, Popliteus, Soleus, etc.)

The hock is semi-flexed. The digital joints are also automatically flexed because of the hock, even though the flexor muscles of the digit are paralysed. (Compare this with the symptoms of External poplitial paralysis.) The limb can still bear weight even though the hock and digits are semi-flexed, because the hock· is fixed by the tendoachilis. During progression the limb is brought to the ground at each step with a characteristic "tapping" sound. The limb is lifted from the ground in a swift and jerky fashion somewhat resembling stringhalt.

Obturator Paralysis

The obturator nerve supplies the adductor muscles of the hind limb (i.e. Adductor parvus, Adductor mangnus, Pectinius, Gracilis) and therefore in paralysis of this nerve there is abduction of the limb.

The common cause of obturator paralysis is trauma caused to the nerve during parturition or due to a fracture of the pelvis. In cows the first symptom noticed is a failure to adduct the affected limb-following the act of parturition.

---

*Paralysis of the External poplitial nerve or the Deep peroneal nerve or the Anterior tibial or the Peroneal nerve.

**Paralysis of the Tibial nerve or the Posterior tibial nerve or the Internal poplitial nerve.

Questions

1. Define paralysis. What general treatment will you adopt in paralysis of the hind limb in a dog?

2. Describe the causes, symptoms, treatment and prognosis of radial paralysis.

3. Write an account of facial paralysis in the horse.

4. Discuss the incidence of paralysis of the extremities in horses and describe the symptoms and treatment of unilateral facial paralysis.

5. What is paraplegia? What are the causes, symptoms and treatment in a middle-aged dog?

6. Describe the facial symptoms which are easily detected in paralysis of the third, sixth and seventh cranial nerves. Give the line of treatment and prognosis in case of facial paralysis.

7. What is "dropped elbow"? Describe the etiology and incidence and the line of treatment recommended for dropped elbow condition in canine patients.

8. Write an essay on the incidence, diagnosis and general lines of treatment adopted for clinical cases of peripheral motor paralysis in animals.

9. Write a short notes on Shoulder slip.

CHAPTER 30

Intra-articular Injection of Corticosteroids

Corticosteroids make tissue cell less susceptible to irritation and hence exert non-inflammatory action. Reduction in inflammatory effusions, relief from pain and improvement in lameness are ordinarily seen within twenty-four to seventy-two hours after intra-articular injection. If necessary injections are repeated at three to four day intervals up to four or five injections. If infection is present, combine with antibiotics. Cortisone as such is not suitable for intra-articular injection as it needs conversion into hydrocortisone in the liver. A few of the preparations used are:

Preparations

CORTICOSTEROIDS

1. *Hydrocortisone acetate*: Horse and Ox 50 to 100 mg.
     Dog   5 to 25 mg.

Available: "Efcorlin injection" (Glaxo) 25mg per ml solution, 5 ml vials.

2. *Prednisolone*: Dose same as Hydrocortisone acetate.

Available: "Predsolan soluble" (Glaxo), vials of 25 mg with 1 ml water for injection; "Deltacortil Intramuscular or Intra-articular" (Pfizer) 1 ml ampoules containing 25 mg.

ANTIBIOTICS

1. *Penicillin G sodium*: ("Crystapen" Glaxo)—3 to 12 lakh units in the dilution of 3 lakhs per ml.
2. *Dihydrostreptomycin*: 0.5 to 3g. as 5 g. per ml solution.
3. *Neomycin*: 200 to 800 mg as 200 mg per ml solution.

Technique

The injection should be done with utmost aseptic precautions. The skin at site should be shaved and disinfected. A local anaesthetic solution may be injected subcutaneously. A needle of 22 BWG thickness and 2 to 2½ inches long is desirable. For horse and ox a thicker needle (up to 18 BWG) may be chosen depending on the size of the joint. For hip and shoulder joints in large animals the needle should be about 4 inches long. When the needle enters the synovial cavity a sucking sound can sometimes be appreciated and synovial fluid also may escape through the needle. The escape of synovia confirms the correct position of the needle. It is advisable to aspirate an equal volume of synovial fluid prior to the intra-articular injection, especially when the quantity to be injected is large or when there is excessive distension of the cavity.

Sites in the Horse

1. *Navicular Bursa*: Standing position. From the hollow of the heels the needle is directed forwards through the median plane and parallel to the coronary band.

2. *Coffin Joint* (*coronopedal joint*): Standing position. Immediately above coronary band and slightly lateral or medial to the midline on the anterior aspect of the foot. After skin puncture needle directed downwards more or less vertically. (This joint has communication with navicular bursa and flexor tendon sheath in the pastern region.)

3. *Pastern Joint*: Standing position. Medial or lateral aspect of limb. Palpate the tubercle on the lateral (or, medial) aspect of the distal extremity of ossuffraginis. Above this tubercle and between this bone and flexor tendon is the site.

4. *Fetlock Joint*: Into the volar pouches of the joint. In front of and above the proximal sesamoid (either on the lateral or medial aspect of the limb) and in the space between the large metacarpal bone and the suspensary ligament.

5. *Carpal* (*Knee*) *Joint*: Flex the joint to widen the interspaces between articulating bones. Palpate on the anterior aspect of knee. Inject either into the space between the radius and upper row of carpal bones or into the space between the upper and lower rows of carpal bones.

6. *Elbow Joint*: Standing position. Palpate the lateral tube-

rosity of the radius to which the lateral ligament of elbow is inserted. Site is 1½ inch above this tuberosity either in front or behind the ligament.

7. *Shoulder Joint*: Locate the centre of the upper border of the lateral tuberosity of humerus. Skin puncture is made at this point and the needle is directed medially to enter the joint cavity.

8. *Hock Joint*: (Bog spavin). The supero-antero-internal aspect of hock where the distended synovial capsule can be felt.

9. *Stifle Joint*: Standing position. Immediately above proximal extremity of tibia between the anterior and lateral patellar ligaments.

10. *Hip Joint*: Locate the centre between the superoanterior extremity and the posterior summit of the trochanter major. Make skin puncture above this point and direct the needle antero-medially to enter the joint capsule.

Sites in the Ox
Similar to the horse, but note the following anatomical differences :

1. The navicular joint in cattle is not accessible;

2. Since there are two digits, the phalangeal joints also are paired for each limb;

3. The shoulder joint is relatively smaller in size. The lateral tuberosity of the humerus is more prominent and its upper border is almost in front of the joint proper when the animal is standing.

Sites in the Dog
1. *Carpal Joint*: Flex the joint and palpate the most suitable site for injection between the articulating bones, which will be on the medial or anterior aspect of the joint.

2. *Elbow Joint*: Recumbent position. Flex the joint fully, puncture through the tendon of triceps muscle immediately above the olecranon process of ulna and direct the needle to touch upon the supracondyloid fosa of the humerus. Withdraw slightly and direct the needle at a steeper angle to reach into the joint. Confirm position by aspirating synovia.

3. *Stifle Joint*: Recumbent position; joint semiflexed. Antero-

lateral or antero-medial approach on either side of the anterior
ligament of patella. Needle is directed slightly upwards until it
touches on the trochlea of femur and is then withdrawn slightly
to aspirate synovia and confirm the position of the needle.

4. *Hip Joint*: Recumbent position. Needle is introduced
anterior to the great trochanter of femur and is directed medially
and forward towards the acetabulum. The dorsal rim of acetabulum can be felt. Easy puncture into the hip joint is facilitated
by outward *rotation* of the femur; but while injecting the solution
relax the synovial capsule by resuming inward rotation.

CHAPTER 31

Surgical Conditions Affecting the Locomotor System

Difficulty in locomotion which causes an abnormal gait is called *lameness*. Lameness is not a disease but only a symptom of structural or functional disorder. It may affect one or more limbs.

Examination for Lameness

For the diagnosis of lameness, the animal may be first observed *at rest* and then *during progression* to locate the lame limb. Afterwards a *detailed examination of the lame limb* is conducted to locate the actual seat of lameness. If possible the diagnosis is confirmed by radiography.

1. *Observation during Rest*: Deformity of a part or whole of a limb, abnormal positioning of a limb like abduction, adduction, etc., are to be observed to detect fracture, dislocation, rupture of tendons, paralysis, etc. "Pointing" of a limb is one of the symptoms of lameness especially in a fore-limb. Another example of symptom noticed at rest is "dropped elbow" resulting from paralysis of radial nerve.

2. *Observation during Progression*: The horse is trotted by an assistant with the leading rope sufficiently slackened. The horse is first led in a straight track away from the observer for a distance of about 30 yards and is then turned and brought back.

While the horse is being trotted, see whether the limbs are carried in a straight line or are adducted, abducted or circumducted during progression. Also look for any deviation in the long axis of body during movement. Observe also from the sides in order to find out variation in the length of the stride and diminished flexion of joints.

While the animal is being trotted, the movements of its head and hind quarters (croup) should receive special attention as they are important symptoms of lameness. The movements of the head when the animal is coming towards the observer and the movements of the croup when the animal is going away from the observer are taken notice of.

A horse lame in one of the forelimbs *raises the head* whenever that particular limb is made to bear weight and *drops the head* (*nods the head*) whenever the sound limb bears weight. If a horse is equally lame on both forelimbs the head movements may not be very distinct; the gait may be "pottery" or "stilted" and the strides of both limbs are shorter than normal. If the lameness of both forelimbs are of unequal severity the nodding of the head may be observed as in lameness of only one forelimb. The quarter of the affected side is raised and the opposite quarter is lowered in most cases of hind limb lameness, an exception to this general rule being hock lameness.

When both hind limbs are lame they are carried stiffly and the croup movements are not reliable for diagnosis of lameness. In this case there is much difficulty in "backing" the animal.

The head movement (nodding) seen in lameness of one of the forelimbs may however be seen in case of lameness of the opposite hind limb also so that a horse lame on one hind limb may be suspected to be lame on opposite fore-limb. This is called *Cross Lameness*. Correct diagnosis in cross lameness is made by observing the croup movements also. When one fore-limb and the opposite hind limb are lame the condition is called *Diagonal Lameness*.

In certain types of forelimb lameness difficulty is observed in "turning" and difficulty in "backing" the animal in hind limb lameness.

3. *Detailed Examination of the Lame Limb*: The detailed examination of the lame limb is carried out so as to locate the exact seat of lameness. The various bones, joints, tendons and tendon sheaths, etc., should be palpated. Local inflammatory lesions may be detected by swelling, excessive warmth or evidence of pain on palpation. The limb is then lifted from the ground to test the flexion and extension of various joints and also to examine the foot. Very often the foot may be the seat of lameness and therefore a thorough examination of the foot is important The shoe should be removed. Disproportionate wear of the shoe (either at its toe or quarters) may itself give some

clue to diagnosis. The hoof is cleared and the different parts of the foot, like the wall, sole and frog are carefully examined. A hoof-tester or hammer may be used to detect any painful lesion in the foot. The different parts of the lame limb are also compared with the opposite limb to detect gross abnormalities, if any.

4. *Other Procedures to Confirm Seat of Lameness*: (a) Blocking the nerve supplying the area of a suspected seat of lameness may aid diagnosis in the case of certain painful lesions. When pain is avoided by this type of regional anaesthesia, lameness is relieved temporarily.

(b) Taking a radiograph of the affected part of limb helps to confirm the lameness.

General Symptoms of Shoulder Lameness

The main features of shoulder lameness are marked raising of the head when weight is born on the limb, restricted movement of the scapula and shoulder joint, shortened stride (taking short steps), stumbling: because of the limb being insufficiently raised from the ground, circumduction of the limb, dragging of the toe, increased lameness on uneven or soft ground. Lameness is increased when trotted uphill. Disuse atrophy of the muscles of the scapular region (supra and infra-spinatus muscles) is seen in chronic cases.

General Symptoms of Elbow Lameness

Elbow lameness is uncommon. The head is raised when the lame limb touches the ground and is dropped (nodded) when the sound limb bears weight, as in other types of forelimb lameness.

General Symptoms of Knee Lameness

The limb is carried forward with slight circumduction because of the incomplete flexion of knee joint. Lameness is increased going downhill.

General Symptoms of Fetlock Lameness

There is limited flexion and/or extension of the fetlock joint. A sinking or dropping of the fetlock may be noticed in rupture of flexor tendons and/or suspensory ligament. Contraction of the flexor tendons or suspensory ligament shows an upright pastern.

General Symptoms of Hip Lameness

The affected quarter is carried higher than normal. There is difficulty in advancing the limb and tendency to carry the limb in a stiff manner. The stride is shortened. Circumduction and dragging of the toe may be noticed and this symptom is called *swinging leg lameness*. There may also be *supporting leg lameness*, i.e., the animal tries to avoid weight bearing on the limb. During progression there is tendency towards "diagonal movements" i.e., moving away from the lame side. Lameness is pronounced when the animal is backed. Keeping the toe of the affected limb turned outwards when the animal is standing, is a characteristic symptom of coxitis (inflammation of hip joint).

General Symptoms of Stifle Lameness

The general symptoms are somewhat similar to hip lameness but the raising of the affected side quarter (croup) is not so pronounced in stifle lameness.

General Symptoms of Hock Lameness

This is the most common type of lameness in the hind limb in the horse. There is imperfect flexion of the hock, dragging of the toe and shortening of the stride. Dragging of the toe causes excessive wear of the hoof at the toe.

Splints

A typical splint is an exostosis on the splint bones (small metacarpals or small metatarsals) as a result of localised osteoperiostitis. Exostoses on portions of large metacarpal and large metatarsal bones, away from fetlock joint are also called splints. Splint is a typical example of an osteoperiostitis.

INCIDENCE

It is common in the fore-limb, in young horses below the age of five, that are newly put to work. Horses used for fast work on hard ground are mostly affected. The common seats of splint are the inner aspect of the fore-limb and the outer aspect of the hind limb.

VARIETIES

1. *Simple splint* which is a single exostosis on the splint bones.

2. *Chain splint* consisting of several small exostoses arranged in a row along the small metacarpal/metatarsal bones.

3. *Knee splint* (knee spavin), a splint on the upper third of the splint bone approaching on the knee joint.

4. *Rod splint* (*Peg splint*) which is an exostosis on the posterior aspect of the cannon bone, between that bone and the suspensory ligament.

5. *Jack splint* (*Bump*) which is a very large exostosis on the metacarpal bone.

6. *Spongy splint* which is a more or less uniform thickening of the splint bones usually due to some metabolic disease.

ETIOLOGY

Predisposing causes: Certain horses seem to have hereditary predisposition. Bad conformation, abnormal shape of the limbs, bad quality of bones, work at a very young age, are other predisposing factors. Excessive paring of horn on one half of the foot while shoeing, defective shoeing etc., may also act as predisposing factors.

Exciting causes: Exciting cause is concussion. In young horses the splint bones are comparatively mobile as the interosseous ligament is not ossified. The splint bones because of their articulation with the carpal bones are subjected to slight movement whenever weight is borne on the limb and then the interosseous ligament is stretched. Excessive concussion may overstretch and sprain the interosseous ligament and consequently a localised osteoperiostitis develops at tlle respective point of attachment of the ligament to the bone. Sprain of the suspensory ligament may also bring about localised osteoperiostitis of the metacarpal bones.

SYMPTOMS

There is at first symptoms of acute inflammation and lameness. The inflammatory symptoms subside when exostosis develops. In some cases exostosis may form without exhibiting initial symptoms of acute inflammation. Characteristic features of *splint lameness* are: (1) Imperfect flexion of the knee especially if the exostosis extends into the joint. (2) Marked lameness while trotting, though not much pronounced while walking. (3) Marked lameness on hard ground. (4) Lameness exaggerated while going downhill than on level ground. (5) Slight abduction of the limb during progression. (6) Lameness not improving with exercise. (7) The gait may be pottery.

DIAGNOSIS

From symptoms. Palpate the splint bones both in the standing position and with the limb flexed at the knee and lifted.

PROGNOSIS

Rod (peg) splint causes permanent lameness. Knee splint is incurable. In young animals (below six years) splint is a definite unsoundness. In older animals presence of exostosis without lameness is not usually considered as unsoundness.

TREATMENT

1. Needle-point firing and blistering (with Biniodide of mercury 1 in 20) may be tried. After applying the blister a piece of lint is placed over it and bandaged. Vesicles are formed and they heal in about two to three weeks. Afterwards massaging the area, applying a bland oil and mild exercises are indicated for about six weeks.

2. In the acute inflammatory stage periosteotomy is sometimes advised to let out the inflammatory exudate, followed by application of a pressure bandage to suppress the exudation. Periosteotomy should be done with aseptic precautions to safeguard against infection and further complications.

3. When the exostosis is very large it may be surgically removed.

4. Median and ulnar neurectomies may be tried in cases which do not show any improvement.

Sore-shin (*Buck Shin*)

Sore shin is an osteoperiostitis involving the anterior aspect of the large metacarpal or metatarsal bones.

Sore = a painful lesion; *shin* = the front portion of the metacarpal or metatarsal region.

INCIDENCE

Almost exclusively seen in young horses aged below three years that are newly put to work. Common in race horses under training. More common in the forelimbs. Rarely seen in hind limbs.

CAUSES

Direct trauma or severe concussion as may occur during galloping.

SYMPTOMS

Diffuse painful swelling on the anterior aspect of metacarpal region, usually on its lower third. Pain and severe lameness in the beginning stage when there is collection of inflammatory exudate under the periosteum. Later mineralisation of the exudate forms exostoses. No lameness after exostosis has been formed.

PROGNOSIS

Favourable, provided rest and treatment are given in the early stage. In other instances lameness disappears but the value of the animal is reduced because of the exostoses.

TREATMENT

Rest. Cold and astringent applications during the acute inflammatory stage. A blister may be helpful in some cases. If the swelling is excessive periosteotomy may be done with proper aseptic precautions and a pressure bandage may be put.

Ring Bone (*Phalangeal Exostosis*)

Exostosis on the phalangeal bones is called ring bone. A typical ring bone is an osteo-arthritis involving the inter-phalangeal joints.

INCIDENCE

More common in young horses. A hereditary predisposition probably exists.

CLASSIFICATION

Classified as true ring bone and false ring bone. In *true ring bone* the exostosis is at the interphalangeal joints. A *false ring bone* is an exostosis on the shaft of a phalangeal bone, i.e., away from the interphalangeal joints. Ring bone is also classified as *high ring* bone and *low ring* bone. A high true ring bone is an exostosis involving the suffragino-coronal joint and a low true ring bone involves the corono-pedal joint. High false ring bone is an exostosis on the shaft of os-suffranginis. Low false ring bone is an exostosis on the shaft of os-corona. Periarticular ring bone is exostoses around the phalangeal joints.

ETIOLOGY

Predisposing causes: Hereditory predisposition, defective confirmation, poor quality of bone, uneven weight bearing on the limb due to defective shoeing, use of calkins, etc. Rickets may be a contributing factor.

Exciting causes: False ring bone is usually the result of direct trauma and articular ring bone results from concussion. Periarticular ring bone arises from sprain of articular ligaments. A fissured fracture of the os-suffraginis or os-corona may also cause a ring bone.

SYMPTOMS

False ring bone usually commences as an osteo-periostitis with pain and lameness until an exostosis develops. Exostosis away from the joints may not cause lameness but may cause mechanical interference because of its size and may get struck by the opposite foot during progression. Articular ring bone causes severe lameness. Lameness may not be much during walking but is pronounced during trot and is more uphill. Periarticular ring bone is seen more commonly on the lateral aspect of the suffragino-coronal joint and may not cause lameness. Low ring bone, whether articular or periarticular, causes lameness because of the pain caused by pressure exerted within the hoof. In low ring bone a hard, bony swelling may be noted in the region of the coronet.

DIAGNOSIS

From the symptoms (the presence of exostoses and lameness).

PROGNOSIS

An animal with ring bone is considered unsound. Articular and low ring bones are more serious. In false ring bone lameness may vanish when the acute symptoms subside.

TREATMENT

Rest is essential in the acute stage. Blistering is not likely to be beneficial. Needle-point firing may be tried. Neurectomy of both plantar nerves (or of median nerve and external plantar nerve) is advisable to make the animal useful for work.

Pyramidal Disease (*Extensor Process Disease; Buttress Foot*)

The pyramidal process or extensor process of the ospedis gives attachment to the extensor tendon. Pyramidal diseases is an osteoperiostitis and consequent exostosis involving the pyramidal process.

ETIOLOGY

It is usually caused by a sprain of the extensor tendon at the point of its insertion to the process. It may also result from direct trauma.

INCIDENCE

More common in the hind feet.

SYMPTOMS AND SEQUELAE

Lameness. The inflammation is followed by exostosis which gives rise to an enlargement of the anterior aspect of the hoof in the coronet region. In chronic cases the shape of the foot is altered. The exostosis stimulates the coronary band in the toe region leading to the formation of a thick ridge of excess horn growth at the toe. This gives a V-shape to the foot instead of its normal U-shape. The condition is spoken of as *buttress foot* (*Buttress* = an additional support projecting from the surface). Lameness becomes more and more pronounced as the disease progresses.

DIAGNOSIS

From lameness and the appearance of the foot.

TREATMENT

No satisfactory treatment. Neurectomy may be tried.

Bobba Bone (*Cab-horse Diseases*)

Bobba bone is an exostosis on the supero-antero-internal aspect of the first phalanx which can be felt in level with the tuberosity on supero-postero-lateral aspect of the same bone. Rarely it may be accompanied by a dry arthritis of the fetlock joint.

INCIDENCE

Seen in heavy draft horses. Mostly affects horses over middle age.

CAUSES

Sprain of the lateral ligaments of the fetlock joint. Concussion resulting from work on hard roads.

SYMPTOMS

There is slight lameness. In the initial stages symptoms of acute inflammation are sometimes seen but the disease is usually recognised only when the exostosis has been developed.

TREATMENT

There is no satisfactory treatment. If the exostosis is large, surgical treatment may be tried. Neurectomy is indicated if lameness is severe.

Racing Joint

Racing joint is osteoarthritis and consequent exostosis affecting the distal extremity of the large metacarpus and proximal extremity of os-suffraginis.

INCIDENCE

Met with in young horses newly put to work.

SYMPTOMS

Lameness and pain due to inflammation.

TREATMENT

Cold and astringent applications, pressure bandages, etc. in the acute stage. When exostosis has been formed, no treatment is effective. Neurectomy may be tried.

Rarefying Ostitis of Os-pedis

This is not a common condition. The disease is characterised by a sudden increased vascularity of the os-pedis. This is followed by rarefaction of bone due to the depletion of its mineral content. The bone appears porous.

ETIOLOGY
Not known.

SYMPTOMS
Lameness.

DIAGNOSIS
Diagnosis is difficult. The disease is suspected when the foot lameness cannot be attributed to any other disease. Radiography may confirm it. The dark shadows of vessels in the radiograph indicate increased vascularity.

TREATMENT
Nil. Neurectomy also is *not* advisable.

Navicular Disease
Navicular disease is a chronic ostitis of the navicular bone, associated with navicular bursitis and inflammation of the plantar aponeurosis.

INCIDENCE
More common in light horses than in heavy horses. Common in horses about seven years old. Young horses, donkeys and mules are only rarely affected. More common in the fore-feet.

ETIOLOGY
Predisposing causes: Heredity. Abnormal conformation of foot, e.g., upright and narrow foot, contracted foot, foot having small frog etc. Excessively sloping pastern and long toe favours development of navicular disease by shifting more weight on the posterior region of the limb. Defective shoeing which inhibits the physiological action of frog, use of calkins, thick-heeled shoe, etc. are other predisposing factors.
Exciting cause: Severe and repeated concussion.

PATHOLOGY

There is inflammation of the navicular bone and the navicular bursa. Exostosis may develop. Friction of exostosis on the flexor tendon may cause sprain of the tendon. There may be adhesions formed between the tendon and bone. Sometimes there is rarefaction of navicular bone and it may fracture easily.

SYMPTOMS

Pointing of the foot at rest. In the initial stage lameness is intermittent and the animal goes without lameness after period of rest. As the disease progresses lameness becomes more pronounced. The stride is shortened, the toe is dragged, and there is stumbling. The gait may be "pottery" or "stilted". A "groggy gait" or "shuffling gait" is rather characteristic. When the horse is turned, the animal "screws" on the fore-limbs rather than having them lifted normally.

SEQUELAE

In chronic cases changes in the foot are marked by contraction of heels, concavity of the sole, etc. The foot becomes "boxy" (i.e., contracted and high at the heels with very concave soles). There may be atrophy of the frog. Bulging of the hollow of the heels due to enlargement of the navicular bursa may be seen. Rarely, however, a foot affected with navicular disease may not show any abnormality in shape.

DIAGNOSIS

Diagnosis is made from the symptoms. The animal may evince pain when pressure is applied on the central third of the frog. Digital nerve block and radiography are helpful for confirming the diagnosis.

PROGNOSIS

Unfavourable.

TREATMENT

Rest. Wall of the hoof may be thinned and grooved to facilitate expansion of foot. A light shoe may be worn. Neurectomy (*digital* neurectomy) is indicated to prolong the usefulness of animal. (see page 615).

Side Bones

Ossified lateral cartilages of the foot are called side bones.

INCIDENCE

Ossification of the lateral cartilage is more commonly noticed in the fore-feet.

ETIOLOGY

(1) Hereditory predisposition. (2) Natural tendency of cartilages in contact with bone to ossify. (3) Bad conformation. (4) Defective shoeing. (5) Concussion. (6) Direct injury to the cartilage resulting in inflammation and subsequent invasion of cartilage with osteoblasts.

SYMPTOMS

Lameness may or may not be present. In horses having good open feet and doing only slow work, side bones do not usually cause lameness.

DIAGNOSIS

In the initial stages difficult because at this stage the palpable portion of the cartilage might not have ossified. When ossification is complete, diagnosis is easy.

TREATMENT

If there is no pain or lameness treatment is not advised. If side bones are causing lameness the quarters of the hoof may be grooved or thinned. This facilitates expansion of the foot and relieves pain. Partial removal of the cartilage is recommended only if it has become very prominent and unsightly. The operation is not likely to be much beneficial. Digital neurectomy may be tried to relieve lameness.

Quittor

Quittor is a condition resulting from necrosis of the lateral cartilage and is noticed by the presence of sinus openings in the coronet region. The fore or hind feet may be affected.

ETIOLOGY

(1) Infection getting into the cartilage through an oper

in the coronet region, e.g., tread injuries. (2) Necrosis of skin in the pastern region due to constant accumulation of mud. (3) Suppuration extending from neighbouring lesions like suppurating corn, sandcrack, penetrating wounds of the foot, etc.

SYMPTOMS

The coronet appears swollen and one or more sinus openings may be noticed in the region. These sinus openings arise from the necrosed portion of the cartilage.

COMPLICATIONS

(1) Septic arthritis of the corono-pedal joint due to extension of the lesion. (2) Necrosis of the ospedis. (3) Necrosis of the sensitive laminae or the plantar cushion. (4) Gangrene of the skin of the affected region.

PROGNOSIS

Guarded. Many cases however respond favourably to treatment. Quittor in the hind limbs responds to treatment better than of the fore limbs because the lateral cartilages are thinner in the hind limbs.

TREATMENT

On general principles as for sinuses. Surgical treatment consists of removal of lateral cartilage.

1. Irrigation of the sinus tracts with antiseptic lotions to remove pus and necrotic tissue. But this may cause spread of the lesion to surrounding tissues because it is difficult to remove the fluid completely.

2. One of the following solutions may be injected into the sinus tracts to control bacterial infection and facilitate separation of necrotic tissue: Corrosive sublimate in alcohol (1 in 10), zinc chloride solution (5 to 10%), zinc sulphate solution (5 to 10%).

3. A solid caustic like silver nitrate or corrosive sublimate is powdered and introduced through the sinus openings. This is called *Coring*. The caustic facilitates separation of the necrotic tissue ·by forming an eschar or *Core*. This has got only limited use because, to be effective the powder should reach all necrotic tissue.

4. Applying a red-hot iron through the sinus openings.

The effectiveness of this treatment depends on whether the necrotic tissue comes in contact with the red-hot iron.

5. A combination of treatment with red-hot iron and use of caustics.

6. A seton passed through the opening in the coronet and through the wall of the hoof in level with the bottom of the suppurating tract, provides good drainage and helps quicker healing.

7. The operation for removal of cartilage (excision of the lateral cartilage) is done under general anaesthesia. The horse is cast and secured in lateral recumbency with the affected side of the foot above. A tourniquet is applied above the fetlock. The cartilage is exposed by "stripping" the corresponding portion of the wall of the hoof. The portion of skin in the pastern region also is reflected along with the stripped piece of horn so as to expose the cartilage completely.

The stripping of the horn is done as follows. First make a groove extending from the coronet to the planter aspect of the foot, in level with the anterior border of the cartilage. Then make a similar groove in level with the posterior border of the cartilage. Join the lower extremities of these two grooves by a third groove made along the white line on the planter aspect of the foot. Hold the demarcated piece of horn at its lower border with pincers and lift it upwards. To reflect the corresponding piece of skin in the pastern region, two incisions are made continuous with the vertical grooves on the hoof.

The exposed cartilage is removed by using a sage knife. All the necrosed tissues are removed and haemorrhage is controlled. The reflected piece of skin is kept in place after cutting away the portion of horn below its coronary border, leaving the coronary band intact. A bandage is applied. The dressing is changed next day and thereafter on alternate days. Healing takes four to six weeks or more.

Corns

A *corn* is a contusion (bruise) of the sensitive laminae at the angle formed between the wall and the bars of the hoof. This region of the foot is called *seat of corn*. A contusion on the sole is known as "bruised sole"; and a contusion on the frog as a "bruised frog".

Corns are more common in the fore-limb, mostly on the inner aspect.

CLASSFIICATION

1. *Dry corn*: In this there is only slight capillary bleeding resulting in echymosis or staining of overlying horn.

2. *Moist corn*: In this there is collection of inflammatory exudate beneath the horn and the horn appears to be soaked in moisture.

3. *Suppurating corn* (*Festered corn*): Suppuration is caused when infection gains entrance through any small fissure in horn and pus collects underneath. The horn appears more or less translucent.

4. *Complicated corn*: The pus tries to migrate upwards following the line of least resistance, and escapes through small opening at the coronet region. During the course of migration of pus, infection may extend to the plantar aponeurosis, plantar cushion, lateral cartilage, portion of os-pedis, etc. Portions of these structures coming in contact with pus may show partial necrosis.

ETIOLOGY

Predisposing causes: Faulty conformations of foot like upright walls, turned-in toes, wide, spreading foot with low, weak heels, atrophy of frog, contracted heels, etc., interfering with the anti-concussion mechanism.

Exciting causes: Bad shoeing is the major exciting cause of corns. Corns are only very rarely seen in unshod feet. As examples of bad shoeing the following may be mentioned. Excessive paring away of the horn at the seat of corn and easing of the horn at the heels, causing a space between the shoe and the foot. (For easing of the shoe, a special shoe which is thinner at its posterior portions is used. Though this shoe has the advantage of reducing pressure at the heels its major disadvantage is the likelihood of gathering foreign particles like small stones which may cause bruised sole or corn.) Cutting away at the bars or "opening the bars". "Close fitting" of the shoe usually done at the inner side, to prevent brushing. Delayed shoeing which causes the shoe to move forward causing the heel edge of the shoe to press at the seat of corn. The heel portion of the shoe causing excessive pressure at the "seat of corn", especially during fast work on hard grounds.

SYMPTOMS
Pointing. Lameness, varying according to the severity of the lesion. Going on toe.

DIAGNOSIS
The hoof is cleaned and is carefully examined at the seat of corn. Pain is evinced when the "seat of corn" is gently tapped with hammer. The horn at this region may appear moist and translucent. In dry corn, a reddish colouration may be seen due to the presence of blood collected underneath. Suppurating corn presents a yellowish, moist appearance because of pus.

PROGNOSIS
If treated early, prognosis is favourable. In suppurating corn prognosis is guarded. A well-established corn is an unsoundness.

TREATMENT
(1) Remove the shoe. (2) Pare away the horn at the seat of corn to relieve pressure at this point and use a seated-out shoe. (3) Rest is essential. (4) In the case of suppurating corn a conical portion of horn may be excavated to facilitate drainage of pus. (5) Foot-bath and antiseptic dressings. (6) In complicated corn stripping of the wall may be necessary to evacuate the pus.

Sand Crack
A sand crack is a fissure in the wall of the hoof parallel to the horn tubules, extending from the coronet to the plantar border. It is usually met with in the toe region of the hind feet and the inner quarter of the fore-feet.

CLASSIFICATION
1. Complete sand-crack, when the fissure is extending from the coronet to the plantar border.
2. Incomplete, when it extends only for a short distance.
3. Superficial, when the fissure involves only part of the thickness of the wall of the hoof.
4. Deep, when it involves the entire thickness of the wall.

5. Straight or sinuous according to its course.

6. Recent or old, depending on duration.

7. Simple or complicated, depending on the degree of damage to the sensitive tissues. In complicated sandcrack there is pus formation and the suppuration may spread on to surrounding tissues.

ETIOLOGY

(1) Hereditary predisposition. (2) Thinness of the wall. (3) Excessive rasping of the wall. (4) Alternate drying and moistening of the horn. (5) Injury to the coronet. (6) Violent extension of the corono-pedal joint causing the os-corona to press forcibly against the coronet.

SYMPTOMS

The fissure can be easily detected after cleaning the hoof. In complicated sandcrack there may be effusion of blood, serum or pus. Lameness is due to pinching of the sensitive laminae. Spasmodic lifting of the limb during progression is seen because of the pain. No lameness is seen if the fissure is superficial.

DIAGNOSIS

The sandcrack or fissure in the wall can be easily recognised after cleaning the hoof. Discharges may or may not be present.

TREATMENT

Treatment consists of (a) preventing the edges of the sandcrack pinching on the sensitive laminae, (b) promotion of new horn, and (c) the treatment of complications, if any.

(a) The following measures may be adopted to prevent the edges pinching on the sensitive laminae: (i) Use of a shoe having no bearing surface at the fissure. A flat shoe seated out at this level may be used or a portion of the bearing surface of the wall at this level may be removed to avoid it coming in contact with the shoe. (ii) Bandaging the hoof. This is not much helpful to prevent movement of the edges but prevents the entrance of dirt into the fissure. (iii) Application of *clasps*. Clasps are applied using sandcrack forceps, after making a groove on either side of the fissure with a red-hot iron. Clasps when properly applied are effective for immobilisation, but they are likely to fall out easily.

(iv) By using horseshoe nails instead of clasps. Horseshoe nails may be driven transversely through the lips of the sandcrack to serve as clasps. These nails are driven through grooves made on either side of the fissure. The excess length of nail at either end are cut and removed and the stumps are flattened and levelled with a hammer. Nails cannot be used for fissures on the quarters of the hoof because the wall is thinner here. (v) A small wooden piece introduced into the fissure may be efficient to prevent pinching of the sensitive laminae but it may fall off easily. (vii) Thinning the horn at the edges.

(b) *Promotion of secretion of newhorn*: A blister may be applied to the coronet region to stimulate growth of new horn.

(c) *Treatment of complications*: Complicated sandcrack is treated as follows: Pus and necrotic tissue removed by thinning the horn and cleaning. Antiseptic foot baths are given and foot dressing is applied. To remove pus and necrotic tissue portion of the horn at the wall may be stripped.

Transverse Crack

A transverse crack on the wall of the hoof results from injury to the sensitive laminae and lack of growth of horn at that level for a short period.

TREATMENT

Thinning of the horn may be done to avoid it pinching on the sensitive laminae. Complications, if any, are treated on the same lines as mentioned above.

Laminitis (*Founder*)

Laminitis (Founder) is the inflammation of the sensitive laminae of the foot. It is more common in the fore-foot. Ordinarily one or two feet may be affected. Sometimes all the four feet are affected. The symptoms are produced by a derangement of the vasoconstrictor nerves, thereby causing a congestion of the laminae.

ETIOLOGY

Predisposing causes: Heavy body weight, flat, spreading feet.

Exciting causes: Laminitis in the horse may occur due to any of the following causes. (1) Enterotoxaemia resulting from over eating, excessive intake of grains like barley and wheat or highly proteinaceous feeds. (2) Drinking of cold water immediately after hard work. (3) Concussion, especially due to fast work on hard ground. (4) Overwork. (5) Toxaemia resulting from pneumonia, metritis, retained placenta, etc., e.g., post-parturient laminitis in the mare if the placenta is not thrown out within twenty-four hours after parturition, and (6) Superpurgation.

Laminitis may be acute or chronic.

Acute Laminitis

SYMPTOMS

1. The animal becomes dull and has an anxious expression. When only one fore foot is affected the horse points it while standing. When both fore-feet are affected, they are kept forward so as to bear weight on heels and the hind limbs are also advanced forward to support the body weight. When both hind feet are affected they are placed forward so as to bear most weight on the heels and the forelimbs are placed slightly backwards in order to further relieve weight-bearing on the hind feet. When all four feet are severely affected the horse lies recumbent on the side.

During progression the gait is characteristic, the heels being first brought to the ground to avoid bearing weight in the toe region. When more than one foot is affected the animal appears to be walking like a "cat on hot bricks".

2. The temperature is elevated (103° to 106° F).

3. Pulse is frequent (70 to 120 per minute), strong in the early stages and later weak due to exhaustion.

4. Respirations are accelerated.

5. Conjunctiva is injected.

6. Local symptoms of acute inflammation are noticed in the hoof. The hoof feels very hot. Pulsation in the digital arteries is full and throbbling. There is pain on percussion of foot.

The acute symptoms of laminitis usually subside within four to twelve days and may be followed by gradual recovery or may develop into chronic laminitis. But very severe cases (called peracute laminitis) may terminate fatally.

In the severe form of acute laminitis there is an intensification of the symptoms due to profuse exudation and haemorrhage into the sensitive laminae. Haemorrhage is due to rupture of the distended vessels resulting from the pressure of body weight conveyed through the ospedis. The collection of blood or exudate causes severe pain and the animal lies prostrate, sweating profusely. It may groan with pain. Occasionally in certain cases the blood or exudate may escape through the coronet region. This may be followed by gangrene because of infection gaining entrance into the inflammed tissues. The onset of gangrane may show a temporary relief from pain and give a false hope of recovery. But cases in which gangrene has set in are usually fatal.

DIAGNOSIS

Diagnosis is easy from the symptoms.

PROGNOSIS

Depends on the severity of the attack. Prognosis is usually favourable when only one foot is affected. What all the four feet are affected, it is guarded.

TREATMENT

1. *Cold applications*: Ice packs, keeping the foot in cold water, etc.

2. Inducing purgation (except in cases where laminitis is due to superpurgation, metritis or pneumonia) may have a favourable effect. Drugs used for this purpose are Arecoline hydrobromide ¼ to 1½ grains S/c; Pilocarpine Nitras 2 to 3 grains S/c; Eserine (Physostigmine) ½ to 2 grains S/c; Carbacol (M & B) 4cc. S/c; Esmodil (Bayer) 4 cc. S/c; etc.

3. *Administering anti-histaminic drugs*: These drugs are very effective in bringing about symptomatic relief, e.g., Anthisan (M&B), available as 5% solution, vials of 10 cc to 30 cc. Anthisan is given intramuscularly or by slow intravenous injection. Or, Adrenaline (1 in 1000) 5 cc may be given I/m.

4. *Administering corticosteroid*: Intravenous injection of corticosteriods are helpful in the acute stage. Hydrocortisone 100 to 600 mg. diluted in 500 to 1000 cc of 10% glucose solution or in isotonic saline may be administered by slow I/V injection, e.g., Efcorlin soluble (Glaxo). vials of 100 mg with 2 cc of diluent.

5. Glucose-saline solution is administered to counteract toxaemia.

6. Put the animal on a laxative diet containing bran, linseed, green grass etc. Mag. Sulph and Pot. Nitras may be added to the drinking water for laxative and diuretic effects.

7. *Ligation of the digital artery*: This is an old method of treatment which is not recommended nowadays.

8. Blocking the plantar of nerves may be done to relieve pain.

9. Febrifuges like salicylates.

10. Largactyl 5% solution 10 to 15 cc may be given I/M to reduce temperature.

11. Jugular phlebotomy may be done to reduce the general blood volume and thereby to relieve congestion in the sensitive lamine. About 1 to 2 gallons of blood can be removed from a horse.

12. *Auto-haemotherapy*: Frank (1959) has mentioned this to be beneficial in the early stages of the disease. 80 to 120 cc. of blood is drawn out from the animal through the jugular vein and is injected into the *same* animal I/M. The injections may be repeated two or three times at an interval of one or two days.

Chronic Laminitis

Symptoms and Sequelae

The foot changes its shape as a result of chronic laminitis. The changes are caused by the rotation of the os-pedis on its horizontal axis and sinking of its anterior planter border on the sole, which indirectly pulls down the coronary band. The following alterations in the shape of the foot are noticed consequently.

1. The anterior portion of the sole becomes flat or convex. This is called *Dropped sole*. The sensitive laminae of the sole undergoes pressure atrophy and fails to secrete new horn due to compression by the os-pedis. So when the horn of the sole wears off there may be *perforation* of the sole anterior to the frog. This exposes the sensitive tissues to infection and necrosis and consequently a serous or purulent discharge may be noticed.

2. There is excessive growth of horn in the toe region and

the foot is enlongated antero-posteriorly, because of the stimulation of the coronary band.

3. The rings or rugae on the wall representing horn growth becomes more prominent because of the increased secretion of horn.

4. Immediately below the coronet the growth of horn is more vertical because of the stretching downwards of the secreting papillae of the coronary band, and therefore the anterior portion of the hoof has an upright appearance near the coronet.

5. The white line of the foot becomes more prominent and thick due to separation of the wall and the sensitive laminae and deposition of abnormal horn between them. The separation of horn is widest at the centre of the toe and may measure 2 to 3 inches. The space between the wall and sensitive laminae in the toe region appears more or less vacant except for the scanty deposition of abnormal horn.

6. As the horse puts more weight on the heels during progression, the toe is pushed forwards and upwards and as a result of this the lower portion of the anterior aspect of the hoof approaches a horizontal direction.

Diagnosis

From the abnormal and characteristic alteration in the shape of the foot, viz., the convexity of the sole, the space formation between the wall and the sole at the White line, etc.

Prognosis

Unfavourable. The abnormality persists and recurrent attacks of subacute laminitis may occur.

Treatment

1. Remove all the excess horn at the quarters and toe. When new horn grows downwards in the toe region the space between it and the sensitive laminae might become less.

2. The deformities are corrected to a certain extent by shoeing. Apply wide-webbed (broad) shoe which is well seated out to protect the sole.

3. A strip of leather may be placed between the shoe and the foot, so as to prevent the sole touching the ground.

4. A thin metal plate may be fitted between the shoe and the foot to cover and protect the sole.

5. The horse generally goes better on a long-heeled shoe (a shoe whose heels project slightly backwards).

6. If the sole is perforated, antiseptic foot baths (eg., formalin 10%) and foot dressing (eg., triple sulph foot dressing containing: Cupri Sulph + Ferri Sulph + Zinc Sulph) are recommended. After the perforation has healed, cover the sole with tar and tow and protect it with a thin metal plate fitted between the foot and the shoe.

Seedy Toe

Seedy toe is a condition characterised by the separation of the wall and the sensitive laminae of the foot. The interspace may contain soft abnormal horn.

ETIOLOGY

The cause is not clear. Apparently due to chronic laminitis. Wide, spreading feet are more susceptible.

SYMPTOMS

A part or whole of the foot may be affected. Lameness is not seen if only a small portion of the foot is affected. When the affected area is tapped with a hammer a hollow sound is heard.

PROGNOSIS

Depends on the depth and area of the lesion. When a large area is involved and there is lameness, a long time is taken for the recovery.

TREATMENT

The abnormal horn between the sensitive laminae and the wall can be removed after paring away portion of the wall in that region. A blister may be put in the coronet region to stimulate formation of new horn.

Keratoma

Keratoma is a tumour consisting of horny tissue, growing from the inner aspect of the wall of the hoof. When the plantar aspect of the foot is examined, the white line of the foot appears pushed inwards by the tumour. The pressure of the tumour on the sensitive laminae and the os-pedis causes lameness. Prognosis is not favourable because the tumour may recur even after surgical removal.

TREATMENT

If there is not much pain or lameness, the shoe is applied in such a way as to cause minimum bearing on the affected region. If pain and lameness are severe only surgical removal of the tumour is likely to be beneficial. Extirpation of the tumour is accomplished after exposing it by stripping the wall.

Canker

Canker is a chronic, hypertrophic, moist, eczemaious, dermatitis involving the foot (CHMED). The frog, sole and wall of the foot are affected.

INCIDENCE

Canker is more common in the hind feet. Heavy draft horses are more commonly affected.

ETIOLOGY

1. Constant work in mud; dirty, unhygienic condition of stable etc.

2. No specific organism is found to be responsible for the condition.

3. Heredity may be a predisposing factor.

SYMPTOMS

The horn in the affected areas becomes separated in flakes and is moist as though soaked in oil. In long-standing cases the sensitive lamina is exposed. The sensitive lamina shows hypertrophic changes and becomes covered with vegetations or finger-like hypertrophic papillae and foul-smelling caseous exudate. The lesions may be covered with horn, constituting what are known as *ergots*. The lesion is not very painful and lameness is not marked except in very severe cases where the os-pedis is exposed.

PROGNOSIS

There is no tendency for spontaneous cure. The lesion is progressive. Response to treatment is slow and takes about six weeks for cure. Afterwards the horse should be given at least 2 weeks rest before it is worked.

TREATMENT

1. Remove the loose horn.
2. Clean and dress the foot with antiseptic powder. After about twenty-four hours take away the dressing and remove the loose flakes of horn. An antiseptic dressing like triple sulph foot dressing (i.e., Cupri Sulph + Ferri Sulph + Zinc Sulph) is applied.
3. After the diseased horn has completely sloughed away a less irritant antiseptic like iodoform with zinc oxide is preferable
4. The affected portion of sole is protected by a metal or leather sole.
5. Administration of arsenic as a skin tonic is also advisable.

Thrush

Thrush is a degenerative condition of the horny frog. It commences from the central lacunae (sulcus) of the frog and extends to the lateral lacunae and the entire frog.

INCIDENCE

Common in heavy draft horses than in light horses. More frequent in contracted feet wherein the frog is inactive. Hind feet are more commonly affected.

ETIOLOGY

1. Work in muddy roads, housing in soiled and moist flooring. The horn gets soaked in urine and faeces and becomes brittle and comes away in flakes.
2. Neglect of cleaning (pricking) the frog regularly.

SYMPTOMS

There is shedding of the horn of the frog and a foul-smelling, greyish or blackish discharge is present. The affected hoof may be surrounded by flies. But there is *no* vegetative growth or hypetrophy as in canker. Usually no lameness.

TREATMENT

Clean the frog and apply antiseptic foot dressings. House the animal in a clean stable and avoid its standing on moist flooring. Thrush easily responds to treatment.

Cracked Heels (*Dermatitis Eczematosa*; *Scratches*)

An *acute* inflammatory condition of the skin of the posterior aspect of the pastern. Fissures and vesicle formation causes severe pain. An exudate sticks to the hair in the region.

TREATMENT

Clean with soap and water and dry. White lotion dressing twice daily until the inflammation subsides a little. Then a dressing made up of equal parts of Tincture iodine + Liq ferri. perchlor + Glycerine, twice daily or zinc oxide ointment twice daily. Tannic acid + Salicylic acid (each 5%) in alcohol is stated to be good if the discharge is profuse.

Grease Heel (*Dermatitis Verrucosa;* "*Grapes*")

A chronic inflammation of the skin on the posterior aspect of pastern, sometimes extending on to the fetlock, hock and knee. Thickening of the skin, pain and a foul smelling discharge sticking on to the skin are noticed. In long-standing cases wart-like growths called *grapes* are seen. The condition is not easily cured. Prognosis is guarded.

TREATMENT

Thorough cleaning and drying of the skin. The "grapes" are removed by thermocautery. Any of the following antiseptic solutions may be used for cleaning: Zinc sulphate (5 to 10%), Alum (5 to 10%), or Creolin (2 to 3%) and a dressing (e.g. zinc ointment) may be applied after drying the skin.

Coronitis*

Coronitis or inflammation of the coronary band may involve the whole of the coronary band or only a portion of it.

Villitis; Dermatitis of the coronary band

ETIOLOGY

Unknown. It is sometimes caused by direct injury to the coronary band. (See also Gangrenous Coronitis on next page.)

SYMPTOMS

Overgrowth of horn due to excessive stimulation of coronary band and also thickening of skin close to it. Subsequently there may be formation of fissures on the hoof and ulcers on the skin.

TREATMENT

Consists of removing the excess horn and applying an emollient foot dressing like mixture of tar and shark liver oil,etc.

Treads

Treads are injuries inflicted at the coronet of the foot, either by the shoe of the opposite foot, or when horses are worked in pairs, by the foot of adjacent horse.

TREATMENT

Remove the cause by corrective shoeing. See also general treatment for wounds.

Broken Knee

Wounds or traumatic injuries caused in front of the knee are in general called "Broken knee". These wounds if deep may cause open joint.

TREATMENT

On general principles for treatment of wounds. In addition a protective bandage, and a "knee cap" may be applied to the affected knee.

Gangrenous Coronitis

The condition results in sloughing of a portion of coronet. It may be due to infection by Bacillus necrosis. Treatment on general principles.

Evulsion (Avulsion) of Hoof

Separation of the horny covering of the hoof exposing the sensitive laminae is called *evulsion of the hoof.*

ETIOLOGY

(1) Suppurative lesions beneath the horn, e.g., foot and mouth disease in cattle. (2) Degenerative changes sometimes following neurectomy. (3) Traumatic injury.

SYMPTOMS

The sensitive laminae are exposed. There will be severe bleeding if the case is due to a recent traumatic injury. Pain may not be very marked.

PROGNOSIS

Prognosis is unfavourable if it is due to neurectomy. In traumatic cases prognosis may be considered favourable when properly treated. It will take about *nine months* for the horn to replace itself completely. Rarely lameness persists even after new horn is formed because of some hypersensitivity in the subcoroneal tissue.

TREATMENT

If the bleeding is severe, a tourniquet is applied above the 'etlock until the wound is dressed. The wound is cleaned with an antiseptic lotion like Perchloride of mercury (1 in a 1000) followed by an anodyne antiseptic dressing like Iodoform or BIPP. A bandage is applied. A leather boot may also be put over the bandage. The dressing is changed daily or once in every two or three days, i.e., whenever the bandage becomes wet with the discharges. After a thin layer of horn tissue has been formed, tar dressing can be applied and is sufficient. (See also page 35, 42)

Section of Suspensory Ligament and Flexor Tendons

This condition usually results from traumatic injuries. e.g., accidentally kicking the limb against a sharp object. The structures cut may be either the suspensory ligament or one of the flexor tendons. Sometimes there is section of the suspensory ligament as well as one or both the flexor tendons.

SYMPTOMS

The symptoms will vary according to the structure that has been severed. When the superficial flexor (F. perforatus) only is cut there is slight dropping of the fetlock. Marked lowering of the fetlock is noticed if the suspensory ligament is cut. When the deep flexor (F. perforans) is divided, the phalangeal joints are in an excessively extended state with the result the toe is directed upwards and the plantar aspect of the foot is facing forwards.

If all the three structures are divided, the fetlock is almost touching the ground and the pastern is horizontal.

PROGNOSIS

The prognosis is guarded. The severity will depend upon whether one, two or all the three structures are divided and whether there is an infection. Possible complications are necrosis of tendons and purulent synovitis of the flexor tendon sheath. However, many cases of complete healing have been recorded. The deformity may sometimes persist after healing.

TREATMENT

The wound is treated in the usual manner. The ends of the tendon may be sutured if possible. A bandage is put. A special shoe (Swan necked shoe) is put to support the fetlock. In favourable cases healing takes place in about four weeks. A thick-heeled shoe or a shoe with calkins is put thereafter to relieve the tendons. After about two months the patient is able to bear weight on the affected limb though the fetlock may appear abnormally low for sometime. This deformity may later get corrected to a certain extent by the cicatrical contractions.

Rupture of Flexor Tendons

The rupture may be primary, secondary, partial or complete. *Primary rupture* may happen during galloping or jumping due to over-stretching of the tendon. *Secondary rupture* is a result of degeneration or necrosis of the tendon as may result from a double plantar neurectomy. Excessive weight-bearing on one limb due to severe lameness in the opposite limb may act as predisposing factor. Other predisposing factors are natural weakness of the tendon, weakening of the tendon due to debilitating disease, working a horse in unfit condition when it is exhausted or fatigued.

SYMPTOMS

The first symptom is usually seen during gallop or after a

jump from a height or immediately after an accidental slipping. Suddenly the horse goes lame followed by severe local inflammation. The deformity due to the rupture of the tendons is similar to what has been described under the section of tendons. The gap between the broken ends can sometimes be palpated. Later this space gets filled with blood clot.

PROGNOSIS

If the rupture is due to degeneration or disease of the tendon prognosis is unfavourable.

TREATMENT

Incomplete rupture is treated like sprain of tendon. Complete rupture is treated as for section of tendons. Healing may take about six weeks and about two to three months rest is necessary before the animal is put to work. Suturing the ends of ruptured tendon is not advocated for fear of introducing infection.

Rupture of Suspensory Ligament

Rupture of suspensory ligament is of common occurrence in the race horse. The affected horse is commonly spoken of as *broken down.*

The rupture is caused by excessive strain of the ligament during galloping or jumping. The horse stops suddenly and refuses to bear weight on the affected limb. When the animal is made to keep the foot flat on the ground, the fetlock appears very much lowered. On palpation of the suspensory ligament the gap caused by the rupture may be detected.

Sometimes the flexor tendons are also ruptured along with the suspensory ligament. In some instances only one branch of the suspensory is ruptured, more commonly the inner branch.

TREATMENT

As for rupture of flexor tendons.

Sprain of the Flexor Tendons (*Sprained Tendons: Tendinitis*)

The term "sprained tendons" denotes sprain of the superficial or deep flexor tendons, their check ligaments or the suspensory ligament. (See also Addendum on page 654)

INCIDENCE

The condition is more common in the forelimb than in the hind limb.

Sprain of the suspensory ligament and superficial flexor tendon and its check ligament is common in animals doing fast work. Sprain of deep flexor tendon and its check ligament is more common in heavy draft horses.

Note: The suspensory ligament and the flexor tendons are relaxed during flexion of the fetlock and interphalangeal joints and are tensed during extension of these joints. As the foot is brought to the ground during progression there is a momentary period when the phalangeal joints are flexed but the fetlock joint is extending. At this moment prior to the stretching of the superficial flexor tendons, there is increased tension on the suspensory ligament. Therefore if the foot is brought to the ground with great force, there is chance for sprain of suspensory ligament. This is possibly the reason for the frequent occurrence of sprain of suspensory ligament in fast working animals. Immediately before the foot is lifted from the ground during progression there is full extension of the coronopedal joint and relatively more tension on the deep flexor tendon as compared to the superficial flexor or the suspensory ligament. This tension will be more in the case of heavy draft horses and hence there is greater chance of sprain in such animals.

CHIEF SITES OF SPRAIN

1. The superficial flexor tendon may be sprained at the level of its check ligament (radial check ligament), at the upper or middle portion of the metacarpal region or at its points of insertion. The characteristic swelling of the posterior aspect of the metacarpal or metatarsal region resulting from tendinitis and peritendinitis is referred to as *bowed tendon*.

2. The deep flexor tendon may be sprained at the level of its check ligament, middle portion of metacarpal region or the posterior aspect of pastern region.

3. The suspensory ligament is usually sprained just above its bifurcation or in its middle part.

ETIOLOGY

The *predisposing causes* are unfit condition; defective conformations (like sloping pastern, oblique hoof, slender fetlock, calf knees, etc.); fast work (like galloping); heavy draft; slippery grounds; muscular fatigue; bad quality of tendons (e.g., soft, "gummy" tendons), diseases of tendons, etc. The *exciting cause* is undue stretching.

SYMPTOMS

In *acute case* there is pain, swelling and lameness. The swelling becomes pronounced two to three days after the accident. It may be diffuse, extending over the entire metacarpal region, or may be localised at the level of the sprain. Palpation of the suspensory ligament or the flexor tendons reveals pain. Pain and lameness are more marked when the lesion is close to the joints (knee, fetlock or pastern joints). At rest the limb is kept with fetlock and phalangeal joints slightly flexed, so as to relax the tendons.

In *chronic sprain* the pain and lameness are slight. The lameness may be intermittent. There may be enlargement and thickening (induration). Chronic sprain may become acute when the horse is put to work. Sprain at the level of the synovial sheath may sometimes cause synovitis in addition to tendinitis.

DIAGNOSIS

Palpate the tendons after flexing the joints and lifting the limb. The seat of the lesion is the point where pain and swelling are most evident.

PROGNOSIS

The prognosis is guarded. Prognosis depends on the severity of the sprain. When there is extensive damage to the tendon fibres, the same are replaced by fibrous tissue. In such cases knuckling may result due to cicatrical contractions. Complications like synovitis of the tendon sheaths may also result from tendinitis.

TREATMENT

Corrective shoeing may be adopted to preserve the normal slope of the pastern. Rest is necessary. In the acute stage cold and astringent applications, moist hot fomentations, pressure bandages, injection of corticosteroids (Hydrocortisone acetate,

50 to 100 mg into the tendon tissue etc. may help reduce inflammation. After the acute stage has passed massaging the area is beneficial. Counter-irritation with blisters or by firing (thermo-cautery) is advocated in chronic cases. Superficial line-firing in the form of transverse lines is usually adopted for tendinitis. Deep needle-point firing is also effective but it may give rise to more of scar tissue.

Sesamoiditis

Inflammation of the proximal sesamoids is sometimes seen in the horse. The fore-limbs are usually affected. The inflammation may be acute or chronic. There may be ulceration of the sesamoid bones.

ETIOLOGY

Similar to sprain of flexor tendons and suspensory ligament.

SYMPTOMS

There is swelling in the region of the sesamoids and lameness. The symptoms resemble those of sprained flexor tendons. The acute inflammation subsides after a varying period. Exostoses on the inner aspect of the sesamoid bones cause lameness. Neurectomy may be helpful in such cases to make the animal useful for work.

Rupture of Tendo-achilis

Rupture of the gastrocnemius muscle or its tendon (tendo-achilis) has been met with in the horse, cattle, dog and cat.

ETIOLOGY

(1) Excessive strain on the tendon during jumping or while pulling heavy draft. (2) External violence. (3) Due to malicious injury. Malicious cutting of the tendon is called *hamstringing*. The tendo-achilis and portion of the superficial flexor tendon situated close to it are usually cut simultaneously.

SYMPTOMS

The hock and all joints below it are flexed. The affected limb is not able to bear weight.

TREATMENT

In small animals like dogs and cats suturing may be tried. Keep the hock extended by putting *plaster of Paris* bandage. Healing and re-union of the tendon takes four to six weeks and will depend on whether the hock has been properly immobilised in the extended position.

PROGNOSIS

In small animals like dogs and cats recovery usually takes place if properly treated. In large animals healing is difficult when the tendons are completely cut.

Contraction of Achilis Tendon (*Spastic Paresis of Hind Limbs*)

ETIOLOGY

Not known.

SYMPTOMS

Marked contraction of tendo-achilis, quadriceps extensor cruris muscle and the adductor muscles of the thigh, with the result the limb is extended and slightly held backward adducted. It may appear shorter and only the toe may touch the ground. Sometimes the spasms subside and the limb may be used without much difficulty. In very marked cases the limb may move like a pendulum during progression.

DIAGNOSIS

Differentiate from Gonitis and subluxation of patella.

TREATMENT

No satisfactory treatment. Tenotomy of the tendo-achilis plus cutting half the thickness of the superficial flexor tendon immediately above the tuber calcis (through a small skin incision) has been tried but without much benefit.

Knuckling

An excessively flexed condition of the fetlock joint is called *knuckling*. It is due to the contraction (shortening) of the flexor tendons.

VARIETIES (DEGREE) OF KNUCKLING

(1) If the contraction is slight the pastern assumes a somewhat vertical position; (2) in more severe types the fetlock is pushed forwards almost in level with the hoof; (3) in the extreme degree of knuckling (the fetlock and phalangeal joints are flexed so much that) the pastern is pushed forward and may even touch the ground.

ETIOLOGY

Knuckling may occur congenitally. In adult animals it is due to cicatrical contraction of the flexor tendons following tendinitis. Improper weight-bearing on the limb due to contracted foot, ring bone, dry arthritis, etc. may cause knuckling.

SYMPTOMS

The fetlock is flexed to a varying degree depending on whether one or both flexor tendons are affected. If only the superficial flexor tendon is affected, the foot can be placed flatly on the ground but the fetlock is flexed. When the deep flexor is affected, the fetlock and interphalangeal joints are flexed. Knuckling causes stumbling during progression. If the pastern is touching the ground, "open joint" of the fetlock or pastern may be produced.

PROGNOSIS

In the young animal below one year knuckling of a slight degree may get corrected when the animal grows. In adult animals prognosis is usually unfavourable.

TREATMENT

In *young animals* the correction of the deformity can be tried by putting a plaster cast for sometime. The plaster cast is applied in such a way that the foot is allowed to touch the ground and bear weight. As the condition improves, a shoe having its toe thickened and projecting forward is applied. Friebel's extension apparatus also can be tried. The Friebel's apparatus consists of a metal covering for the hoof to which can be fitted two stiff iron bars. When applied, these iron bars come along the anterior aspect of the limb and help to keep the fetlock and phalangeal joints in an almost normal position.

In adult animals tenotomy of the superficial or deep flexor tendon (plantar tenotomy) may be tried. For details see operative surgery. (See page 618).

Shivering

Shivering is an involuntary contraction of muscles thereby causing irregular movements of certain parts of the body. Shivering is sometimes seen in the horse affecting the hind limbs and tail. Less frequently shivering of forelimbs or regions like lips, eyelids and cheek are seen.

ETIOLOGY

Not definitely known. May have some hereditary predisposition. The exciting factor may be the effect of toxins on the nervous system, as it is frequently seen after strangles, influenza or pneumonia.

SYMPTOMS

There is shivering of the affected limb especially when the animal is backed or when the affected limb is picked up. The leg may be held semi-flexed and raised from the ground and kept abducted. There may be varying degrees of the disease, very slight to pronounced shivering. In well-marked cases the animal may have difficulty to get up from the ground. Such animals may show bruises and abrasions over knee and fetlock.

TREATMEN

There is no treatment for shivering. In milder cases the animal may be used for work but stress and excitement makes the condition worse.

Stringhalt

Stringhalt is an involuntary overflexion and lifting of a limb during progression. Usually it is seen only in hind limbs. Stringhalt is considered to be an unsoundness though the animal can be used for work.

ETIOLOGY

The etiology is obscure. Possible causes are articular lesions of hock or stifle, some reflex irritation in the flexor muscles of the hock (flexor metatarsi, lateral digital extensor, etc.), nervous lesions of the sciatic nerve causing overstimulation of flexor muscles.

SYMPTOMS

The characteristic flexion of the limb is recognised only during progression. The symptoms is more pronounced after a period of rest.

DIAGNOSIS

Diagnosis is made from the symptoms. Stringhalt is different from shivering. Unlike shivering, stringhalt is noticed only during progression.

TREATMENT

Peroneal tenotomy (Boccar's Operation) gives relief in certain cases. The tendon of peroneus muscle (Lat. digital extensor) is cut below the hock on the lateral aspect of the metatarsus where it joins with the tendon of anterior digital extensor. (See operative surgery.)

Gonitis

Gonitis or inflammation of the stifle joint, may be acute or chronic. It is more common in bullocks than in horses.

Acute Gonitis

Acute Gonitis is usually caused by trauma. Overextension of the stifle joint, e.g., due to slipping, is sometimes responsible for the condition.

INCIDENCE

Occasionally noticed in work bullocks and breeding bulls.

SYMPTOMS

The symptoms of acute synovitis and arthritis are present. The joint is swollen and painful. There is incomplete flexion (stiffness) of the joint during progression, there is shortening of the stride, and dragging of the toe.

TREATMENT
General treatment for acute inflammation.

Chronic Gonitis
It is common in bullocks, heavy draft horses, and breeding bulls.

ETIOLOGY
Not well understood. Excessive strain on the joint may be an exciting factor. It may also be due to rheumatism or toxins.

SYMPTOMS
Symptoms appear gradually and in the initial stages are not pronounced. During rest the horse repeatedly flexes the stifle and keeps the limb slightly raised from the ground. There is dragging of the toe during progression and sometimes the stifle may get fixed in the extended position. Boggy enlargement of the stifle joint due to distension of the joint capsule is also seen. Pain may be evinced on palpation of the joint. There is erosion of aricular surfaces and crepitation may be heard on flexion of the joint due to friction between eroded surfaces.

PROGNOSIS
Gonitis is incurable.

TREATMENT
Treatment is not effective. Firing and blistering may be tried.

Curb
Normally, the posterior aspect of the hock (in the horse) when viewed from a side conforms to a straight line connecting the point of the hock and the back of fetlock. When there is a backward curvature at the lower portion of the hock due to some enlargement or inflammation of underlying structures, the condition is described as a curb. A curb is therefore noticed on the *postero-inferior* aspect of the hock. The enlargement usually is due to sprain of the calcaneocuboid ligament, though sprain of the superficial or deep flexor tendons at that level may also cause it. The calcaneocuboid (plantar tarsal) liga-

ment is the ligament connecting posterior aspect of oscalcis, cuboid and external small metatarsal bones.

ETIOLOGY

Predisposing causes: (1) Hereditary predisposition. (2) Defective conformation of the hock in which the oscalcis is inclined slightly forwards and thereby increases strain on the ligament ; Tied-in hock in which the hock is narrow at its lower portion, etc.

Exciting causes include overstretching of the ligament during jumping, pulling heavy draft, etc.

SYMPTOMS

The enlargement on the postero-inferior aspect of the hock. Lameness may or may not be present. Lameness characterised by putting less weight in the heel region of the foot and "going on toe". No lameness after about three weeks, but the local enlargement may persist.

PROGNOSIS

In young horses with normal hocks a curb may sometimes disappear without treatment. Curb has a tendency to recur, especially in horses with deformed hocks. Curb is considered to be an unsoundness.

TREATMENT

In the *acute* stage rest and cold and astringent applications. A shoe with thick heels. In *chronic* stage iodine ointment, blistering, firing, etc. may be tried.

Spavin*

An exostosis in the hock region below the level of the tibio-tarsal articulation is called *spavin*. Spavin is a typical example of an osteo-arthritic disease. In the majority of cases the exostosis is seen on the postero-infero-internal aspect of the hock in front of the chestnut. This area is therefore spoken of as the *seat of spavin*. The exostosis in this region involves the cunei-form parvum and the upper extremity of the inner small

---

*Bone spavin; Osteo-periostitis and chronic arthritis of the hock joint.

metatarsal bone. When the seat of exostosis is higher up it is called *high spavin*. If on the anterior aspect of hock, *anterior spavin*. If exostosis is very large, *jack spavin*. Typical spavin lameness with no exostosis seen outside is referred to as *occult spavin*.

ETIOLOGY
  Predisposing causes: (1) Heredity; (2) Defective conformation of hock like tied-in-hock (=hock narrow in its lower part), cow hock (=both hocks close together as in cow), sickle-shaped hock, etc. (3) Young age, (4) Over-working.
  Exciting causes: (1) Violent movements as may occur during rearing, jumping, accidental slipping, etc. (2) Deficiencies in diet and improper Ca : P ratio. (3) Rheumatism. (4) Trauma, concussion.

SYMPTOMS
  (1) Presence of the exostosis. (2) Lameness. Spavin lameness is characterised by (i) imperfect flexion of hock, (ii) Dragging of the toe, (iii) circumduction, (iv) taking longer steps, (v) lowering of hip when the limb is advanced, (vi) lameness is most marked when the animal is worked immediately after a period of rest and lameness diminishes when the animal is exercised for sometime, (vii) during rest the hock is sometimes kept in a state of spasmodic flexion, (viii) atrophy of the gluteal muscles is seen in very chronic cases.

DIAGNOSIS
  From the symptoms. To detect the exostosis compare the affected hock with the opposite one. Look at the hocks from in front, from behind and from the sides. A radiograph will be helpful to find out the extent of exostosis. Spavin test may be conducted to find out whether lameness is present. [Spavin test is conducted as follows. Lift the affected limb and keep it holding with the hock flexed for about two minutes. Then release the limb immediately and trot the animal. If spavin is present lameness becomes evident.]

PROGNOSIS
  Spavin is an unsoundness, though the lameness may disappear in certain cases. The exostosis already formed persists.

Occult spavin is more serious. Anterior spavin and high spavin mechanically interferes with the flexion of the hock.

Treatment

The object of treatment is to bring about local ankylosis. Needle-point firing and blistering hastens the ankylosis. Cunean tenotomy may be performed to bring about ankylosis. (See Operative Surgery.) Anterior and posterior tibial neurectomies are performed as a last resort when other treatments are ineffective.

Bog Spavin

Bog spavin is a swelling noticed on the *supero-antero-internal* aspect of the hock because of the distension of the joint capsule of the tibio-tarsal articulation (Bog=spongy).

Etiology

Predisposing cause: Deformities of the hock. *Exciting cause*: Constant hard work.

Symptoms

Bog spavin does not usually cause lameness and pain is absent. It does not affect the usefulness of the animal unless the distension is very large and mechanically interferes with the movement of the joint. In rare cases there is an acute synovitis causing pain and lameness.

Treatment

Blistering, needle-point firing, aspiration and injection of an irritant antiseptic solution into the joint, etc.

Blood Spavin

Blood spavin is a varicose condition of the internal saphena vein in the region of the hock. The swelling is noticed on the *antero-internal* aspect of the hock.

Treatment

Treatment is not attempted.

Kumri (*Kamree or Kamri*)

Kumri is a chronic disease of horses causing loss of strength in the hind limbs.

ETIOLOGY

The actual cause of the disease is not known. The etiological agents suggested are the following: (1) Schistosome affecting the spinal cord, (2) Trypanosomes, (3) Larval stages of setaria.

SYMPTOMS

While standing, the hind limbs are kept wide apart and the fore-limbs are placed backwards to share the body weight. There is weakness and incoordination. The limbs are carried stiffly and the toe is dragged. Because of the abducted movement of both the hind limbs, hind quarters show a characteristic swinging gait and the loin region does not go straight. Pressure over the loins may cause wincing and crouching. The animal has difficulty in backing. The disease is progressive in its course and complete paralysis may set in.

TREATMENT

There is no specific treatment. Some cases are reportedly cured by the use of tartar emetic, Antrypol, etc.

REFERENCES

Malkani, P.G. (1933). *Kumri Ind. Vet. J.*, 9, 184-192.

Iliac Thrombosis

Arteritis and consequent thrombosis of the terminal portion of the posterior aorta gives rise to certain characteristic clinical symptoms in the horse. The thrombus may be located either proximal to or distal to the iliac quadrification of the abdominal aorta or in any one of the iliac arteries. When the thrombus is situated proximal to iliac quadrification the blood supply to both the hind limbs are affected; when it is situated in iliac vessels of one side only the hind limb of that particular side is affected. The thrombus may occlude the vessel partially or completely. When the occlusion is only partial the limb would get a limited blood supply and no uneasiness is felt during rest or mild exercise. But when the animal is given work there is pronounced distress for want of adequate blood supply to the affected limb. The animal suddenly goes lame and begins to struggle due to severe pain. Sweating may be noticed all over the body *except* over the affected limb. The superficial veins of the affected limb appear in a collapsed condition and the limb itself is cold as compared to other parts of the body. The thrombus can be located on rectal examination and pulsation in the vessel is quite distinct proximal to the thrombus while it is feeble or absent distally. In partial occlusion a tremour is felt due to the thin stream of blood passing the thrombus.

PROGNOSIS

Prognosis is unfavourable because there is no satisfactory treatment for the condition.

TREATMENT

Treatment is useless. The following treatments have been tried.

1. Administration of potassium iodide.

2. Massage of the aorta per rectum to dislodge the thrombus. This is sometimes likely to be dangerous because of the possibility of embolism.

3. Frequent and systematic exercise to encourage formation of collateral circulation. The animal is given exercise every day until it just begins to show the symptoms of lameness. This is repeated for a number of days.

Lameness in Cattle

Most cases of common lameness in cattle is due to some trouble in the foot. The next common seat of lameness is the stifle. Many of the conditions causing lameness in the horse described above are also met with in cattle. Some of the other conditions seen in cattle are: Tendersole, Foul-in-the-foot, Interdigital vegetative dermatitis, Pappilloma of foot, Elongated hooves, Coxitis, etc.

Tender Sole in Cattle

This is a contusion of the sole of the foot. Cattle walked for long distances by road, especially heavy-bodied ones are affected.

SYMPTOMS
Lameness; tendency to lie down most of the time; pointing.

DIAGNOSIS
From the symptoms. On examination after cleaning of the foot, the sole appears reddish due to underlying contusion. If the contusion is severe, the sole appears moist due to collection of inflammatory exudate.

PROGNOSIS
In mild cases recovery takes place if the animal is given rest for a few days. Possible complications in severe cases are necrosis, sinus formation and shedding of the hoof.

TREATMENT
Rest the animal. If necrosis and sinus formation are evident provide drainage and apply antiseptic dressings.

Foul in the Foot in Cattle*
A chronic condition caused by Fusiformis necroforus leading to necrosis and ulceration of the foot.

ETIOLOGY
The causal organism, Fusiformis necroforus, enters into the tissues through some open wound in the interdigital space. The chance of infection is enhanced by moist, dirty surroundings.

SYMPTOMS
There is severe lameness. Anorexia and rise of temperature also may be seen. Uncomplicated cases may recover in a few days. Otherwise involvement of pedal joints or other complications develop.

TREATMENT
Foot baths of copper sulphate (2% to 5%) is advised. Sulphonamides and broad spectrum antibiotics are found useful. Sulphamezathine $33\frac{1}{3}\%$ solution I/V is reported to be good. To prevent the lesion extending or when one of the digits is badly

*Foot-rot in cattle; Necrotic pododermatitis.

damaged, it may be advisable to amputate the digit. (For details see Operative Surgery.)

Inter-digital Vegetative Dermatitis in Cattle

Growth seen in the interdigital space due to hyperplasia of the skin and subcutaneous tissues in the region. This condition is sometimes wrongfully referred to as corn.

INCIDENCE
Breeding bulls are more frequently affected, especially in the hind limbs.

ETIOLOGY
The cause of the condition is not known. Possibly due to some hereditary factor.

SYMPTOMS
Lameness and the excess tissue in the interdigital space can be noticed. If the tissue is large sized the digits are pushed apart and when this deformity is present lameness is more severe and persistent.

TREATMENT
Surgical removal of the excess tissue. A mild antiseptic dressing powder is put and a bandage is applied. Repeat dressing about once a week. Avoid soiling with urine and manure.

Papilloma of Foot in Cattle

Papillomas are sometimes seen developing on the posterior aspect of the pastern and may sometimes extend to the bulbs of the heels. They cause lameness. Treatment consists of surgical removal and proper treatment of the resulting wound. The tumour tissue should be completely removed to prevent recurrence.

Elongated Hooves

Due to lack of proper wear the hooves may become overgrown. This is a condition commonly seen in breeding bull. One or more foot may be affected. Lameness and deformity of the claw are noticed. The toe and quarters of the hoof are elongated and the affected digit may be turned in.

TREATMENT
Trim away the excess horn tissue.

Coxitis in Cattle (*Inflammation of the Hip Joint*)

ETIOLOGY
Inflammation of the hip joint in cattle and horses (draft animals) are usually caused by pulling heavy loads or by accidental slipping.

SYMPTOMS
At rest the limb is kept extended with the *toe turned outwards*. During progression lameness is noticed when weight is borne on the affected limb.

PROGNOSIS
Usually unfavourable.

TREATMENT
1. Blistering and firing of the hip.
2. Injection of corticosteroids can be tried.

Foot Rot in Sheep
This is similar to "foul-in-the foot" in cattle. In sheep the disease is of a contagious nature and the lesions are more severe.

Inflammation of the Biflex Canal in Sheep
Biflex canal in sheep is a narrow cutaneous channel in the pastern region which opens downwards about ¼ inch above the interdigital space. Biflex canal is present only in sheep. It is absent in goats.

The biflex canal sometimes gets inflamed due to accumulation of dirt and foreign matter. The inflammation may lead to abscess formation and necrosis.

TREATMENT
On general principles.

Interdigital Cyst or Interdigital Abscess in Dogs

This is fairly common condition in long-haired breeds of dogs like cocker spaniels, golden retriever, Irish setters, etc.

ETIOLOGY

No specific organism has been identified, but the condition is apparently due to bacterial infection.

SYMPTOMS

There is marked pain and the dog lifts and carries the leg during progression. It may frequently lick the affected part. On examination, a reddish cystic swelling is recognised on the paw. If untreated, the cyst ruptures spontaneously in a few days and heals, but may reappear again.

TREATMENT

Open the cyst. Touch with Tincture iodine, or silver nitrate sticks and then apply a bandage.

Fracture of Pes in the Dog

If there is fracture of the phalangeal bones (pes) in the dog, filleting operation may be performed to remove the broken pieces of bone. (See Operative Surgery for details.) (page 575).

Bumble Foot in Poultry

This is characterised by formation of cold abscess on the foot. It is more common in heavy breeds of poultry like R.I.R., Plymouth rock and New Hampshire. Older birds are mostly affected.

ETIOLOGY

Not definitely known. Trauma may be one of the reasons. Mycobacterium tuberculosis, Staphylcocci, etc. have been isolated from the lesions.

TREATMENT

Open the abscess and drain out the pus. Touch the cavity with Tincture iodine. Apply a protective bandage. On subsequent days the wound may be dressed with Mag. Sulph-Glycerine paste or Penicillin-Streptomycin ointment.

Questions

1. Name the diseases of the foot of the horse. Describe one in detail.

2. Discuss the etiology, symptoms, prognosis and treatment of sprained tendons in the horse.

3. Write short notes on: (1) Occult spavin, (2) Down in the hip (see chapter on fractures), (3) Bowed tendon, (4) Pyramidal disease, (5) Sore shins, (6) Bumble foot, (7) Filleting, (8) Side bone, (9) Curb, (10) Racing joint, (11) Seedy toe, (12) Thrush, (13) String halt, (14) Sand crack, (15) Knuckling in calves, (16) Navicular disease, (17) Bog spavin, (18) Foul in the foot, (19) Split pastern, (20) Spondylitis.

4. Discuss the surgical pathology and symptoms of equine laminitis and outline the treatment.

5. How does shivering differ from stringhalt? Give symptoms and treatment of stringhalt.

6. What is tendinitis? In which animal is it common? What treatment would you adopt in a recent case?

7. Define navicular disease. Describe the symptoms, diagnosis and prognosis of the condition.

8. Define the term sprained tendons. Give the etiology, symptoms, treatment, and prognosis.

9. Describe the etiology, symptoms and treatment of acute laminitis in the horse.

10. What is break-down in the horse? What are the structures involved in this condition? Describe the symptoms and treatment briefly.

11. What are the clinical symptoms associated with navicular disease? Describe the surgical pathology and mode of diagnosis?

12. Write an essay on the etiology, incidence and treatment of acute laminitis? What are its sequelae and to what extent could they be overcome?

13. Name the common diseases of the foot of horses and cattle which cause chronic lameness and describe the treatment adopted for navicular diseases in horses and laminitis in cattle.

14. What are the different forms of locomotor disability met with in working animals? Describe the common clinical forms with special reference to differential diagnosis.

15. Discuss the etiology and incidence of ruptured tendons and describe the process of repair under proper surgical management.

16. Describe the etiology and incidence of laminitis in horses and cattle and discuss the sequelae and the value of treatment followed.

17. Name the diseases of the foot of horses and cattle where the symptoms noticed may be considered as typical of acute or chronic inflammation. Describe also the prognosis and treatment of one typical example to represent each of the two clinical groups.

18. Give few examples of clinical forms of osteoarthritis in large animals. State how you will differentiate common forms of osteoperiostitis from the former and describe treatment adopted in both the clinical forms commonly encountered.

19. Write briefly on the pathogenesis of foul in the foot in cattle. Describe the clinical symptoms noticed, diagnostic methods adopted and treatment recommended.

20. Enumerate the various abnormal conformations of the foot which may affect the anti-concussion mechanism. Give a few examples of which such deformities may predispose.

21. What is thrombosis? Give the symptoms, diagnosis and prognosis of iliac thrombosis.

CHAPTER 32

Neurectomy

Neurectomy is the division and removal of a piece of nerve. It is usually done on a sensory nerve to relieve pain. Neurectomy of a nerve (like the median nerve, ulnar nerve, plantar nerve, anterior tibial nerve, posterior tibial nerve, etc.) is indicated in certain cases of lameness in which there is pain. Generally such neurectomies are advisable only in cases of lameness due to chronic conditions which are *not of a septic nature* and which do not respond to any other methods of treatment or in which other methods of treatment are not practicable. The object of neurectomy in such cases is to remove the pain caused to the animal by such diseases and thus provide symptomatic relief of lameness.

Indications

By neurectomy it should be possible to remove pain and to improve the usefulness of the animal. If not, there is no purpose in doing it Neurectomy is thus indicated in certain cases of splints, ring bone, navicular disease, etc. In diseases causing structural alterations in tissues (e.g., laminitis, canker of the foot) neurectomy is *not* likely to be beneficial and is therefore contra-indicated.

Technique

The techniques for various neurectomies are described in Operative Surgery. Neurectomy is generally done under general anaesthesia. If deep anaesthesia is not obtained a local analgesic is in addition injected around the nerve before cutting it. The following points may help to identify the nerve during a neurectomy and differentiate it from a tendon, an artery or a vein. The nerve is striated longitudinally and has pale grey colour unlike a tendon which has a shining white appearance. The nerve can be stretched far outside the wound and when released it may remain limp in the incision. The pulsation and pinkish colour will differentiate an artery from the nerve. A vein has a bluish or purple colour. A blood vessel when lifted with a tenaculum will become pale at the spot due to displacement of blood contained in it.

The nerve is first divided proximally and then distally.

Disadvantages of Neurectomy

1. Oedema may be caused shortly after neurectomy because of the interference with the trophic nerve supply which control the tone of blood vessels. When they are severed local vascular dilation and oedema may be caused. After twenty-four to forty-eight hours the oedema usually subsides due to the setting up of collateral circulation. Massaging of the region may promote quicker establishment of collateral circulation.

2. Degenerative changes. If the oedema persists gelatinous degeneration of tissues in the region may set in which may also cause shedding of the hoof. If the oedema persists for about seven days or more the operation is considered to be a failure because degenerative changes may follow.

3. Since the animal does not feel any pain it is likely to use the limb less carefully and traumatic injuries may be caused.

4. Wounds in the affected region may take a long time to heal because of the lack of adequate blood supply and the oedema.

5. Amputation neuroma. A nodular enlargement called amputation neuroma may be formed at the proximal cut end of the nerve due to the regenerative growth of the nerve fibres from that end. These newly growing fibres just club together because they are unable to reach the distal cut end. Pressure and friction on the amputation neuroma during movement of the part produces pain and lameness. The development of an amputation neuroma can be prevented by properly crushing the cut ends or injecting absolute alcohol $\frac{1}{2}$ to 2 cc into each cut end. (For Neurectomies of different nerves, see pages: 506, 587, 609, 614, 615, 616, 617).

Questions

1. Write short notes on: Amputation neuroma.

2. Define neutectomy. What are the general indications for neurectomy? Describe the general technique, after-treatment and operation.

CHAPTER 33

Surgical Conditions Affecting the Vertebral Column and Spinal Cord

Fracture of the Vertebral Column

Fracture of the vertebral column is of common occurrence in the horse and the condition is spoken of as *broken back*. The last four thoracic and the first three lumbar vertebrae are more commonly involved. The transverse processes, the arches or the bodies of vertebrae may get fractured.

ETIOLOGY

(1) Struggling when cast. (2) The animal falling on its head by accident, for example, during a race. (3) Violent muscular efforts during galloping.

The fracture usually happens when a horse is being cast or subsequently when it struggles after being secured, due to the muscular contractions produced by arching the spine or by bending it laterally. The arching of spine is more likely to happen if the head is not properly controlled while casting. (The head should be held upward.)

The fracture may be noticed only sometime after the animal has got up if it happens to be a *deferred fracture*.

DIAGNOSIS

If there is involvement of the spinal cord due to the fracture, there is complete paralysis posterior to the seat of fracture (paraplegia). Loss of sensation in the paralysed areas may also be noticed. Faeces and urine may be passed involuntarily.

PROGNOSIS

If the dorsal spinous processes of the vertebrae only are fractured recovery may follow. In other cases prognosis is guarded. When paraplegia is present the case is hopeless.

TREATMENT

If a deferred facture is suspected the animal should be tied with a short rope to give rest and to prevent lying down and avoid making the fracture complete. Necrosed pieces of bone, if any, interfering with proper healing may be removed if possible. Euthanasia is advisable in cases with paraplegia.

Intervertebral Disc Disease

(Enchondrosis Intervertebralis; Herniation of the intervertebral disc; Protrusion of the intervertebral disc; Extrusion of the intervertebral disc.)

ANATOMICAL CONSIDERATION

Intervertebral discs are situated between the bodies of adjacent vertebrae. The intervertebral disc is in contact dorsally with the conjugal costarum ligament and the dorsal longitudinal ligament and ventrally with the ventral longitudinal ligament. The dorsal longitudinal ligament stretching over the vertebral bodies is situated along the floor of the vertebral canal and the ventral longitudinal ligament has a similar position on the ventral aspect of the vertebral bodies. In the thoracic region the conjugal costarum ligament connects the heads of the respective pair of ribs on either side and goes across the vertebral canal between the dorsal longitudinal ligament and the respective intervertebral disc. The intervertebral disc has central gelatinous portion called the nucleus pulposus and a peripheral fibrous portion called annulus fibrosus.

Herniation of the intervertebral disc is seen in dogs and cats. It is commonly met with in Dachshunds.

PATHOLOGY

Intervertebral disc disease is a degenerative process of the intervertebral disc involving either the annulus fibrosus or the nucleus pulposus. Degeneration and weakening of the annulus fibrosus causes protrusion of the nucleus pulposus when pressure is exerted on it. The nucleus pulposus bulges upwards through the dorsal longitudinal ligament. This condition is called herniation of the intervertebral disc. Sometimes there is separation of the fibres of the dorsal longitudinal ligament at that point causing extrusion of the nucleus pulposus through the dorsal longitudinal ligament and its escape into the vertebral canal.

ETIOLOGY

Herniation of the disc is caused by the compression of the disc during movements of the vertebral column. The predisposing factor is the degeneration of the annulus fibrosus. Herniation occurs in those portions of the vertebral column which are subjected to maximum movement, viz. the cervical and thoraco-lumbar regions.

SYMPTOMS

The symptoms are caused by the pressure exerted by the protruded portion of the disc on the spinal cord and spinal nerves. Protrusion of the cervical discs (second cervical to the first thoracic) usually exerts only slight pressure on the spinal cord but the pressure on the spinal nerve roots may cause oedema of the nerves. Protrusion of the discs from between first thoracic (T-1) and tenth thoracic (T-10) is not likely to affect the spinal cord because of the presence of the conjugal costarum ligament. The frequency of occurrence of disc protrusions in different regions of. the vertebral column is as follows: *Most frequent*: between eleventh and twelfth thoracic. (T-11 and T-12) and between second and third lumbar (L-2 and L-3). *Less frequent*: between second cervical and first thoracic (C-2 to T-1) and between T-11 to L-5. *Rare*: other regions.

1. *Symptoms of cervical disc protrusions*: There is hypersensitiveness over the neck and forelimbs. The neck is held rigid and the head is kept lowered. Pain is a prominent symptom, especially when the head is manipulated and lifted upwards. The gait is cautious with a slow stilted movement of the limbs. If the spinal cord is involved the flexion reflex and extensor thrust are sluggish in the forelimbs. (Flexion reflex is the reflex flexion of the limb when the web of the foot is pinched. Extensor thrust is the reflex extension of the limb when the foot pad is pressed.)

2. *Symptoms of protrusion of the thoraco-lumbar discs*: The back is arched and there is reluctance to move quickly. Lameness of one or both hind limbs with slight incoordination may be the first symptom noticed. Pain may not be prominent.

Sluggish flexor reflex, extensor thrust and pateller reflex indicate spinal cord involvement. Chronic paraplegia is seen within a few days. Incontinence of urine may be noticed. Paralysis seen in thoraco-lumbar disc protrusions may set in suddenly or only gradually. The bladder and rectum may also be affected causing either incontinence or retention of urine and faeces. Involvement of middle and posterior lumbar discs causes *flaccid* paralysis whereas involvement of anterior lumbar dics causes *spastic* paralysis (=paralysis in extension).

DIAGNOSIS

A radiograph may be taken for confirmation. A lateral view of the vertebral column shows narrowing of the space between vertebral bodies at the seat of disc protrusion.

PROGNOSIS

Guarded. When the symptoms are slow in onset prognosis is generally favourable. Cervical disc protrusions are less serious than thoraco lumbar disc protrusions.

TREATMENT

Administration of corticosteroid, massage, electrotherapy, and other general treatment for paralysis. Surgical treatment consists of making a dorsal approach to vertebral canal and the removal of the protruding portion of the pulpus nucleosus either by performing *a laminectomy* or *hemilaminectomy*, or by *fenestration* of the intervertebral disc through a thoraco-abdominal approach. Laminectomy is the removal of the dorsal spinous process with its *laminae* on either side, of the concerned vertebra of the intervertebral disc. Hemilaminectomy is removal of the laminae of one side only.

Ossifying Pachymeningitis of Dogs

This is a condition characterised by progressive ossification of the spinal cord.

INCIDENCE

The disease is met with in aged dogs; mostly in large breeds like Grea` Danes, Collies, Alsations (German shepherds).

SYMPTOMS

Initially there is stiffness of the spine and weakness. There is flexion of the head and hypersensitiveness of one or both forelimbs. Progressive paralysis develops within a few months. Muscular atrophy is common. Retention of urine or incontinence of urine occurs late in the course of the disease.

TREATMENT

Treatment is of little benefit. Euthanasia is advised.

Spondylitis

This is a chronic type of arthritis and anchylosis affecting the vertebral column. Met with in cattle, dog and horse. The articular cartilages situated between the vertebrae (inter-vertebral discs) get degenerated and destroyed and fibrous adhesions are formed between adjacent vertebral bodies. These fibrous adhesions are later converted into bony fusion due to a proliferative type of osteo-periostitis resulting in anchylosis of vertebral joints. The exostoses that are formed exert pressure on the spinal cord. The joints affected in spondylitis are usually of the loin region.

SYMPTOMS

The first symptom noticed is stiffening of the muscles of the back and hind limbs. The hind limbs are rigid for a few seconds when the animal starts to move and the toe is dragged along the ground for a short distance. Then the limb is suddenly jerked forward. After a few steps the gait becomes normal. Within about a year the symptoms become more severe (the stiffness in the limbs remaining for a longer period) and is later on followed by complete paralysis of the hind limbs.

PROGNOSIS

Unfavourable.

TREATMENT

No satisfactory treatment.

Torticollis

Torticollis or distortion of the neck is sometimes seen in the horse due to the animal falling with the head and neck under the body. There may be subluxation of one or more joints of certain cervical vertebrae or spasm of certain cervical muscles. Unilateral paralysis of some of the muscles in the region of the neck may also be present. The head is kept lowered, slightly twisted and turned to a side. There is also severe pain in the initial stage.

Correction of the subluxation, if any, can be attempted after the local inflammation and pain subsides to a certain extent. Splints can be applied on either side of the neck by way of immobilisation.

Kyphosis (*Roach Back*)

Kyphosis is an upward curvature of the vertebral column.

Scoliosis

Scoliosis is a curvature of the vertebral column to a side.

Questions

1. Write short notes on: (1) Spondylitis, (2) Ossifying pachymeningitis.
2. Give a brief account of "herniation of the disc" in dogs.

CHAPTER 34

Hernia

A *hernia* is the protrusion of an organ or tissue through an opening. The opening may be one caused by a tear in the abdominal wall or diaphragm or it may be a natural opening like the inguinal canal or femoral canal. A hernia is different from a prolapse. In a prolapse the protruded tissue is exposed outside whereas in a hernia it is covered by the skin.

ETIOLOGY

Predisposing causes: (1) Imperfect closure of an embryonic defect, e.g. imperfect closure of umbilicus predisposing to an umbilical hernia, imperfect formation of the diaphragm predisposing to a diaphragmatic hernia. (2) Weakness of the abdominal wall due to contusions, local inflammation, etc.

Exciting causes: (1) Increase in the intra-abdominal pressure due to straining from constipation, diarrhoea, during parturition, violent coughing, gastric or intestinal tympany. (2) Direct violence due to falling on a blunt object.

PARTS OF HERNIA

A typical hernia has a *hernial ring,* through which the contents have migrated and the *hernial* sac. The *hernial sac* encloses the *hernial contents* and consists of the neck, body and fundus. The neck is that portion of the hernial sac close to the hernial ring, the fundus is the lowest part and the body is the portion between the fundus and neck. The hernial sac is formed by the parietal peritoneum.

Portions of visceral organs (e.g., intestines, omentum, liver, spleen, bladder, uterus) usually form the hernial contents. The sac may sometimes be empty.

CLASSIFICATION

1. A hernia may be congenital (=present at birth) or acquired;

2. It may be external, internal or interstitial. In an external hernia the contents have protruded through the abdominal wall and come close to the skin. In internal hernia the contents have moved from one body cavity into another (e.g. diaphragmatic hernia). In interstitial hernia the contents are situated between the abdominal muscles. An external hernia may sometimes have an interstitial diverticulum.

3. According to the location a hernia may be called: Umbilical hernia; Inguinal hernia; Scrotal hernia; Diaphragmatic hernia; Perineal hernia; Ventral hernia; Femoral hernia; etc.

4. According to the hernial contents: Enterocele (containing portion of intestines); Epiplocele or Omentocele (of omentum), Enteroepiplocele (of intestine and omentum); Gastrocele (of stomach); Vesicocele (of bladder); Hepatocele (of liver); Hysterocele (of uterus); etc.

5. *Reducible* hernia or Irreducible hernia, according to reducibility or not of contents: A hernia may become irreducible because of adhesions, incarceration or strangulation.

SYMPTOMS

Physical symptoms include presence of the hernial swelling. The swelling varies in size and shape. On manipulation it has a characteristic consistency depending on the contents. For example, the consistency is elastic in enterocele and doughy in epiplocele. The swelling may increase in size while coughing. *Functional symptoms* are ordinarily absent in reducible hernia. Colic is seen in incarcerated hernia. Severe pain, rise of temperature and colic are pronounced in strangulated hernia.

DIAGNOSIS

1. By palpating the hernial ring in reducible hernias. In the case of umbilical hernia, the hernial ring can be easily felt if the animal is placed in dorsal recumbency and palpated.

2. By the nature of its contents. Auscultation will reveal

gurgling or bubonic sound in an enterocele. On palpation the contents feel doughy in epiplocele while enterocele will have an elastic consistency.

DIFFERENTIAL DIAGNOSIS
A hernia should be differentiated from abscess, tumour, haematoma and cyst. Abscess, tumour, and cyst develop slowly whereas a hernia is of sudden occurrence. In a developing abscess there are symptoms of local inflammation and it does not fluctuate under the skin. An abscess has a tendency to point. In cold abscess the contents may crepitate when the pus is inspissated. In a haematoma the collection of blood may feel like free fluid or may give a slight crepitating sound on palpation. A cyst fluctuates uniformly and has no tendency to point and pain and functional symptoms are absent. The presence of a hernial ring confirms a hernia. Exploratory puncture and/or radiography may also be done for confirmation.

PROGNOSIS
Guarded. Prognosis is favourable in many cases when properly treated. Congenital hernias like umbilical and inguinal hernias may disappear spontaneously within one year after birth.

POSSIBLE CHANGES IN A HERNIA
The following changes may occur in a case of hernia: (1) Adhesions, (2) Hydrocele of the sac, (3) Incarceration, (4) Torsion and (5) Strangulation.
1. *Adhesion*: Adhesion may take place between the sac and contents, making reduction difficult or impossible. The fibrous tissue poliferation close to the hernial ring may cause constriction due to cicatrical contractions.
2. *Hydrocele of the sac*: Collection of fluid within the sac (hydrocele) is caused by exudations from the hernial contents. A constricted hernial ring favours such exudations.
3. *Incarceration*: An incarcerated hernia is a hernia wherein the hernial contents have become very voluminous so that they cannot be reduced. For example an enterocele may become incarcerated either due to more and more of intestinal, segments entering into the hernial sac or as a result of accumulation of

intestinal contents (food materials) within the lumen of the herniated segment. The accumulating food materials become hard masses as water gets absorbed from them and these hard masses make reduction of hernia very difficult. They may also cause partial or complete obstruction of the bowel segment and thus favour further accumulation of food materials.

4. *Torsion*: Torsion or twisting of the hernial contents within the hernial sac interferes with the blood supply to the tissue and may lead on to gangrene, toxaemia etc.

5. *Strangulation*: Compression caused by the hernial ring causing interference with the blood supply to the hernial contents is called strangulation of a hernia. When a hernia is strangulated soon after the time of its occurrence it is spoken of as an *acute hernia*, e.g., strangulated inguinal hernia in race horses.

A hernia gets strangulated due to constriction of the hernial ring which may also be due to additional contents being pushed into the hernial sac. In a strangulated hernia the constriction at the hernial ring interferes with blood supply to the hernial contents (and if it is an enterocele retention of bowel contents). The vascular compression at the hernial ring interferes with the blood supply and venous drainage and causes congestion and oedema. The oedematous portion of bowel has a deep blue colour due to venous congestion. Blood and mucous escape into the lumen and blood-stained effusions take place from the peritoneal surface. Gangrene sets in gradually and the hernial contents appear black and the peritoneum loses its shining lusture. Pathogenic organism from the gut pass through the intestinal wall and death happens from toxaemia/septicaemia/peritonitis.

GENERAL PRINCIPLES OF TREATMENT FOR HERNIA

1. *Reduction and retention by bandage*: The hernia is reduced by local manipulation and bandage is applied around the abdomen to prevent its return. An "elastoplast" bandage is better to avoid interference with breathing. The bandage is retained for two to three weeks.

This method of treatment is effective in some cases of umbilical hernia.

2. Application of blisters or injection of irritant solutions close to the hernial ring after reducing the hernia causes inflammatory swelling which is sometimes sufficient to prevent recur-

HERNIA 279

rence of a small hernia and to facilitate closure of the hernial orifice. The solutions commonly employed for the purpose are Sodium chloride 5% to 15%, Zinc chloride 5% to 10%.

3. A ligature or a hernia clamp or a set of through-and-through mattress sutures may be applied at the base of the hernial sac after reducing the hernia to facilitate sloughing of the sac and simultaneous closure of the hernial ring. This method also may not be effective in some cases.

4. *Radical operation for hernia*: The hernial sac is incised and the hernial contents are returned through the hernial ring. The hernial sac is ligatured at its neck, amputated, and its stump is pushed through hernial ring. The borders of the hernial ring are then freshened and sutured together and closed. Suturing of the hernial ring is called *herniorrhaphy*. If the hernial ring is very large suturing its edges is not possible. In such cases *hernioplasty* is performed by covering the gap with facia lata or stainless steel wire-mesh and suturing it to the borders. After closing the hernial ring the skin edges are also sutured, after removing any excess skin.

HERNIAS ENCOUNTERED IN ANIMALS

1. *Umbilical hernia*: In foals, pigs, calves, and pups.
2. *Ventral hernia.* Horses and cattle.
3. *Inguinal hernia*: Bitches, horses, bulls, and male and female pigs.
4. *Diaphragmatic hernia*: Pups, adult dogs, and horses.
5. *Perineal hernia*: Uncastrated, old, male dogs.
6. *Pelvic hernia (Gut tie)*: Bullocks (steers).
7. *Femoral hernia (Crural hernia)*: Not common in animals.

In *cattle* umbilical hernia and ventral hernia are more common. Inguinal hernia and gut-tie in bullocks are met with only occasionally. Other hernias are very rare. Similarly, the frequency of occurrence in other species are: *Horses*—Umbilical hernia, Inguinal hernia, and Ventral hernia; *Dogs*—Umbilical hernia in pups, Perineal hernia in male dogs, and Diaphragmatic hernia. *Pigs*—Umbilical hernia and Inguinal hernia.

Umbilical Hernia (*Omphalocele; Exomphalos*)

A hernia situated in the umbilical region. The contents usually consist of omentum or intestines.

INCIDENCE

Occurs in all domestic animals, more commonly in foals; pigs, calves and pups.

ETIOLOGY

Predisposing cause: Usually congenital. Imperfect closure of the umbilicus. *Exciting causes:* compression of the abdomen during birth, straining due to constipation or diarrhoea.

DIAGNOSIS

Hernial swelling at the umbilicus. Differentiate from abscess, haematoma, urachal cyst due to persistent urachus (pervious urachus), etc. The hernia can be usually reduced after putting the animal on its back and then the hernial ring can be felt.

TREATMENT

(1) In the case of foals and calves below one year and puppies below six months spontaneous recovery may take place when the animal grows. Recovery may be accelerated by reducing the contents and putting an "elastoplast" bandage. In favourable cases the hernial ring closes up within two to three weeks. Laxative diet is preferable during this period to prevent any straining due to constipation. (2) Other methods of treatment like injection of irritant solutions, ligation and application of clamp, etc. may be tried as already described. An aluminium clamp with leather straps is used in calves. (3) Radical operation is advised for cases which are not likely to respond to the above methods of treatment. The operation is preferably done under general anaesthesia. The skin over the hernia is incised by an elliptical or linear incision: (If the peritoneal sac is present it is separated from the skin by blunt dissection. Then incise through the peritoneum.) The contents are reduced through the hernial ring and the edges of the ring are freshened and sutured. If the hernial ring is circular, suturing is made easier by removing a triangular piece of tissue from either end and converting it into an elliptical shape. "*Double breasting*" is sometimes prefered for closing the hernial opening. This is done by suturing the respective pairs of superficial and deep muscle sheaths of the rectus abdominis muscle so that the muscle bellies of either side will

slightly overlap each other at this point. Another method of suturing the hernial ring is by "overlapping stitches". If the edges cannot be brought together a piece of sterile stainless steel wire mesh cut to the required size and shape can be sutured and fixed in position to cover the gap of the hernial ring.

After the hernial ring has been properly closed the skin edges are also sutured, after removing any excess skin.

Inguinal Hernia (*Bubonocele*) (Bubon. Gr. =groin)

[The *inguinal canal* is an oblique passage through the poste-. rior part of the abdominal wall between the two oblique muscles. The entrance into the inguinal canal from the abdominal cavity is called the *internal inguinal ring* (abdominal inguinal ring) and the outer opening of the canal is called the *external inguinal ring* (subcutaneous inguinal ring). The internal inguinal ring is bounded anteriorly by the thin margin of the internal oblique muscle and behind by the inguinal ligament (Poupart's ligament). The external inguinal ring is a slit-like opening lateral to the prepubic tendon in the aponeurosis of the obliqus Abdominis Externus muscle. The inguinal canal in the male contains the spermatic cord, tunica vaginalis, the external cremaster muscle, the external pudic artery (and inconstantly a small satellite vein) and the inguinal lymph vessels and nerves. In female it contains the external pudic vessels and nerves. In the bitch it also lodges the round ligament of the uterus. The internal inguinal ring is longer than the external and is directed from the lateral edge of the prepubic tendon towards the tuber coxa. Its length is about 6 to 7 inches in the horse. The external inguinal ring is directed from the edge of the prepubic tendon outward, forward and slightly ventrally. Its length is about 4 to 5 inches in the horse.]

An *inguinal hernia* is the passage of part of the abdominal viscera (usually omentum or intestine) into the inguinal canal.

If a hernia occurs not through the inguinal canal, but through a tear in the abdominal wall close to the inguinal canal, it is spoken of as an *atypical inguinal hernia*.

If the contents of an inguinal hernia have come up to the scrotal sac a *scrotal hernia* (Oscheocele) results.

INCIDENCE

Common in the bitch than in other animals. Also met with in castrated horses, stallions, bulls, and male and female pigs.

ETIOLOGY

The hernia is usually congenital. *Possible exciting cause*: accidental slipping causing stretching of the hind limbs outwards which may dilate the inguinal canal.

SYMPTOMS

The hernial swelling, if small, may not be recognised easily. In small animals it is better to examine after raising the forelimbs making the animal stand on hind legs.

Abduction of the hind limbs is one of the symptoms and is called *broad stepping*. When inguinal hernia occurs in horses during racing the animal suddenly stops and evinces severe pain. The testicle of the affected side is seen pulled upwards due to contraction of cremaster muscle. Due to the pain the animal frequently makes kicking movements with the limb of the affected side. This is described as the animal trying to "kick off the pain". In acute cases severe colicy pains are envinced. In chronic cases of scrotal hernia the corresponding testicle becomes atrophied due to pressure. Stallions and bulls used for breeding purpose are reluctant to serve. In bitches there may be difficulty in defecation as more of the visera gets pushed through the hernial sac during straining.

PROGNOSIS

Congenital hernias occurring in young animals often disappear within one year. When surgical treatment is properly conducted prognosis is generally favourable. Prognosis is guarded or unfavourable when the hernia is the strangulated type.

DIAGNOSIS

The hernial swelling is recognised close to or including the scrotum. The swelling can be easily differentiated from a sarcocele (=a hard tumour of the testicle), hydrocele, cyst, enlarged lymph node, scirrhous cord, etc. A sarcocele is a hard swelling on the testicle. The characteristic wave-like feeling of fluid in hydrocele is different from the feeling of hernial contents.

Drawing up of the testicle of the affected side accompanied by symptoms of continuous abdominal pain, is an almost pathognomonic sign of strangulation of an inguinal hernia. In large animals diagnosis may be confirmed by rectal examination and in small animals by radiography or fluoroscopy.

TREATMENT

(i) *Treatment of small animals* (e.g., bitch): In the bitch the uterus or the urinary bladder usually forms the content of the inguinal hernia. The uterus (if the animal is not pregnant or is only in the early stage of gestation) may be reduced and a supporting bandage may be put to prevent recurrence of the hernia. Reduction of the urinary bladder is quite easy if the urine is aspirated.

The radical (surgical) treatment consists of performing laparotomy either through the linea alba or through a paramedian or pararectal incision close to the hernia. The hernial contents are reduced by gentle pressure from outside, combined with traction exerted with fingers introduced through the incision. Afterwards the torn portion of the inguinal ring is sutured. If necessary, ventropexy (hysteropexy or cystopexy as the case may be) may be done to prevent recurrence. Fixing portion of any abdominal organ to the abdominal wall is called *ventropexy*. The fixation can be easily done with one or two sutures.

For completing the operation for hernia the laparotomy wound is closed in the usual manner.

(2) *Treatment in large animals* (e.g., horse): Expectant treatment for congential hernia in young animals below one year unless there is strangulation or incarceration. Castraction by the covered method in the case of male animals not needed for breeding purpose. The spermatic cord (with its tunics) is ligatured and severed after reducing the hernial contents. The cut stump is then pushed as far up into the inguinal canal as possible. The inguinal canal and scrotum are then packed with sterile gauze and retention sutures are put on the skin. The gauze packings will cause local inflammatory swelling and will thus prevent any prolapse of viscera. The gauze packs are removed after twenty-four to forty-eight hours.

(3) In male animals that are to be used for breeding, the operation is done as follows. Incise the skin close to the external

ring and expose portion of the tunica vaginalis containing the spermatic cord and the hernial content. Reduce the hernia and put purse-string suture around the tunica vaginalis as far high as possible in order to prevent return of the hernial contents, and to constrict the lumen of the tunica. vaginalis so as to make it sufficient for the passage of the spermatic cord only. The skin incision is closed as usual. If there is difficulty in reducing the hernia during the course of this operation, the hernial ring (i.e., the ingunial ring) may be enlarged with a curved scalpel properly directed and protected with fingers or with a herniotome. Afterwards the enlarged portion can be sutured. The knife should be turned outward and forward, care being taken to avoid injury to the external pudic artery. Enlarging of a hernial ring is called "kelotomy". A portion of omentum that is difficult to be reduced can better be amputated; reduction of an enterocele is made easier by aspirating accumulation of gas in it or sometimes by enterotomy.

Diaphragmatic Hernia in Dogs

A diaphragmatic hernia is caused by the passage of abdominal viscera into the thoracic cavity, through a tear or a congenital defect in the diaphragm.

INCIDENCE

Diaphragmatic hernia is very rare in animals. It is seen in dogs more frequently than in other species. (Diaphragmatic hernia in buffaloes is stated to be common in some northern parts of India.)

ANATOMICAL CONSIDERATIONS

The diaphragm is a muscular partition between the thoracic and abdominal cavities. It is attached to the 8 to 13th ribs at their costochondral junctions and to the sublumbar region by its crura. The central areas of the diaphragm are tendinous. The posterior aorta, posterior vena cava and the oesophagus pass through it. Herniation is usually noticed close to these structures or at the costal attachments of the diaphragm. The weakest portion of the diaphragm where it gets torn is close to the posterior vena cava, because the vein collapses when the part is subjected to pressure. The costal margin constitutes another weak portion. The portion close to the oesophagus constitutes the third weak portion. The abdominal organs in contact with the diaphragm are the liver and the stomach. Liver of the dog is in contact with the entire right side and part of the left side of the diaphragm. The left dorsal portion of the diaphragm is related to the stomach. The hernial content is usually portion of omentum, stomach or liver; very rarely the intestines. The extent of herniation depends on the size and location of the tear. Sometimes there is gradual development of a hernia through a small tear, due to the negative pressure in the thoracic cavity, the bellowing action of the abdomen during respiration and due to the peristalsis of the digestive tract.

ETIOLOGY
1. Due to a congenital defect in the diaphragm. 2. Due to trauma e.g., getting run over by an automobile, falling from a height, etc.

SYMPTOMS
In congenital cases the symptoms may not be noticed until the pup is about six months old and starts feeding on solid foods. Abdominal breathing, peculiar cough, tendency to tire easily, unthriftiness, tucked up abdomen and tendency to vomit after feeding, are seen. Other symptoms are: The animal is unwilling to move and remains most of the time in the standing or "sitting on the haunches" position. Difficulty and pain while walking down from a height. Chronic stomach disorders. Respiratory distress if the stomach is full and is causing pressure on the lungs. When the chest is ausculcated gurgling sounds may be heard. Cardiac sounds may be subdued or misplaced either forward or to the side. Respiratory sounds may be absent on the affected side. Immediately after feeding the respiratory distress is more pronounced. Conditions like hydrothorax aspiration-pneumonia, cardiac diseases, foreign body in the oesphagus etc. which may also cause respiratory distress must be eliminated in arriving at a diagnosis.

DIAGNOSIS
A lateral and a ventro-dorsal radiograph of the thorax may help confirm the diagnosis.

TREATMENT

Surgical treatment. After reducing the hernia the tear in the diaphragm is sutured. There are two methods of approach to the diaphragm, viz., the thoracic approach and abdominal approach. In either of these methods it is necessary to provide positive pressure ventilation of the lungs. For this, a cuffed endotracheal tube (*Magill's endotracheal tube*) is introduced into the trachea and the tube is then connected to a respiratory pump. The volume and rate of air entering the lungs can be adjusted according to necessity. (See also chapter on thoracotomy in this book.)

Thoracic approach. The sixth or seventh intercostal site may be chosen, starting a little lateral to the sternum and extending dorsally for about 2 to 3 inches. (see also thoracotomy page 296).

On entering the thoracic cavity care is taken to prevent injury to lungs. The wound edges are retracted by proper retractors. The respiration pump is so adjusted that the lungs will be inflated to only about half their normal capacity. The hernia is reduced and the tear in the diaphragm is sutured with No. 1 chromic catgut. Closure of the intercostal incision is made by placing sutures around adjacent ribs. When the intercostal wound is sutured in this manner, the negative pressure in the pleural cavity should be re-established. This is achieved by inflating the lungs to their full capacity immediately before tying the last intercostal suture. The skin edges are united by apposition sutures.

Abdominal approach: After establishing positive ventilation of the lungs, a laparotomy incision is made through the linea alba from a little behind the Xiphoid cartilage towards the umbilicus. The hernia is reduced, the tear in the diaphragm is sutured and the abdominal wound is closed in the usual manner. Before disconnecting the respiration pump air in the pleural cavity is aspirated to re-establish the negative pressure. This is done by introducing a proper sized inoculation needle through the intercostal space and using a 50 c.c. syringe.

"Gut Tie" in Bullocks*

This type of hernia is formed by the passage of a portion of

---

* *Intra-abdominal hernia; Pelvic hernia; Peritoneal hernia.*

intestine either through a tear in the fold of serous membrane suspending the spermatic cord in the sublumbar region or through a "hernial ring-like" passage formed between the spermatic cord and the lateral abdominal wall by the adhesion of the cut end of the spermatic cord to the abdominal wall.

INCIDENCE
In bullocks only. A very rare condition.

ETIOLOGY
The adhesion of the cut end of the spermatic cord to the abdominal wall after castration predisposes to herniation. The hernia occurs only on the *right* side, the occurrence on the left side being prevented by the presence of rumen.

SYMPTOMS
Clinical symptoms are usually absent unless there is strangulation. When there is strangulation the animal becomes uneasy and shows signs of intestinal obstruction and colic. (Frequent lying down and getting up, looking towards the flank, attempting defecation, etc.) Small pellets of faeces or simply mucous, may be passed. In some cases the symptoms are noticed for a few days followed by spontaneous relief but recurring after a variable period.

DIAGNOSIS
Pain is evinced if pressure is exerted on the right flank. The herniated portion of bowel may be palpated per rectum. It gives the characteristic feeling of distended bowel wall and can be palpated close to the pelvic inlet, on the right side. The tensely stretched abdominal portion of the spermatic cord on the medial aspect of it also can be palpated.

PROGNOSIS
Guarded. When there is strangulation prognosis is unfavourable.

TREATMENT
By making the animal jump down from a height or by

making it walk rapidly down a steep incline, the herniated
bowel may sometimes get reduced. Manipulation per rectum
may also be tried. The rational method of treatment is to
perform laparotomy and cut the portion of the spermatic cord
to release the herniated bowel. The right flank (para-lumbar
fossa) is the site chosen for laparotomy. The hand is introduced
through the laparotomy wound and the spermatic cord is severed
with a protected knife like the *Ankers scalpel* (a curved, blunt-
pointed knife with a long handle). The laparotomy incision is
closed in the usual manner.

Perineal Hernia in Dogs

Perineal hernia is seen in old, uncastrated male dogs. It is
caused by the protrusion of viscera through a defect in the
supporting structures of the pelvic outlet. The supporting structures of the pelvic outlet are together spoken of as the pelvic
diaphragm. The pelvic diaphragm is constituted by the medial
coccygeal muscle, the sphincter ani muscles, the obturator internus
muscle and the perineal facia. The medial coccygeal
muscle (Ilio-schio-pubo-coccygeus muscle) originates from the
shaft of ilium, ischeum and pubis and is inserted on to the ventral
aspect of the first few coccygeal vertebrae. It is a fan-shaped
muscle. The obturator internus muscle originates from the floor
of the pelvis around the obturator foramen. The sphincter ani
internus muscles surround the anal opening.

The tear through which herniation occurs is actually caused
by the separation of adjacent muscles, viz., the posterior border
of medial coccygeus, the sphincter ani internus and obturator-
internus.

The hernia may occur on one or both sides. (Unilateral or
bilateral hernia.) The hernial contents are usually covered only
by the perineal facia and the skin as the hernia is often
retroperitoneal. The contents may be any of the following: (1)
the retroperitoneal areolar and fatty tissue, the appearance of
which in a chronic case may resemble omentum; (2) a
diverticulum of the rectum; (3) the prostate; and (4) the urinary
bladder.

ETIOLOGY

Uncastrated male dogs are predisposed to this type of hernia. The exciting factor is straining. Chronic constipation, diarrhoea and enlargement of anal glands are certain conditions which might cause straining.

SYMPTOMS

A fluctuating swelling is noticed lateral to the anus, in the region between the base of the tail and the tuber ischii. The swelling may be seen on one or both sides. It may disappear temporarily when manipulated locally after raising the animal from behind. Systemic disturbances are rare. If the bladder is included in the hernia there may be retention of urine due to kinking of the urethra and symptoms of uraemia are noticed. Exploratory puncture will confirm the presence of the bladder.

TREATMENT

Surgical repair is performed under general anaesthesia. The dog is laid on the operation table in the ventral recumbent position with the hind part raised by cushions or by small sand bag pillows. The anus is temporarily closed by pursestring sutures.

After cleaning and preparing the site, a sufficiently long cutaneous incision is made on the hernial swelling from below the base of the tail towards the tuber ischeii. The skin edges are retracted and the perineal facia is incised. At about the junction of the lower and middle third of the incision the internal pudic vessels and nerve are recognised as a cord. This cord may be ligatured as this will facilitate easier manipulation of deeper structures during the operation. However, when the operation is to be done on both sides see that this neurovascular cord is severed only on one side because if cutting is done on both sides paralysis of the rectum may be caused.

Reduce the hernia. Recognise the gap in the pelvic diaphragm which forms the hernial ring. The hernial ring, perineal facia and the skin are sutured separately as follows in three layers.

Suturing the hernial ring: The suturing is started from above by uniting the posterior border of the medial coccygeus muscle to the sphincter ani internus muscle. This suturing is continued up to about the 3 O'clock position and thereafter the sutures are placed to unite the sphincter muscle to the medial surface of the sacro-sciatic ligament up to about 4 or 5 o' clock position. Beyond this the sutures are placed uniting the internal sphincter muscle to the obturator internus muscle on the pelvic floor, and completed.

Suturing the perineal facia: The lateral cut edge of the perineal facia is sutured on to the border of the sphincter ani-externus muscle.

Suturing the skin: The skin edges are united after removing the excess skin, if any.

Note: The sutures of perineal facia and skin may be combined, if so desired.

The purse string suture on the anus is removed. If the suturing is not done correctly the anus will appear pulled towards a side. Castration is advisable to prevent recurrence of hernia. *Cystopexy* may be done, if necessary in the case of a vesicocele. This is done by fixing the urinary bladder to an incision on the linea alba. Similarly, *rectopexy* (fixing the rectal wall to the flank) can be done if the rectum has herniated. For fixing an organ to the abdominal wall one or more sutures are placed through the wall of the organ (without including its mucus coat) and through the parietal peritoneum and abdominal muscles. *Ventropexy* (cystopexy, rectopexy, etc.) is, however, necessary only in hernias that are likely to re-occur.

Ventral Hernia

A ventral hernia is caused by the migration of viscera through a tear in the abdominal wall. (Even if the hernia is situated on the lateral aspect of abdomen it is called a ventral hernia.) The rupture of prepubic tendon is also a ventral hernia.

INCIDENCE

More commonly met with in cattle and horses. In horses, they occur usually close to the ribs.

ETIOLOGY

(1) External violences. e.g., kicks, blows, horn thrusts due to butting by cattle, falling on blunt objects, etc. (2) Increased

intra-abdominal pressure as may occur during later stages of pregnancy or parturition, tympanitis etc.

SYMPTOMS

The hernial swelling is very prominent. Systemic symptoms are usually absent. The contents of the hernia are usually omentum or intestines or both. The hernia may be reducible or irreducible. Strangulation is rare in ventral hernias.

DIAGNOSIS

Diagnosis is easy as the hernial ring can be felt in most cases.

PROGNOSIS

Guarded.

TREATMENT

Measures like application of bandages are rarely successful. Application of clamps and ligatures may be helpful in a few cases where the hernial ring is small. Radical operation is not always effective because of the hernial ring being very large, or due to the chance of rupture of the scar tissue.

Radical operation: The operation is performed under general anaesthesia. Pre-operative starving of the patient for twenty-four to thirty-six hours is necessary. After preparation of the skin in the usual manner, an elliptical or linear cutaneous incision is made. The skin edges are retracted and are separated from the peritoneal sac up to the hernial ring. The hernial contents are reduced. The peritoneal sac is ligatured (or sutured) close to the hernial ring and is amputated distal to the ligature. The ligatured stump after amputation is pushed into the abdomen. The hernial ring is freshened and sutured preferably by overlapping sutures. The skin is sutured by vertical mattress suture.

Post-operative-care: Over distension of the abdomen is prevented by moderate feeding and a laxative diet. Rest for a few months after the operation is necessary. Tear of the scar tissue during parturition and re-occurrence of the hernia sometimes happen in cows.

Crural Hernia (*Femoral Hernia*)

This is a very rare condition in veterinary practice. It is recognised as a swelling on the inner aspect of the thigh between the sartorious and gracilis muscles due to the protrusion of abdominal viscera through the femoral canal.

The contents protrude between the Pouparts ligament and sartorious muscles, lifting the facia covering the sartorius and gracilis muscles.

ANATOMICAL CONSIDERATIONS

The upper or abdominal opening of the femoral canal (the femoral ring) lies behind the internal inguinal ring and is bounded posteriorily by the anterior border of pubis and laterally by the tendon of Psoas minor muscle.

The femoral canal is bounded anteriorly by the sartorius, posteriorly by the pectineus and laterally by the ilio-psoas and vastus medialis. Its medial wall is formed by the femoral facia and the gracilis.

The muscles referred to are briefly described below.

1. *Psoas minor*: Origin: Bodies of the last three thoracic and first four or five lumber vertebrae and the vertebral ends of sixteenth and seventeenth ribs. Insertion: The psoas tubercle on the shaft of ilium.

2. *Ilio-psoas* (Psoas major and lliacus muscles combined):

(a) *Psoas major*: Origin: Ventral surface of transverse processes of lumbar vertebrae. Insertion: Trochanteric minor of femur by a common tendon with iliacus muscle.

(b) *Iliacus*: Origin: Ventral surface of ilium. Insertion: Trochanteric minor of femur by a common tendon with Psoas major.

3. *Sartorius*: Origin: Iliac facia and tendon of Psoas minor. Insertion: Medial patellar ligament and the tuberosity of tibia.

4. *Gracilis*: Origin: Middle third of pelvic symphysis, the prepubic tendon and accessory ligament and ventral surface of pubis behind the prepubic tendon. Insertion: The medial patellar ligament, medial surface of the crural facia.

5. *Pectinius*: Origin: Prepubic tendon, accessory ligament and anterior border of pubis. Insertion: Middle and medial border of femur near the nutrient foramen.

6. *Vastus medialis*: Origin: Medial surface of the femur, from

its neck to the distal third. Insertion: The medial border of the patella and its cartilage and the proximal part of the medial patellar ligament, tendon of Rectus femoris.

7. *Inguinal ligament*: Inserted to the pubis close to the insertion of the prepubic tendon and also to the tuber coxa.

SYMPTOMS

Interference with the normal gait of the animal. The affected limb is carried forward in an abducted fashion during progression. i.e., circumduction is noticed.

TREATMENT

Not usually attempted. Radical operation can be done. The skin is incised over the swelling and to facilitate reduction the incision may be extended upward, if necessary. Care is necessary to prevent injury to the femoral vessels. After return of contents into the abdomen re-herniation is prevented by suturing Poupart's (Inguinal) ligament to the Sartorious muscle.

Questions

1. Describe the etiology, symptoms, treatment and prognosis of perineal hernia in the dog.
2. Write an account of gut-tie in cattle.
3. Define hernia. Describe the symptoms and treatment of an irreducible adherent umbilical hernia in a calf of eighteen months.
4. Describe the surgical technique, including anaesthetic used for the treatment of scrotal hernia in the bull.
5. Write an essay on abdominal hernia in animals with special reference to classification, incidence and treatment.
6. Classify hernias. Describe the incidence of external hernia in the dog and the line of treatment for inguinal hernia in the female of the species.
7. Describe the relative incidence of umbilical and inguinal hernia in calves and dogs. Describe the line of treatment for umbilical hernia in grown up heifer calves.
8. Name the surgical affections of new-born calves and foals. Briefly indicate their symptoms and suggest suitable remedial measures.

CHAPTER 35

Thoracotomy in Small Animals

Thoracotomy is the opening of the thorax for surgical interference.

Sites

1. *Intercostal site*: Commonly done for diaphragmatic hernia at sixth intercostal site (i.e., between the sixth and seventh rib).

2. *Intercostal site, with resection of adjacent ribs*: Resection of adjacent ribs is done to get better retraction of the thoracotomy wound. One of the ribs is cut in level with the lower commissure of the intercostal wound and the other rib in level with the upper commissure of the wound.

3. *Transverse thoracic or "trans-thoracic" site*: This is done along the ventral aspect, cutting across the sternum and the incision extending through corresponding intercostal spaces of either side. The two vessels running parallel to the sternum on either side (namely, the internal thoracic artery and vein of each side), should be ligatured prior to cutting the sternum.

Technique

Before discussing the technique for throracotomy, it is necessary to understand as to what happens when the pleural sac is opened.

1. *Collapse of the lung of that particular side*: In the normal states, as there is no air in the pleural cavity, the alveoli of the lungs are in close contact with the chest wall because the pressure of air inside the lungs keeps the lungs distended. The tendency of the lungs to collapse on account of its natural elasticity is counteracted by the pressure of air inside the lungs. When the pleural sac is opened, air enters the pleural cavity, and this counteracts the force of air inside the lungs. The force on

account of natural elasticity of lungs is, therefore, not counteracted by force of air inside the lungs and the result is collapse of the lung.

Note: In the dog, even though the mediastinum separating the right and left side is complete, the entry of air into the pleural sac of one side also affects the lung of the other side because the mediastinum is very thin. In the horse the mediastinum is incomplete and there is free communication between the pleural cavities of both sides. In cattle, the mediastinum is complete and firm and the opening of pleural sac of one side do not seriously affect the functioning of the lung of the other side.

When the lung collapses, most of the blood which normally reaches the lungs from the heart (through the pulmonary artery) passes on the pulmonary vein, without getting a proper chance for oxygenation in the lungs. This is called *pulmonary arterio-venous shunting*.

2. *Mediastinal movement*: During inspiration, the mediastinum moves towards the unopened side of the thorax due to entry of atmospheric air through the wound in the thorax and on expiration it moves in the opposite direction. As a result of this the volume of air entering the lung of the unopened side is much reduced.

This mediastinal movement also impedes the venous return to the heart.

3. *Paradoxical respiration*: In the normal state (when the thorax is unopened), the thorax expands during inspiration and contracts during expiration. The lungs also correspondingly expand and collapse and, because of air pressure inside the lungs, the outer surface of the lungs is in close contact with the thoracic wall both during inspiration and expiration.

When the chest wall of one side is opened, air enters the pleural cavity of that side and the pressure of this air (atmospheric pressure) counteracts the pressure of air inside the lungs (which is also the atmospheric pressure); the result is collapse of the lung due to its own inherent elasticity. These changes occurring as a result of pneumothorax (entry of air in the pleural sac), may be illustrated as follows:

	In the normal state	*After opening the thorax and thereby causing pneumothorax*
Forces from inside the lung trying to keep it expanded	Atmospheric pressure	Atmospheric pressure
Opposing forces from outside the lung	Elastic recoil of lungs	Atmospheric pressure from air entered the pleural sac plus elastic recoil of lungs
Result	Collapse of the lung is prevented by atmospheric pressure	Collapse of the lung due to elastic recoil as the forces of atmospheric pressure inside and outside neutralises

During inspiration when more air enters the pleural cavity the lung of the affected side *collapses*, even though the lung of the normal side inflates. Similarly, during expiration when air in the pleural sac is partially expelled, the lung of the affected side to some extent inflates; though the normal lung at that time is deflating. This phenomenon in which a lung or a portion of it deflates during inspiration and inflates during expiration, is called *paradoxical respiration*.

4. *Pendulum air and dead space in the lungs*: During inspiration, the air pressure in the main bronchus of the affected lung is greater than the air pressure in the trachea as well as air pressure in the main bronchus of the normal lung. This causes free movement of air from the affected lung to the opposite normal lung in preference to the outside air coming through the trachea. So only a smaller quantity of fresh air enters the normal lung at each inspiration.

During expiration the affected lung expands while the normal lung collapses. This facilitates entry of air from the normal lung into the affected lung, in addition to the fresh outside air coming from the trachea.

The air shifting in this manner from one lung to the other and back has been called *pendulum air*.

The pendulum air passing from one lung to the other has the effect of increasing the dead space in the lungs. (The *dead space* of the lungs means the space or area of lungs which is not exposed to fresh air for normal gaseous exchanges to take place.)

5. *Controlled respiration*: The abovementioned effects caused by paradoxical respiration and pendulum air can be abolished during thoracotomy by controlled respiration. Controlled respiration can be induced by exerting pressure on the reservoir bag of the anaesthetic apparatus for each inspiration and relaxing the compression to induce expiration. (Another method is by using the respiration pump.)

If the rate followed in the controlled respiration is the same as the normal respiratory rythm of the animal, it is called *assisted respiration*.

In view of the above possibilities, special techniques are to be employed to assist respiration, or to maintain respiration in a controlled manner, during a thoracotomy operation.

Closure of the Chest after Thoracotomy

Before tying the last stitch to close the thoracotomy wound, inflate the lungs fully so that all air is emptied from the pleural cavity.

An inoculation needle is introduced into the pleural cavity. This needle carries a rubber tubing and the other end of the rubber tubing is connected on to a simple suction bottle with water seal.

The suction bottle should be kept at least 80 cm below the level of the patient, as otherwise water will be aspirated into the pleural cavity during expiration.

An alternative method of removing any air left in the pleural cavity after closure of the thorax is by suction, using a three-way needle and syringe.

Note: See the technique for thoracotomy in Operative Surgery. See also "thoracic approach" for surgery of diaphragmatic hernia in the previous chapter.

CHAPTER 36

Surgical Conditions Affecting the Mouth

Lampas (*Lampers*: *Palatitis*)

Lampas is an inflammatory thickening of the mucous membrane of the hard palate appearing as a ridge immediately behind the upper incisors.

INCIDENCE

Common in young horses when the incisors are erupting. Only very rarely seen in old horses.

SYMPTOMS

Pain is evinced when biting hard foodstuffs.

TREATMENT

Scarification of the mucous membrane is sometimes practised to relieve the local congestion. But this is unnecessary since spontaneous recovery ensues within a few days. Only soft foods are given to avoid pain while chewing.

Gnathitis

Gnathitis is an inflammation of the inter-dental space in horses due to injury caused by bits. It may be a mild inflammation of the mucous membrane or may involve the underlying tissues like periosteum or bone.

The horse evinces severe pain when the bit is moved. Sometimes there is suppuration and the underlying bone may also be affected.

TREATMENT

The use of the bit should be discontinued till healing takes place. When there is suppuration drainage should be provided. If the bone is affected, the necrosed piece of bone (sequestrum) may have to be removed.

Ranula (Salivary Cyst)

Ranula is a transparent cyst occurring under the tongue close to the phrenum linguae. It is very commonly seen in dogs and less frequently in other animals. It is a retention cyst originating from the ducts of the sublingual salivary gland. Its presence interferes with feeding. There is increased salivation.

TREATMENT

Incise the cyst to drain out the contents. The cyst wall is then touched with Tinct. Iod. to destroy its lining and prevent further accumulation of fluid.

Salivary Fistula

A salivary fistula usually results from a wound in the region of a salivary duct. A fistula of the gland may heal in due course but a fistula involving the duct usually persists because of the constant flow of saliva through it.

TREATMENT

1. Freshening of the fistula and suturing (after the distal portion of the duct has been cleaned of any inspissated mucus by introducing a flexible probe).

2. An artificial opening of the duct into the mouth at the level of the fistula. This is accomplished by perforating the cheek at that level with a trocar and canula and passing a silk thread through it. The two end of the silk thread are tied close to the commissure of the mouth and it is allowed to remain there for a few days until saliva freely flows into the mouth through the artificial opening made. The silk thread is removed at this stage and the external wound on the cheek is sutured.

3. If the above methods are not successful destruction of the salivary gland is indicated to bring about healing of the fistula. Destruction of the gland is brought about either by injection of irritants (Tinct. Iod.) into the gland or by ligation of the duct. Ligation of the duct is made at a convenient site between the fistula and the gland. (See Operative Surgery.) (page 460).

CHAPTER 37

Surgical Conditions Affecting the Teeth

The surgical conditions affecting the teeth may be classified into four types.

(i) Abnormalities of development.
(ii) Abnormalities due to irregular wear of teeth.
(iii) Abnormalities due to alterations in the substance of the teeth.
(iv) Diseased conditions of the alveoli.
(v) Other diseases of teeth.

ABNORMALITIES OF DEVELOPMENT

The developmental abnormalities include: (a) Abnormal number of teeth, (b) Irregularities in the shedding of temporary teeth, and (c) abnormal position and direction of teeth.

(a) *Abnormal number of teeth*: Supernumerary incisors and molars are frequently met with. There may be one or two extra teeth or a complete double row of incisors or molars may be present. Due to lack of wear by not coming in contact with any opposing teeth, these extra teeth show abnormal prominences which cause injury to soft tissues. In these cases they are to be shortened or removed.

(b) *Irregularities in the shedding of temporary teeth*: The temporary teeth may persist for a longer period: This may in turn delay the eruption of the permanent teeth or may alter their direction.

(c) *Abnormalities of the position and direction of teeth*: When the teeth grow in an abnormal direction, they fail to come in contact with their counterparts in the opposite jaw. This causes lack of wear and the teeth become excessively long, causing injury to the soft tissues they come in contact with.

When the upper jaw is much longer than the lower jaw the upper incisors overhang the lower ones. This condition is called *parrot mouth* (brachygnathism). In this condition the lower incisors are likely to cause injury to the hard plate. When the lower jaw incisors are longer, the condition is called *pig mouth* or *sow mouth* (prognathism).

TREATMENT
Periodical shortening of the overgrown teeth is indicated, if they are causing injury to the soft tissues.

ABNORMALITIES DUE TO IRREGULAR WEAR OF TEETH

Sharp Teeth
Sharp teeth are commonly met with in cattle and horses. The sharpness is seen on the outer border of the upper molars and inner border of lower molars. As the upper jaw is wider than the lower jaw the outer border of the upper molars and the inner border of the lower molars extend beyond the tables of the opposing teeth. But under normal conditions there is more or less uniform wear of the tables because of the side to side movements of the jaws during mastication. When the side to side movement of the jaws becomes restricted due to some reason e.g., weakness of masseter muscles, painful lesions in the mouth, etc., the wear at the borders mentioned above is diminished and they become extra sharp. The sharp borders cause injury to the cheek and tongue and also make lateral movements of jaws difficult. The restricted jaw movements so caused further diminishes the wear at the already prominent borders and thus aggravates the condition.

SYMPTOMS
(1) As the sharp borders of the upper molars rub on the cheek and those of the lower molars cause injury to the tongue during mastication, there is pain. (2) There is imperfect grinding of food. (3) The animal may hold the head to one side during chewing. (4) Partially chewed food materials mixed with saliva may drop out of the mouth while chewing (Quidding). (5) Foaming saliva may be seen at the borders of the mouth while chewing. (6) If the mouth is opened and

examined, food materials accumulating between the cheek and molars may be detected. (7) The sharp edges of the teeth can sometimes be palpated from outside or they can be seen after opening the mouth. (8) There may be wounds or ulcers on the tongue and inner aspect of the cheeks. There is loss of general condition of the animal due to improper feeding.

TREATMENT

The mouth is opened by using a mouth speculum or by holding out the tongue through the interdental space and the sharp borders of the teeth are rasped.

Overlapping Molars (*Shears Mouth*)

In this condition the outer borders of the tables of upper cheek teeth and the inner borders of the lower ones becomes so prominent that they overlap like the blades of shears. Sometimes the borders may be so sharp as to injure the opposite gums. Treatment consists of periodic rasping of the sharp edges.

Irregularities of Individual Teeth Due to Lack of Wear

Part of the table surface of a particular tooth may project due to lack of wear. This is commonly called a *dental hook*. Dental hooks may cause injury to the cheek, tongue or the opposite gum. Dental hooks are commonly seen on the first upper cheek tooth and the last lower molar in herbivora.

TREATMENT

Dental hooks can be removed by using tooth shears or may be rasped.

Wave-formed Mouth

In this condition the plane of the tables of the teeth is irregular, certain teeth being very short and their opposing counterpart in the opposite jaw too long. Usually the fourth cheek teeth are affected in this manner. The teeth become short either due to some lack of durability or due to diseases of the alveoli. The difficulty in mastication is caused by the opposing long tooth causing injury to soft tissues.

TREATMENT

To avoid difficulty in chewing, a soft diet may be prescribed. Remove the sharp points and edges of the long tooth, or extract the tooth. If alveolar periostitis is present it should be treated.

Step-formed Mouth

This is also caused by overgrowth of individual molars. It may also result from loss of the opposing tooth. The irregularity in the table surface is much more than in "wave-formed mouth".

TREATMENT

As for wave-formed mouth.

Premature Wear of Teeth

In some individuals the crowns of teeth become worn to the level of gums at a very young age. This causes pain while chewing and also causes alveolar periostitis. There is no treatment for the condition. The wearing of teeth may be retarded by feeding on soft diet.

Smooth Mouth

This is caused by an excessive wear of teeth. The table surfaces of teeth appears very smooth instead of having the normal rough grinding surface. This interferes with proper mastication and the animal loses condition.

There is no treatment. A soft diet may be prescribed.

ABNORMALITIES DUE TO ALTERATIONS IN THE SUBSTANCE OF THE TEETH

Dental Tartar

Dental tartar is greyish brown or greyish yellow deposit seen accumulating on the teeth. It is composed of organic matter, bacteria and minerals like carbonates and phosphates of calcium and magnesium. Accumulation of tartar is common in the dog and cat. In herbivora it is rare and is not of much significance.

In the dog and cat prolonged accumulation of tartar predisposes to gingivitis and alveolar periostitis. There is also an offensive odour (halitosis) from the mouth.

TREATMENT
The tartar is removed with dental scalers. The scalers are used from alveolar border of the affected tooth. If used in the opposite direction they may injure the gum. The tooth is cleaned with dilute hydrochloric acid (1 in 100).

Dental Caries
Caries is a progressive destruction of the tooth substance. It is caused by bacterial activity which is favoured by accumulation of food particles on the tooth. Caries is initially recognised as a dark spot on the tooth. Gradually excavation of tooth substance progresses and when it touches on the nerve tissue there is pain. Symptoms like quidding and offensive odour from the mouth are evident. Accumulation of food in the dental cavity may be noticed. The tooth may fracture during mastication. Alveolar periostitis may be present.

TREATMENT
Removal of the affected tooth.

DISEASES OF THE ALEVOLI

Alveolar Periostitis
Inflammation of the alveolar periosteum (Alveolar periostitis) may be classified into two types: (1) Chronic ossifying alveolar periostitis and (2) purulent alveolar periostitis.

The chronic ossifying type is more common in horses and cattle while the purulent type is seen more commonly in dogs.

Alveolar Periostitis in Horses and Cattle
Chronic ossifying alveolar periostitis: This is characterised by the formation of exostoses on the root of the tooth.

Purulent alveolar periostitis: The periosteum becomes highly vascular and swollen. Pus may collect between the root of the tooth and alveolus. Complications like necrosis of bone and purulent osteomyelitis may also be seen.

ETIOLOGY

Inflammation of the alveolar periosteum is caused by the presence of foreign matter or infection. Accumulation of food materials or tartar, fracture of the jaw involving the alveolus, caries of the tooth, excessive wear of tooth (up to the level of gum), etc. exposes the alveolus to infection.

INCIDENCE

The lower molars are more commonly affected. The 3rd and 4th molars are more often diseased than the other teeth. The incisors are only rarely affected.

SYMPTOMS

(1) Mastication is slow. (2) Food is not chewed in the affected side of the mouth. (3) Quidding. (4) Accumulation of food between the teeth and cheek. (5) A peculiar "carious" smell from the mouth. (6) Receding of the gum. (7) Change in the direction of the affected tooth as it becomes loose.

TREATMENT

Removal of the affected tooth. (See page 472 & 590).

Alveolar Periostitis in Carniovora (*Pyorrhoea*)

Alveolar periostitis in carnivorous animals is usually of the purulent or suppurative type.

ETIOLOGY

The chief cause of the condition is accumulation of tartar. The condition is commonly seen in dogs that are kept on soft food. The lack of proper chewing is supposed to predispose to softening of gum Gingivitis and alveolar periostitis follows invasion of the devitalised gum tissue by micro-organisms.

SYMPTOMS

(1) Halitosis (= foul smell from the mouth). (2) Gum is red, swollen, bleeds easily. (3) Ulcerations on the gum. (4) Slimy discharge may be seen on gum. (5) Accumulation of tartar on tooth. (6) Falling of the affected tooth in due course.

TREATMENT
(1) Removal of tartar. (2) Antiseptic mouth washes. (3) Extraction of the affected tooth if necessary.

OTHER DISEASE CONDITIONS OF TEETH

Shaky Tooth in Dogs
This condition is generally due to the accumulation of tartar. Differentiate also from natural shedding of teeth at appropriate age.

TREATMENT
Remove tartar. Irrigate the mouth with normal saline immediately after each feed.

Some cases may not respond to treatment when in which case removal of the tooth may be advised.

Dental Fistula (*Pus in the Antrum*)
A dental fistula is produced by the communication of the root of a tooth with the outside.

ETIOLOGY
(1) External injury. (2) Alveolar periostitis. (3) Caries of the tooth. A dental fistula (due to external injury) may be caused by fracture of the mandible. Dental fistula affecting the fourth upper cheek tooth in the dog usually results from alveolar periostitis. The root of this tooth is located in the antrum (=maxillary sinus). Hence the condition is popularly called *pus in the antrum*.

SYMPTOMS
In the dog, pus is seen to escape through a small opening on the skin below the lower eyelid. In the horse dental fistula affecting the upper molars may either open into the nasal chambers or maxillary sinus or on the outside skin and discharge may be seen through the nostrils.

TREATMENT
Removal of the tooth and necrosed pieces of bone, if any.

Epulis

Tumours originating from the gums and alveoli are generally called epulis. They are more commonly met with in dogs. These are usually benign tumours and can be removed surgically. The tumour is firm and hard in consistency; may be grey, pink or bright red and is located at the gingival margin.

SYMPTOMS

The animal may frequently rub the mouth with the paws. Impaired appetite (dysorexia), difficulty in mastication (dysmasesia), hypersalivation, oral haemorrhage, difficulty in swallowing (dysphagia), bad odour from the mouth (halitosis; oral fetor), loosening of the teeth, etc. are other symptoms.

Odontoma

Odontoma is a tumour composed of tooth tissue. It usually originates from the tooth. Odontoma is only rarely met with in domestic animals. When the tumour is present extraction of the tooth becomes very difficult or sometimes impossible. Removal of the tooth in case of odontoma is facilitated by removal of the external alveolar plate. (See Operative Surgery.) (pages 472, 528, 530)

CHAPTER 38

Dentition and Ageing

Horse

Deciduous teeth: Upper jaw: 2 (di 3 dc 0 dp 3)
               Lower jaw: 2 (di 3 dc 0 dp 3)
Permanent teeth: Upper jaw: 2 (I 3 C 1 P3-4 M3)
               Lower jaw: 2 (I 3 C 1 P 3 M 3)

Canine teeth are absent in the mare. The first premolar in the upper jaw when there are four premolars, is called a *wolf tooth*. Wolf tooth may or may not be present.

Birth to two weeks: Temporary central incisors present; the temporary premolars erupt.

Two to six weeks: Lateral incisors present.

Six to nine months: Corner incisors present

One year: All temporary incisors present; centrals show wear on their tables; fourth cheek teeth (first molar) erupt.

One-and-a-half years: All temporary incisors well-formed; fifth cheek teeth (second molar) erupt.

Two years: All temporary incisors show wear on their tables.

Two-and a-half to three years: Temporary central incisors shed and permanent centrals erupt; first and second permanent premolars erupt at two-and-a-half years.

Three-and-a-half years to four years: Temporary lateral incisors shed and permanent laterals erupt; third and sixth cheek teeth (last premolar and last molar) erupt at four years.

Four-and-a-half years: Temporary corner incisors shed and permanent corners erupt.

Five years: Permanent corner incisor in wear.

(*Note*: At two years all temporary incisors and at five years all permanent incisors are in wear.)

Six years: Infundibulum (Cup) disappear from the centrals. (*Infundibulum* or cup is a dark depression on the table of the tooth due to an invagination of the crown.)

Seven years: Infundibulum disappears from laterals; seven-year hook on upper corner incisor; the tables of incisors are roughly rectangular up to about seven years. (Rectangular or roughly oval sideways.)

Eight years: Infundibulum disappears from corners; seven year hook disappears at one or both sides and hence called *smooth mouth*. Dental star present on centrals. (A horse above eight years of age is said to be *aged*.) *Dental star* is a mark seen on the table of the tooth in front of infundibulum as age advances.

Nine years: Dental star on laterals.

Ten years: Dental star on corners.

Eleven years: Table of corners round.

Thirteen years: Thirteen year hook on upper corner incisor, dental stars are in the middle of the table surfaces.

Fourteen years: The tables of central incisors become triangular.

Fifteen years: Galvayne's groove comes up to half, table of lateral incisor triangular; dental stars dark and distinct.

Seventeen years: Corner incisor table triangular.

Eighteen years: Central incisor table biangular, or oval antero-posteriorly.

Nineteen years: Lateral incisor table biangular, or oval antero-posteriorly.

Twenty years: Galvayne's groove comes to full length.

Twenty-one years: Corner incisor table biangular, or oval antero-posteriorly.

Twenty five years: Galvayne's groove disappears from about half the length.

Thirty years: Galvayne's groove disappears fully.

A popular poem to tell the approximate age of a horse is given below:

> To tell the age of any horse,
> Inspect the lower jaw, of course:
> The six front teeth the tale will tell,
> And every doubt and fear dispel.
>
> Two middle *nippers* you behold
> Before the colt is two weeks old,

Before eight weeks two more will come;
Eight months the *corners* cut the gum.

The outside grooves will disappear
From middle two in just one year.
In two years from the second pair;
In three, the corners, too, are bare.

At two, the middle *nippers* drop;
At three, the second pair can't stop,
When four years old, the third pair goes;
At five a full new set he shows.

The deep black spots will pass from view
At six years from the middle two,
The second pair at seven years;
At eight the spot each *corner* clears.

From middle *nippers* upper jaw,
At nine the black spots will withdraw;
The second pair at ten are white;
Eleven finds the *corners* light.

As time goes on the horsemen know
The oval teeth three-sided grow;
They longer get project before,
Till twenty, when we know no more.

BISHOPING

Sometimes infundibulum marks are artificially made in an aged horse so as to make it look young. This is called *bishoping* and is a method of cheating adopted in the sale of horses.

The artificial infundibulum marks are made to resemble normal infundibulum marks by staining with silver nitrate. The normal infundibulum marks disappear from centrals by six years. From laterals by seven years and from corners by eight years. The artificial marks on laterals are therefore made deeper than those on centrals but less deep than corners.

Bishoping can be easily detected by noting the shape of the table surface of the tooth. In the young horse the table is roughly oval sideways, whereas in aged animals (above eight years) it becomes triangular. In very old animals the tables become oval antero-posteriorly or circular in shape. It will also be evident that the artificial markings are not lined by enamel unlike the normal infundibulum.

Cattle

Deciduous teeth: Upper jaw: 2 (di 0 dc 0 dp 3).

Lower jaw: 2 (di 4 dc 0 dp 3).

Permanent teeth: Upper jaw: 2 (I 0 C 0 P3 M3).

Lower jaw: 2 (I 4 C 0 P3 M3).

The incisors in the bovine are normally movable or shaky.

Birth to one week: At least the two central temporary incisors are usually present at birth.

Two weeks: Temporary centro-lateral (first intermediate) incisors erupt.

Three weeks: Temporary lateral (second intermediate) erupt.

Four weeks: Temporary corner incisors erupt.

(By the end of one month all temporary incisors are present.)

One year: Indication of wear in temporary central teeth.

One-and-a-quarter years: Indication of wear in temporary centrals and centro-laterals.

One-and-a-half years: Indication of wear in temporary laterals.

Two years: Indication of wear in temporary corners.

Two centrals shed and replaced by permanents.

Three years: Centro-laterals shed and replaced.

Four years: Laterals shed and replaced.

Five years: Corners shed and replaced.

Six years: Commencement of wear on centrals.

Seven years: Commencement of wear on centro-laterals.

Eight years: Commencement of wear on laterals.

Nine years: Commencement of wear on corners.

Ten years: All teeth well-worn.

Dog

Deciduous: Upper jaw: 2 (di 3 dc 1 dp 3)

Lower jaw: 2 (di 3 dc 1 dp 3)

Permanent: Upper jaw: 2 (I 3 Cl P 4 M 2)

Lower jaw: 2 (I 3 C 1 P 4 M 3).

The fourth cheek teeth of the upper jaw and the fifth cheek teeth of the lower jaw are known as sectorial or càrnassial teeth.

At birth: At birth the puppy has no teeth.

Three to four weeks: Temporary canines erupt; first, second and third temporary premolars appear.

Four to five weeks: All temporary incisors and premolars erupt.

Four months: Permanent central and lateral incisors erupt.

Four-and-a-half to five months: Permanent corner incisors and canines erupt.

Five to six months: First, second and third permanent premolars appear; fifth cheek teeth (first molars) appear in the upper jaw.

Six to eight months: Sixth cheek teeth (second molar) present in the lower jaw.

One year: Full set of permanent teeth present. Central incisors full wear as evidenced by wear in their central cusps (tubercles) though the tripartite or trituberculate appearance of their tables are retained.

One-and-a-half years: Cusps worn off lower central incisors.

Two years: Wear in central and lateral incisors.

Two-and-a-half years: Cusps won off lower lateral incisors.

Three years: Wear starts in corners also.

Three-and-a-half years: Cusps worn off upper central incisors.

Four years: Definite wear in all the incisors.

Four-and-a-half years: Cusps worn off upper lateral incisors.

Five years: Cusps of lower corner incisor slightly worn; occlusal surface (table) of lower central and lateral incisors rectangular; slight wear of canines.

Six years: Cusps worn off upper and lower corner incisors. Canines worn blunt. Lower canines show impression of upper corner incisors.

Seven years: Lower central incisor worn down to root so that the occlusal surface is elliptical (biangular) with the long axis sagital.

Eight years: Occlusal surface of lower central incisor is inclined forward.

Ten years: Lower lateral incisor and upper central incisor have elliptical occlusal surfaces.

Twelve years: Incisors begin to fall out.

Cat

Temporary teeth: Upper jaw. 2 (di 3 dc 1 dp 3)

        Lower jaw. 2 (di 3 dc 1 dp 2)

Permanent teeth: Upper jaw. 2 (I 3 C 1 P 3 M 1)

        Lower jaw. 2 (I 3 C 1 P 2 M 1)

Two to three weeks: Temporary central incisors erupt.

Three to four weeks: Temporary lateral and corner incisors and temporary canines erupt.

Four to six weeks: Temporary second upper molars erupt.

Two months: Temporary second upper molars erupt.

Three-and-a-half to four months: Permanent central and lateral incisors erupt.

Fo r to five months: Permanent corner incisors erupt. Permanent second premolars erupt. First molars erupt.

Five to six months: Permanent canines erupt.

Sheep

Dental formula: Same as cattle.

At birth: Usually no incisors.

One week: Temporary central and centro-lateral incisors cut.

Two weeks: Temporary lateral incisors cut.

Four weeks: Temporary corner incisors cut; temporary premolars erupt.

Three months: Four permanent cheek teeth (first molar) erupted.

Seven to twelve months: Fifth permanent cheek teeth erupted.

One-and-a-quarter years: Permanent central incisors cut.

One-and-a-half years: Permanent central incisor in wear; (age described as "two-toothed"); sixth permanent cheek teeth erupted.

One and three-fourth years: Permanent centro-lateral incisors erupt.

Two years: Permanent centro-lateral incisors in wear. ("Four-toothed").

Two-and-a-quarter years: Permanent lateral incisors erupt.

Two-and-a-half years: Permanent lateral incisors in wear. ("Six-toothed".)

Two and three-fourth years: Permanent corner incisors cut.

Three years: Permanent corner incisors in wear. ("Full-mouthed".)

Goat

Dental formula: Same as cattle.

One year: All temporary incisors present.

Fourteen months: Permanent centrals erupted.

Three years: Permanent centro-lateral incisors erupted.

Four years: Permanent laterals erupted.

Five years: Permanent corners erupted.

(*Note*: The standard for ageing of goats given above is applicable to foreign goats. Datt and Sreenivasan (*Ind. Vet. Jour.* 28 (1951): 94-99) have given the ageing of Barbari cross-bred goats as follows, which is probably more suitable for various mixed breeds of goats in Kerala).

Twelve months: Central temporary incisors shed.

Twelve to eighteen months: Central permanent incisors come up.

Fourteen to seventeen months: Centro-lateral permanent incisors shed.

One and a half to two years: Centro-lateral permanent incisors come up.

One and three-fourth to two-and-a-quarter years: Lateral temporary incisors shed.

One and three-fourth to two-and-a-half years: Lateral temporary incisors come up.

Two to two and three-fourth years: Corner temporary incisors shed.

Two-and-a-half to three years: Corner permanent incisors come up.

Pig

Temporary teeth: Upper jaw: 2 (di 3 dc 1 dp 3 or 4)
Lower jaw: 2 (di 3 dc 1 dp 3 or 4)

Permanent teeth: Upper jaw: 2 (I 3 C 1 P 3 or 4 M 3)
Lower jaw: 2 (I 3 C 1 P 3 or 4 M 3)

The canine teeth of the pig are commonly called *tushes*.

At birth: Temporary tushes (canines) and corner temporary incisors present.

One week: Second and third premolars appear in the lower jaw.

Three to four weeks: Second and third temporary premolars appear in the lower jaw.

Four to six weeks: First temporary premolars erupt.

One month: Temporary central incisors erupt.

Two months: Temporary lateral incisors erupt.

Five months: First molar erupts.

Nine months: Permanent corners and permanent tushes erupt.

Ten months: Second molars erupt.

Twelve months: Permanent central incisors erupt.

Eighteen months: Permanent lateral incisors erupt.

Elephant

Deciduous: Upper jaw: di 1 dc 0 dm 3-4

Lower jaw: di 0 dc 0 dm 3-4

Permanent: Upper jaw: I 1 C 0 M 3.

Lower jaw: I 0 C 0 M 3.

Note: "In elephants temporary molars (milk molars: deciduous molars) and permanent molars gradually replace one another from before backward throughout life so that there are never more than two back teeth in each segment of the jaw at any one time". Encyclopaedia Britannica Vol. 21, p. 877.

AGEING

1. Turning over or curling over of the upper edge of the ear flaps increase with advancing age: Edge quite straight up to eight or nine years. By twenty-five to thirty years it turns over to the extent of one inch and from thirty to sixty years to about 2 inches or more.

2. Ear flaps of a young animal are not much torn and are flexible. In older animals ear flaps rough, badly torn, tough, and stiff.

3. Head fleshy in young age. Sunken here and there in old age, especially in the cheeks and over the eyes.

4. In young age skin heavily wrinkled and supple. In old age, skin thin, glazed and harsh-to-feel.

5. In old animals diminished bulk and suppleness of muscles, deterioration of feet and nails. Circumference of limbs above fore-feet becomes smaller. Nails split and skin around the nails go rough and warty. Trunk rough and lacking inflexibility. Tip of tail hard and devoid of bristles.

CHAPTER 39

Surgical Conditions Affecting the Oesophagus

Choking (*Obstruction of Oesophagus*)

CAUSES

1. Large size of the swallowed material.
2. Sharp projections or rough surface of the material preventing passage through the oesophagus.
3. Spasm or stricture of the oesophagus.
4. Tumour pressing on the oesophagus.

INCIDENCE

The seat of obstruction may be cervical or intrathoracic. The anterior end of the oesophagus behind the pharynx and the portion of the oesophagus situated between the first pair of ribs (i.e., at the entrance into thorax) are two common seats of obstruction in all species. The posterior third of the oesophagus is narrow in the horse ("funnel shaped") and therefore obstruction in the posterior part of the oesophagus is common in this species. The lumen of the oesophagus of cattle is narrower at its anterior end ("trumpet shaped") and therefore post-pharyngeal obstructions are common in cattle. The oesophagus of the dog is more or less uniformly dilatable.

SYMPTOMS

(1) The animal stops feeding. (2) Food swallowed may return partly through the nostrils. (3) Anxious expression and restlessness. (4) Swallowing (gulping) movements. (5) Vomiting attempts. (6) Salivation. (7) Cough, due to pressure on trachea. (8) Difficulty in breathing. (9) Bulging of oesophagus palpable in cervical obstruction. (10) Oedema of head if there is pressure on the jugular vein. (11) Tympany of rumen in cattle,

In cattle the important symptoms are lowering of the head and salivation. In the dog an anxious expression appears on the face. Salivation and attempts at vomiting are characteristic. In the horse arching of the neck as though attempting to vomit, is usually seen.

DIAGNOSIS

From the symptoms: The seat of obstruction can be ascertained by passing a stomach tube or probang. If the obstruction is partial the animal is able to drink water but there is difficulty in taking solid food. Partial obstruction is common in the dog due to swallowing of bones and can sometimes be diagnosed by what is described as the "meat-ball test". [Meat-ball test: If a piece of meat is offered the dog may as usual gulp the meat piece but because of the obstruction of the oesophagus the same is vomited out.]

Diagnosis of choking in small animals can be confirmed by radiography.

TREATMENT

1. Inject Pilocarpine, Eserine or Arecoline in order to stimulate peristaltic movement of the oesophagus so that the obstructing material may pass on to the stomach. If successful, the effect of the injection is noticed within twelve hours. In the dog, cat and pig apomorphine may be given S/C to induce vomiting.

2. If the obstruction is close to the pharynx, an attempt may be made to remove it by introducing the hand or a suitable forceps through the mouth.

3. Extraction by means of an oesophageal forceps or screw. This is rarely successful. Care is necessary to prevent injury to the oesophagus.

4. Passing the probang to push the foreign body into the stomach. This is often successful if carefully performed without causing injury to the oesophagus.

5. Oesophagotomy. (See pages 476, 533, 597).

Stricture of Oesophagus

Constriction of the oesophagus may result from cicatrical

contraction following injury or inflammation.   Stricture of oesophagus is usually incurable.

Dilatation of Oesophagus (*Ectasia of Oesophagus*)

Dilatation of oesophagus is sometimes seen immediately
above a stricture of the oesophagus because of accumulation of
food materials. The dilatation may be uniform or may be in
the form of a diverticulum affecting only one side of the oesophagus. Sometimes the outer coats of the oesophagus may
rupture due to dilation and the mucous coat may protrude
through it, similar to a hernia. This is called an *oesophagocele*
(*Jabot*). An oesophagocele may also be caused by local injury
as may happen during careless use of probang.

INCIDENCE

Dilatation of oesophagus and oesophagocele are met with in
all species. More commonly in horse and cattle.

SYMPTOMS

(1) Accumulation of food materials in the dilated portion
causes obstruction of the oesophagus. (2) While feeding regurgi-
tation through the mouth or nose may be noticed. (3) Liquids
may be taken normally. (4) If the cervical region is affected, the
swelling can be palpated. (5) No pain usually. (6) Difficulty in
respiration if much pressure on trachea. (7) The contents of the
diverticulum may pass on to the stomach in small quantities and
then the animal feeds normally for sometime till there is obstruction. (8) Progressive debility.

TREATMENT

Feeding on semi-liquid diet. Surgical teatment is not usually
successful but may be tried. Oesophagotomy may be performed
at the seat of the diverticulum. The excess mucous membrane
that is protruding is trimmed and sutured. Then the muscular and
aerolar coats also of the oesophagus are sutured. Give only semi-
liquid feed until healing is complete.

Paralysis of the Oesophagus

SYMPTOMS

Difficulty in swallowing. Swallowed food materials are returned through the mouth and nose. No satisfactory treatment.

Impaction of Crop in Birds

The crop (ingluvius) in birds may get impacted with food materials like grains, grass etc. Sometimes this condition is predisposed by the presence of the parasite, Trichostomum Contortum which perforates the mucous membrane of the oesophagus and paralyses the muscular coat.

SYMPTOMS

The distended crop can be palpated at the base of the neck towards the right side. The bird appears dull and off feed with its beak open. A discharge from the beak also may be noticed.

TREATMENT

(1) Part of the contents can be expelled by gently massaging the crop. (2) If the impaction is severe, the crop may be opened surgically to remove the contents (Ingluviotomy). The mucous membrane and skin are sutured as separate layers. (See also page 418).

CHAPTER 40

Surgical Conditions Affecting the Stomach

Traumatic Reticulitis (*Traumatic Gastritis in the Bovine*)

Traumatic reticulitis is caused by the penetration of the wall of the reticulum by foreign bodies. These foreign bodies usually consist of metallic objects like wires, needles, nails, etc. that are accidentally ingested along with feed.

SYMPTOMS

(1) Digestive disturbance is noticed when the object penetrates into the wall of the reticulum. (2) Rumen motility reduced or absent. (3) Impaction of rumen. (4) Suspension of rumination. (5) Tympany may develop. (6) Repeated attacks of anorexia. (7) Reduction in milk yield. (8) Progressive deterioration in general condition. (9) Stiffness in gait and frequent lying down and getting up. (10) Pulse and respiration accelerated. (11) Pain may be evident on pressing the reticular area. (12) Sometimes the foreign body may cause traumatic pericarditis. When there is traumatic pericarditis engorgement of jugular vein, prominent jugular pulse, oedema of dewlap and chest, etc. may be seen. (13) Very rarely a sharp foreign body from the reticulum penetrates through the abdominal wall. This causes a local abscess. Such abscesses can usually be successfully treated after removal of the foreign body.

DIAGNOSIS

From the symptoms: Metallic foreign bodies in the reticulum can be detected with a metal detector. Leucocytosis and neutrophilia with left shift are usually present in traumatic reticulitis. There may, however, be cases in which the leucocyte counts are normal. An exploratory rumenotomy may be done to confirm diagnosis, if necessary.

TREATMENT
Removal of foreign bodies by performing rumenotomy.
(See page 485).

Foreign Bodies in Abomasum

This is a condition seen in calves and lambs. The usual cause of obstruction is hair balls, the seat of obstruction being the pyloric portion of the abomasum. Due to the obstruction the abomasum may get impacted with food materials.

SYMPTOMS
When there is obstruction there is acute tympany. There is eclampsia or fits. Confirmatory diagnosis can be made by an exploratory laparotomy.

TREATMENT
Abomasotomy. (See page 487.)

Displacement of Abomasum

This is a condition met with in cows. The abomasum is pushed towards the left side along the floor of the abdomen.

ETIOLOGY
The cause of displacement is not clearly understood. The abomasum is relatively more movable than the rumen. reticulum or omasum. So it can be forcefully made to change its position when there is undue pressure from neighbouring organs like a pregnant uterus. When displacement takes place in this manner, the abomasum is pushed forwards, downwards and towards the left side. The portion of abomasum so displaced gets compressed by the weight of the rumen.

SYMPTOMS
Symptoms are usually manifested during the last few weeks of pregnancy or after parturition. There is no specific symptom. General dullness and loss of appetite are seen. Symptoms may resemble acetonemia. Sometimes acetonemia may co-exit with displacement of abomasum. A peculiarity seen in some cases is that after one or two days of anorexia the animal may start feeding normally, because the anorexia causes reduction in the rumen

contents and therefore the weight of rumen pressing on the abomasum is relieved with the result the function of the abomasum is restored to a certain extent. Some of these cases may recover spontaneously if the abomasum shifts back to its normal position when compression on it is relieved in this manner.

A somewhat characteristic symptom of displacement of abomasum is the asymmetrical appearance of the anterior portion of the right and left sides of the abdomen. When the abdomen is viewed from behind, left antero-ventral aspect of the abdomen close to the costal arch appears somewhat distended (as compared to the corresponding area on the right side), due to the displaced position of the abomasum.

DIAGNOSIS

The condition is to be differentiated from acetonemia, traumatic reticulitis and torsion of the abomasum.

1. A simple case of acetonemia will respond to the administration of glucose, whereas displacement of abomasum will not.

2. Use of a "metal detector" and blood counts may assist differentiation from traumatic reticulitis.

3. Torsion of abomasum gives rise to more severe and acute symptoms than displacement of abomasum.

4. The contents of the displaced abomasum can be aspirated for a laboratory test by exploring through the ninth intercostal space on the left side with a long inoculation needle and syringe. If there is no displacement of abomasum, only rumen contents can be aspirated from this site. The reaction of abomasal contents will be between ph 6.0 and 6.5 and that of rumen contents between ph 6.5 and 7.0.

TREATMENT

(1) Starving the animal for one or two days may be tried with a view to help natural recovery. Glucose may be given parenterally to avoid chances of acetonemia. (2) Correction of the displaced abomasum may be attempted after casting the animal and securing it in dorsal recumbency. Pressure is exerted with the palm of the hand over the left antero-ventral aspect of the abdomen so as to push the abomasum towards the right side. (3) Part of the rumen contents may be removed after perform-

ing rumenotomy so that reduction in the weight of rumen may facilitate correction of abomasum. (4) Performing laparotomy in the right flank and trying to correct the position of the abomasum by introducing the hand through the laparotomy incision. If necessary, another laparotomy may be conducted simultaneously in the left flank to enable an assistant to push the abomasum from that side. The animal is to be controlled in the standing position for the operation.

Torsion of Abomasum

Twisting of the abomasum along its long axis is called torsion.

SYMPTOMS

The symptoms exhibited in a case of torsion of abomasum are more acute than in displacement of abomasum. (1) Colic, kicking at the belly with hind limbs, etc. are noticed. (2) Faeces may be passed in small quantities or there may be complete cessation of defecation. (3) Temperature above 102°F. (4) Pulse 94 to 100 per minute, weak and accelerated. (5) Reduction in the rate of rumen movements. (6) The right abomasal area may appear distended due to tympany of abomasum. (7) Rectum is more or less empty.

TREATMENT

Laparotomy is performed through the right flank. Accumulation of gas, if any, in the abomasum may be aspirated to facilitate correction. Correction may be difficult and sometimes impossible.

Abomasal Ulcers

Ulceration of the mucous membrane of the abomasum causes bleeding and digestive disturbances. The faeces appear blackish (dark, tarry) due to the presence of digested blood. Progressive anaemia and hypocalcaemia may also be present. The haemoglobin content of blood becomes very low, about 4 gm per 100 cc (Normal: 8 to 12 gm). Other anaemic changes may also be seen.

The faeces should be examined to eliminate parasitic infection.

TREATMENT

Abomasotomy is performed and bleeding ulcers, if any, are sutured to control bleeding. (See page 487).

CHAPTER 41

Surgical Conditions Affecting the Intestines, Colon, and Rectum

Intestinal Obstruction (*Ileus*)

Ileus is a term used for intestinal or duodenal obstruction. Ileus may be acute or chronic. The obstructions may be complete or incomplete.

INCIDENCE

More common in dogs and cats.

ETIOLOGY

Ileus may be caused by any one of the following factors.

(1) Mechanical obstruction caused by foreign bodies, etc. (2) Coprostatic obstruction produced by accumulation of hard faecal matter. (3) Spasmodic ileus due to spasms of the bowel. Paralytic ileus due to lack of tone of the bowel wall. When the tone of the bowel wall is lost, there is distension of bowel due to the accumulation of gas. Paralytic ileus is seen in peritonitis and sometimes as an after effect of it.

SYMPTOMS

(1) Acute abdominal pain (colic). (2) Abdomen is greatly distended. (3) The abdominal wall is tense. (4) There is vomiting and interference with absorption of fluids, especially in high obstruction. This leads to dehydration and high viscosity of blood. If dehydration is severe death may occur. (5) The urine is scanty and high coloured. Urine may contain indican, albumen and sometimes blood.

PATHOLOGY

The distension of the bowel with gas interferes with its blood circulation. There is devitalisation of the bowel wall and bacterial invasion into blood through the devitalised bowel wall causes septicaemia. There may also be necrosis of the bowel. Absorption of toxin from devitalised and necrosed tissues leads to toxaemia and may cause death of the animal.

DIAGNOSIS

(1) By the symptoms. (2) Palpation of the abdomen. (3) Laboratory examination of urine. (4) Radiograph of the abdomen reveals accumulation of air in the bowel (*air traps*). (5) Exploratory laparotomy.

TREATMENT

The treatment consists of enterotomy or enterectomy. Before surgery the animal should be given saline injections with glucose to counteract dehydration. Enterotomy is indicated in obstructions due to foreign bodies if the affected portion of the bowel is quite healthy. If the bowel wall is devitalised enterectomy will have to be performed.

Whether the bowel is devitalised or not can be ascertained by the following tests: (1) The healthy bowel is pinkish but when devitalised appears bluish. (2) When the bowel wall is normal, pulsation can be felt in mesenteric arteries. (3) Normal bowel wall contracts when gently pinched. For techniques of enterotomy and enterectomy see pages 545, 547. Fluids should be administered post-operatively once or twice daily, depending on need.

Different Methods and Techniques for Enterectomy and Enteroanastomosis

Surgical removal of an intestinal segment is called *enterectomy*. After enterectomy the cut ends of the remaining portion are united by sutures. This is called *entero-anastomosis*. Any of the following methods and techniques may be adopted.

METHODS

1. End-to-end.
2. Oblique end-to-end.
3. Side-to-side or lateral.
4. End-to-side.
5. Telescoping type.

TECHNIQUES
1. With the help of Parker-Kherr sutures. Parker-Kherr sutures are put as temporary stay sutures to close the cut ends until the anastomosing sutures are put. The technique is simple and efficient and does not require any special equipment.
2. By using Rankin forceps. The Rankin forceps has very narrow jaws. They help to keep the cut ends closed until the anastomosing sutures are put. Rankin forceps are used instead of Parker-Kherr sutures.
3. Ordinary hair pins (properly closed with the help of artery forceps by or other means) can also be used in place of Rankin forceps or Parker-Kherr sutures.
4. By using Murphy button. The Murphy button has two pieces. Each of these pieces is to be fitted into one of the cut ends by means of purse-string sutures. Afterwards the two pieces of the button are united when continuity of the lumen of the cut ends is automatically obtained. The button will be discarded in faeces in due course after healing is complete.
5. By using furnis clamp.

Intussusception (*Telescoping of Bowel, Invagination of Bowel*)
Intussusception or Invagination of a portion of a bowel into another is seen in pups and calves. The condition may be seen less frequently in adult animals. Intussusception may be any of the following types.
1. Ileo-ileal i.e., confined to the ileum.
2. Ileo-caecal. Portion of ileum getting into the caecum.
3. Caeco-caecal i.e., confined to the caecum.
4. Caeco-colic. Portion of caecum getting into the colon.
5. Ileo-caeco-colic.
Rarely a telescoping portion of bowel may protrude through the anus.

ETIOLOGY
Increased peristalsis in certain segments of the bowel may cause intussusception. Seen in pups as a complication of distemper, worm infestation, etc.

SYMPTOMS
Vomiting, colic, straining. Passing only small quantities of

faeces, semisolid and blood-stained.   Rectum almost empty. Indican urea (=presence of indican in urine).   In pups the intussusception may be detected by palpation of abdomen. Dehydration is seen.   Jaundice is a complication.

DIAGNOSIS
In pups a radiograph may be taken.   Bismuth meal or Barium meal (2 drachms of the powder per 2 ounces of water or milk) may be used as contrast medium.   In calves diagnosis is difficult. The diagnosis is confirmed by an exploratory laparotomy.   The portion of bowel appears hard and congested.   Folds are evident in the mesentery of the affected bowel.

PROGNOSIS
Guarded.   Sometimes natural recovery is seen in cattle and the invaginated portion of bowel is passed out with faeces.

TREATMENT
Salines are administered to counteract dehydration.   Laparotomy is performed and the invagination is corrected by gentle traction of the bowel that has become telescoped, with simultaneous squeezing of the outerwall of the invaginating portion from the opposite end.   If there is adhesion, enterectomy may have to be performed. (page 547)

Volvulus and Intestinal Torsion
Volvulus is a condition caused either by twisting of the bowel on its mesenteric axis or due to a segment of intestine coiling around and strangulating another segment.   Torsion of intestine is a twisting of bowel on its long axis.

INCIDENCE
The condition has been reported in all species but is more common in the horse.

PATHOLOGY
There is obstruction to the blood flow to the affected portion of the bowel and distension of bowel due to the accumulation of gas.   Sero-haemorrhagic fluid is present in the abdominal cavity.

There may be rupture of the bowel. Focal or generalised peritonitis is present.

SYMPTOMS

In the horse the onset of the disease is sudden. There is colic. Temperature in the initial stages is 103° to 104°F but later it may fall to subnormal. Pulse weak and accelerated. A pulse rate of more than 90 indicates a critical condition and death occurs within forty-eight hours.

In cattle colic, abdominal distension and a varying degree of acetonema are seen. Pulse and temperature alterations are not very characteristic.

In dog the onset of the symptom is very rapid. There is distension of abdomen. Paracentesis of abdomen may reveal plenty of sero-haemorrhagic fluid in the peritoneal cavity.

DIAGNOSIS

Exploratory laparotomy is necessary to confirm the diagnosis.

TREATMENT

Correction of the torsion after laparotomy. Enterectomy is advisable if the portion of the bowel is too devitalised. (page 547).

Bowel Fistula (*Stercoral Fistula*)

A *bowel fistula* or stercoral fistula is an abnormal opening of the bowel discharging its contents. (The word stercoral literally means "of the nature of dung.")

ETIOLOGY

Perforating wound on the abdominal wall and also the intestinal wall. (Wound inflicted from outside; of from inside due to sharp foreign bodies inside the bowel.)

During the healing process the epithelium of the skin and the mucous membrane of the bowel unite and a fistulous tract is established.

SYMPTOMS

Passage of bowel contents (resembling faecal matter) through the wound. The general condition of the animal may not be affected appreciably.

PROGNOSIS

When small, the fistula may heal up spontaneously in about two to three weeks. But when large, it may persist.

TREATMENT

The bowel wall will have to be separated surgically from its attachment to the skin and abdominal wall. Afterwards it is sutured separately as in enterectomy. The wound on the abdominal wall is freshened and sutured as for laparotomy.

If there has been extensive damage to the bowel wall portion of it will have to be removed by enterectomy.

Sometimes an intestinal fistula may communicate the intestine with the uterus or urinary bladder, instead of to the outside. The treatment in such cases will be to perform laparotomy and separate the adhesions and suture the openings in the affected organs separately by inversion sutures, and then suture the laparotomy wound.

Caecal Dilatation in the Cow

ETIOLOGY

1. Heavy grain feeding and consequent decrease in caecal motility.
2. High energy ration producing concentration of undissolved volatile fatty acids decreasing caecal motility.

SYMPTOMS

Loss of appetite (Anorexia), reduction in milk yield and caecal dilatation may develop into caecal volvulus and then the symptoms of complete intestinal obstruction are exhibited.

DIAGNOSIS

Auscultation and percussion are to be conducted in the hollow of the flank of the right side. This area is outlined by the external angle of ilium, twelfth rib and lumbar transverse processes. The auscultation-percussion reveals a characteristic "ping" sound.

A "gas-filled viscus" can be auscultated in the angle between lumbar transverse process and twelfth rib.

On rectal examination, the dilated caecum can be felt extending backwards up to the pelvic inlet.

PROGNOSIS

Guarded.   Death may occur due to gangrene.

TREATMENT

Caecotomy and removal of contents. Portion of the caecum may be extirpated. (See also Addendum on page 338)

REFERENCE

Duelk, Barry E., and Whitlock, Robert A., *Cornell vet.* (1976) **66** (3), 301-308.

Inflammation of the Anal Sac in the Dog (*Anal Adenitis*)

Anal sacs are modified sebacious glands located on either side of the anal opening.   The secretion has a lubricating effect in the anal region thereby assisting the passage of faeces. The glands may at times get inflammed, become swollen, bluish, fluctuating and very painful. It may contain pus and if not attended it may burst and produce an anal fistula.

TREATMENT

Evacuate the contents of the gland and inject into it an irritant antiseptic solution. If this is not successful the gland may be excised surgically. (See page 552).

Congenital Abnormalities of the Rectum and Anus

The anorectal passage is developed from two distinct embryonic layers, viz., the ectoderm and the entoderm.   The following are some of the developmental abnormalities encountered.

1. *Atresia ani et·recti* The anus and the rectum are not fully developed. In *agenesis of rectum,* the rectum is not developed and it ends blindly far anteriorly.

2. (a) *Atresia ani:* Rectum fully developed but the anus is not.

(b) Rectum fully developed but there is a thin membrane instead of the anal opening.

(c) Rectum fully developed but anus is represented only by a small opening.

3. *Recto-vesical* or *recto-vaginal* fistula.

INCIDENCE

The conditions are met with in all species.

SYMPTOMS

As there is obstruction to the passage of faeces there is distension of the abdomen, straining and abdominal pain. The meconium is not expelled and the absence of the anal opening can be detected. If the rectum is fully developed without the anal opening, bulging of the anal region during straining is noticed. On palpation the fluctuation of the rectal cul-de-sac can be recognised. If relief is not afforded the animal dies within four or five days. If there is a partial opening in the anal region for the passage of faeces, the animal may not have much difficulty so long as the faeces remain soft and semisolid. In recto-vaginal fistula, faeces is passed partly through vulva.

TREATMENT

If the anus alone is absent remove a circular piece of skin corresponding to the size of normal anus. Open the rectal culde-sac also and remove the faeces. The corresponding skin and mucus edges are sutured to keep the opening patent.

If the anus and rectum are not fully developed the rectal culde-sac is brought backward to the level of the anal opening made as mentioned above. A circular piece of the rectal end is then removed and the corresponding skin and mucus edges are sutured.

If the rectal cul-de-sac is situated far forward and cannot be brought backwards to the level of the anus, it will be necessary to fix it to an artificial opening made in the flank.

In the case of recto-vaginal fistula it is possible to put inversion suturesseparately for the abnormal openings on the vaginal wall and rectum, through a transverse incision in the perineal region between the anus and vulva. (See also page 496)

Prolapses of the Anus and Rectum

1. Protrusion of the anal mucous membrane through the anal opening is called prolapse of anus. (Prolapsus ani.)

2. Prolapse of the posterior portion of the rectum (which does not have the outer peritoneal covering) is called Prolapsus ani et recti.

3. Prolapsus ani et recti with invagination:

(a) The anterior portion of rectum (or colon) has invaginated into the posterior portion of rectum which has already prolapsed. The invaginated portion, however, has not come out beyond the level of the anal opening so that it is not visible outside.

(b) The prolapse of the rectum combined with invagination of the anterior portion of rectum or colon, wherein the invagination has also come beyond the level of anus.

ETIOLOGY

Predisposing causes: (1) Loss of tone of sphincter ani. (2) Loosening of the rectal mucous membrane. (3) Loosening of the attachment of rectum to perirectal tissue. (4) Very young and very old animals are more susceptible.

Exciting Causes: Straining due to constipation, diarrhoea, parturition. In piglings severe diarrhoea is the usual exciting factor.

SYMPTOMS

In mucous prolapse a reddish hemispherical protrusion in the anal region with transverse folds is seen. If there is prolapse of the anterior portion of rectum or of the colon, the prolapsed mass is cylindrical which in small animals may have a length of three to six inches or more. In cattle and horse it may extend to two to three feet.

DIAGNOSIS

It is necessary to differentiate a simple ano-rectal prolapse from a prolapse with invagination. The trench surrounding the invagination may be recognised by passing a finger or a long flexible probe.

TREATMENT

Reduction of the prolapsed mass and measures to retain it are done if the case is a recent one and if there is not much damage to the prolapsed mass. Otherwise amputation is recommended.

1. Reduction and Retention. The prolapsed mass is cleaned with a mild antiseptic lotion and is lubricated with bland oil and is pushed in through the anus. Epidural anaesthesia is helpful for effecting easy reduction. Any of the following methods are adopted for retaining the prolapsed mass inside.

(a) By putting a purse-string suture around the anus.

(b) By the injection submucously of melted paraffin wax

around the anal opening (Gersuny's paraffin prosthesis). The injection is given immediately prior to reduction of the prolapse. The paraffin solidifies at body temperature and thereby prevents recurrence of prolapse.

(c) For mucus prolapse thermal cauterisation (by using red-hot iron) is sometimes effective in bringing about reduction by cicatrical contractions. Snipping away the protruding folds of mucous membrane is another method which produces the same effect.

(d) If there is tendency for re-occurrence of a rectal prolapse laparotomy and ventropexy (autofixation) may be tried.

2. Amputation may be effected by any of the following methods.

(a) For mucous prolapses, snipping the prolapsed mass and suturing the corresponding edges of mucous membrane.

(b) For larger prolapses amputation by any of the following methods.

(i) Two strong silk threads are passed through the prolapsed mass, one vertically and the other horizontally, and the mass distal to these sutures is amputated. Afterwards the two threads are cut in the centre by pulling them out a little through the lumen, and thus four pieces of silk passing though the rectal wall are obtained. Tie them separately. Insert additional suture if necessary to complete the operation.

(ii) A series of haemostatic mattress sutures are passed around the prolapsed mass anterior to the proposed level of amputation. (A finger or a thick sound passed through the lumen may help passing these sutures.) Amputation is done quarter inch to half inch distal to the suture line.

(iii) A hollow cylinder (like Stockfleth's wooden ring) is introduced into the lumen and a ligature is tied close to the anus around the base of the prolapse. Then amputation is then done distal to the ligature.

(iv) About quarter to half of the circumference of the prolapse is incised first and the corresponding proximal edges are sutured. This procedure of incising and suturing is then carefully extended to the remaining portion of the circumference, taking care to ligature larger vessels wherever necessary. This method is specially advisable in the case of prolapses combined with intussuception.

Ano-rectal Fistula

Ano-rectal fistula is seen more commonly in the dog than in other animals.

CLASSIFICATION

1. *Complete fistula*: Having one opening on the skin in the anal region and another opening on the mucous surface of the rectum.

2. *Incomplete or blind fistula*: Having opening only on one surface, i.e., either on the skin surface or on the mucous surface, called respectively as an external blind fistula and an internal blind fistula.

3. *Simple fistula*: When there is only a single fistulous tract.

4. *Complex fistula*: When the main fistulous tract has side passages or tributaries.

ETIOLOGY

(1) An infected penetrating wound. (2) A deep abscess in the region which opens over the skin or the mucous membrane of the rectum. Sometimes a suppurating anal sac may rupture giving rise to a fistula. (3) The presence of necrosed pieces of bone (ischium or coccygeal vertebrae). (4) Lesions like carcinoma, purulent prostatitis etc.

SYMPTOMS

(1) Presence of pus in the anal region in the case of an external fistula. (2) Presence of pus in the faeces when the fistulous opening is on the mucous membrane. (3) The dog frequently licks the anal region.

DIAGNOSIS

A probe passed through the external opening of the fistula may indicate whether it is a complete or an incomplete one. If the fistula is complete and has a straight course, the other end of the probe can be felt per rectum. If a coloured solution is injected through the external opening it will escape through the anus if the fistula is a complete one. In the case of a blind internal fistula, it might be possible to feel the opening of the fistula on the mucous membrane.

TREATMENT

(1) Injection of an irritant solution into the fistula. The solution destroys the infection, if any, and the callous lining of the fistula, thereby promoting healing. Any of the following solutions may be used. Tincture iodine, Zinc chloride solution (5% to 10%), Copper sulphate (4% to 10%). (2) Application of powdered caustics into the fistulous tract. (3) Enlarging the external opening of the fistula or completely opening out of the fistulous tract and treating as an open wound. Injury to the rectal wall during this operation is prevented by introducing a thick sound or finger into the rectum so as to identify the rectal wall during dissection. In the case of external fistula probe is passed through the cutaneous opening of the fistula till it strikes the sound in the rectum. Afterwards the tissue between the two instruments is incised without injuring the rectal wall. (If the fistula is complete a separate sound in the rectum is not necessary too utline the rectal wall because the other end of a flexible probe passed through the external opening of the fistula can be taken out through the anus.)

After the fistula has been opened, its lining is cauterised with silver nitrate to stimulate healing.

If there is a necrosed piece of bone or foreign body interfering with healing it should be removed.

Rectovaginal fistula (See page 496)

Haemorrhoids (*Piles*)

This is *not* a common condition met with in animals. It is caused by dilatation of haemorrhoidal veins in the rectum.

CLASSIFICATION

(1) External piles situated in the anal opening. (2) Internal piles situated more deeply, i.e., anterior to the ano-rectal junction.

SYMPTOMS

Pain in defecation, sometimes bleeding from rectum, constipation. The "piles" may prolapse each time during defecation.

TREATMENT

A laxative diet should be prescribed. Symptomatic treatment

like application of astringent anodyne ointment, warm enema, etc. may be helpful. Surgical treatment consists of extirpating the affected portion of the veins after incising the mucus membrane and liguturing the vessels. (See also Cryosurgery.) On rectoscopic examination, having the patient in dorsal recumbency, the internal piles can be located at 3,7 and 11 O' clock positions. (i.e., one on left and the other two on right side)

Questions

1. Describe the etiology, symptoms and diagnosis of ano-rectal prolapse seen in dogs. Outline the different methods of treatment employed stating your opinion regarding the practical value of each of these methods.

2. Write an account of anal prolapse in dogs giving the etiology, symptoms, differential diagnosis and treatment of the condition.

3. Describe the causation, diagnosis, prognosis, and treatment of intussusception in the dog.

4. Enumerate the common cause of choking in a cow and describe its symptoms, prognosis and treatment.

5. Describe the cause, symptoms and treatment of prolapse of rectum in a calf.

6. What are the indications for rumenotomy in the ox? Describe the operation.

7. What are the causes of prolapse of rectum in dogs? Describe the radical treatment of recurrent prolapse.

8. What are the causes and symptoms of traumatic reticulitis in a freshly calved cow? Describe in detail the surgical treatment of the condition.

9.. Give the diagnosis of traumatic reticulitis in the bovine outlining anaesthesia and the surgical procedure for its relief.

10. Write short notes on: (1) Sharp molars, (2) Ileus in the dog, (3) Anal adenitis, (4) Dental fistula in the dog.

11. What are the diagnostic symptoms of choking in dogs and cats? How will this be confirmed?

12. What are hair balls? What is their significance in the animals health? Describe briefly the surgical interference you are likely to adopt in such cases.

13. Discuss the indications and contra-indications and the precautions to be taken and the method of making an exploratory puncture as compared to an exploratory incision. Describe the aseptic procedure adopted for making the incision and for closing it to promote healing by first intention.

14. What are the diagnostic symptoms of strangulation in intussusception of bowels in puppies? Describe the treatment to be adopted and the prognosis in cases operated upon within twenty four hours after the onset of first symptoms.

15. Name the common causes of ruminal distension in cattle and describe the surgical treatment of the condition.

16. Describe the etiology, incidence, symptoms and treatment of intestinal obstruction in animals.

17. Discuss the indications for gastrotomy in dog and describe in detail the methods adopted.

18. Describe the radiological diagnosis of intussusception in a dog. What corrective measures can be taken surgically? How will you make prognosis in such cases?

19. What are the seats of choking in cattle, horse and dog? Describe briefly the symptoms, diagnosis and treatment in the dog.

20. Name the common sites of oesophageal obstruction in cattle and dog. Describe the clinical picture shown, method of confirmatory diagnosis and treatment in the dog.

21. Write short notes on: 1) Oesophageal diverticulum, 2) Choking.

22. What are the causes and symptoms of dental fistula in the dog? Describe in detail the operation for the relief of the condition.

23. Name the common surgical conditions affecting the oropharyngeal region of the dog and cat. What is epulis? Describe the methods of examination and of extraction of a canine tooth which is involved.

24. Write an essay on the incidence of alveolar periostitis in animals and describe the sequelae, symptoms and treatment of dental caries.

25. Write short notes on: 1) Dental features in a six year

old stallion, 2) Ranula, 3) Lampas.

26. Write an essay on the prevention of dental diseases in domestic animals and the therapeutic measures recommended in the clinical forms of alveolar periostitis in dog and cattle.

27. What is dropped jaw? Describe the special importance attached to clinical forms of dropped jaw in canine practice and the line of treatment followed in each case.

28. State the indications for performing gastrotomy in calves. Describe the procedure adopted in every detail.

29. Discuss the etiology, clinical symptoms, differential diagnosis and treatment of intestinal obstruction in puppies.

30. Name the common causes of colic in animals. Describe the specific symptoms which may suggest the need for immediate surgical intervention in puppies and the procedure adopted in such cases.

31. Explain the clinical significance of "vomiting" as a symptom of disease. Describe the procedure for obtaining a differential diagnosis in surgical disorders of gastro-intestinal system where emesis is a prominent symptom.

Addendum

Caecectomy (Typhlectomy) in bovine

Perform laparotomy through the right flank. Clamp the base of caecum with intestinal clamps. Ligate the blood vessels supplying the caecum and amputate the caecum. Anastomose the cut ends of ilium and colon by suitable inversion sutures, using 2/0 chromicised catgut. A double layer of Cushing's or Lembert's suture or Schmieden's suture (page 25) covered by Cushing's or Lembert's suture are suitable. The laparotomy wound is closed as usual.

CHAPTER 42

Resection of Fifth Rib in Cattle

This operation involves the cutting and removal of about 5 to 6 inches of the distal portion of the fifth rib of the left side.

INDICATION

The object of the operation is to drain the pus and exudates collected in the pericardial cavity in certain cases of traumatic pericarditis. Also to remove any foreign body in the pericardium or close to it.

The operation, however, provides only temporary relief.

SITE

On the left side of the thorax, over the fifth rib. The skin incision about 6 inches long is made from middle of the rib, downwards.

TECHNIQUE

Prepare the area of skin. Local infiltration anaesthesia is recommended. The anaesthetic solution is injected along the anterior and posterior aspect of the rib and also deeply between the rib and the underlying parietal pleura.

The skin is incised (5 to 6 inches) over the rib. The underlying soft tissues are cut and retracted to expose the rib. An obstetrical wire saw is introduced between the rib and parietal pleura and the rib is cut across at about 5 to 6 inches from its distal end. The cut end of the rib is held and is turned outwards to break it through the costo-chondral junction.

The parietal pleura is now visible. The parietal pleura and pericardium may be adherent due to the local inflammatory process. If so, both these tissues may be incised together. Otherwise the pleura should be incised only very carefully to avoid any sudden interference to the functioning of the lung.

After incising the pericardial sac, the fluids inside it are removed and the cavity is irrigated with sterile normal saline and antibiotics. (See also page 480)

CHAPTER 43

Castration and Vasectomy

The term castration can be used to mean removal of the testicles or removal of the ovaries. But by common usage the term is confined only to the removal of testicles. Removal of ovaries is denoted by the term *spaying* or *oopherectomy*. (The term *ovariotomy* is better used for removal of diseased ovaries rather than normal ovaries.)

Castration (*Removal of Testicles*).

METHODS

(1) Closed method, eg., Burdizzo method.

(2) Open method: (a) Open uncovered method and (b) Open covered method

In closed method no incision is put. The spermatic cord is crushed and this causes thrombus formation in the spermatic vessels. The arrest of blood flow to the testicles caused by the thombosis of the vessels brings about gradual atrophy of the testicles. In the open uncovered method the skin and tunica vaginalis are incised to expose the testicle and spermatic cord. The testicle is then removed by cutting the spermatic cord. In the open covered method the tunica vaginalis is not incised. The testes and spermatic cord are pulled out along with their covering of t.v. and the testicle (covered with t.v.) is removed by severing the supermatic cord as such.

Usual age for castration: Horses are usually castrated when they are about one year old. Calves (beef cattle) sheep and goats when they are about two months old. Pigs about the first week after birth. Cats and dogs usually after sexual maturity (ten to twelve months).

Castration of Dogs

Also called Orchiectomy, Testectomy, Sterilization and Neutering. (See page 557)

Castration of Tom Cat

INDICATIONS

(1) To avoid fighting tendencies. (2) The urine of the male cat has a strong pungent smell and this smell is much less after castration.

AGE

Usually when ten to twelve months old.

ANAESTHESIA

General anaesthesia with ether or with Nembutal.

PREPARATION

Pluck the hairs over the scrotum, wash with soap and water and dry. Apply tincture iodine at site.

TECHNIQUE

Tense the testicle against the scrotal skin. Incise the skin of scrotum (or snip a small piece of skin with scissors) and by blunt dissection separate the skin from tunica vaginalis and pull out the testicle and spermatic cord. Then incise the t.v. and separate the anterior and posterior bundles of spermatic cord. Ligation is done by the two portions of spermatic cord itself. Sever distal to the ligature and remove the testicle. The scrotal wound is not sutured.

Castration of the Horse (*Emasculation*; *Gelding*; *Cutting*; *Neutralising*)

INDICATION

(1) To make the horse docile and capable of being controlled in the presence of mares. (2) Malignant diseases or irrepairable injury to the gland. (3) Scrotal hernia.

AGE

May be done at any age. Usually performed at one year. Sometimes the testicles are not fully descended into the scrotum before one year.

ANAESTHESIA

General anaesthesia or sedation with chloral hydras combined with local anaesthesia.

SITE

Ventral aspect of scrotum. Avoid the scrotal veins while incising.

TECHNIQUE

1. *Open uncovered method*: Expose the testicle and separate the anterior (vascular) bundle and posterior bundle of the spermatic cord. The posterior bundle containing the tunica vaginalis, vas-deferens and cremaster internus muscle which is not very vascular can be severed without any haemostatic precaution. The anterior bundle is severed by any one of the following methods.

(a) By using an emasculator: keep the cord crushed for half-a-minute, then partially release and then crush completely and sever. The Hauseman and Dunn's emasculator is commonly used. (b) By using an ecraseur. (c) By torsion. (d) By castration clamps. (e) By thermocautey, i.e., using the red-hot iron. (f) By ligation. Ligation is the most reliable method.

During castration remove as much of the tunica vaginalis as possible as otherwise a hydrocele or "water seed" might develop due to collection of blood or exudate in its cavity. The spermatic cord also should be severed as far high as possible to prevent the development of "scirrhous cord".

2. *Open covered method*: This method of castration is advisable if there is inguinal or scrotal hernia. (See also Operative Surgery.)

Note: A prophylactic dose of Anti-tetanus serum should be given to the horse before or immediately after the operation. (see also page 602).

Complications of Castration in Horse

If proper care and aseptic precautions are not taken the

following complications are likely to follow.

1. Injuries caused during casting: fracture of the vertebral column, tibia, etc.
2. Haemorrhage: primary, reactionary or secondary.
3. Prolapse of bowel or omentum.
4. Extensive swelling or oedema involving the scrotum and surrounding areas.
5. Malignant oedema.
6. Peritonitis.
7. Tetanus.
8. Abscess formation in the spermatic cord.
9. Gangrene.
10. Abscess formation in the sublumbar lymph glands.
11. Scirrhous cord.

Scirrhous Cord (*Champignon*; *Funiculitis*)

(*Champignon* (Fr.)=mushroom; *Funiculus* (L)=cord)

Scirrhous cord is seen as a complication of castration in pigs. horses and cattle. Thickening of the cord develops due to infection. The infection is usually of Bortryomyces. The lesion may develop within a few days or weeks after the operation.

SYMPTOMS

There is pain. The cut ,portion of spermatic cord is thickened and the scrotal region is swollen. The swelling is somewhat hard. The lesion may involve a variable length of the spermatic cord and the affected portion of the cord may be adherent to the surrounding scortal skin. There is stiffness in gait and abduction of the hind limbs. Small sinus openings discharging pus may be noticed on the skin of the scrotal region. The pus is granular in the case of botryomycosis.

TREATMENT

Penicillin is effective in checking the infection. Surgical treatment consists of cutting and removing the affected portion of the spermatic cord along with the affected portion of the scrotal skin. An elliptical skin incision is made enclosing the base of the scrotum above the level of the sinus openings. The upper edge of the skin incision is reflected by blunt dissection and the underlying layer of tunica vaginalis is recognised. By gentle traction on the spermatic cord, the upper portion of it (where there is thickening) is reached. The spermatic cord is ligatured above this point and is severed distal to the ligature. Control haemorrhage and suture the skin wound.

Castration of the Bovine

INDICATIONS
To make the animal more docile and easily manageable when used as a work animal.

METHODS
(1) Closed method. (2) Open method.

(1) CLOSED METHOD OF CASTRATION IN THE BOVINE USING BURDIZZO FORCEPS

This method is preferred in work cattle because no open wound is produced. The technique is simple. However the effect of castration is observed more slowly (in about one month) than if castrated by the open method.

A Burdizzo castrator (Burdizzo forceps) is used for doing this operation. Two types of this instrument are available, viz., Burdizzo forceps with plain jaws and Burdizzo forceps with cord-stop jaws. The latter type is perferable.

Points to remember in the technique are:

1. The spermatic cord should be held tense against the skin of scrotum and should be placed between the jaws of the forceps and crushed.

2. Avoid crushing the penis by mistake.

3. Do not crush the testicle or epididymis but only the spermatic cord.

4. The crushing lines on the skin of either side should not coincide since it may cause sloughing of the scrotal skin. (Also see other details of the operation (See page 491).

(2) OPEN METHOD OF CASTRATION IN THE BOVINE

INDICATION
Open method is preferred for beef animals as it will bring about quicker weight gain.

ANATOMY

Anatomical difference in the position of testicles in the bull as compared to the horse and dog may be noted.

(For other details see Operative Surgery.)

Castration of Sheep and Goats

Same as for cattle. A smaller sized Burdizzo castrator is used. Sheep are usually castrated when they are about 2 weeks old.

Castration with "Elastrator" Rubber Rings

This method is suitable for lambs, kids and small calves (below three weeks of age). A special forceps called "Elastrator" forceps is used to apply rubber rings around base of scrotum, immediately below the rudimentary teats.

The rubber ring acts as a ligature and gradually (in about one month) the scrotal skin and spermatic cord sloughs distal to the rubber ring.

Castration of Pigs

Pigs may be castrated at any age after the first one week after birth.

SITE

On the posterior aspect of the scrotum. Either a single transverse incision across median raphe to expose both testicles, or two separate vertical incisions.

The open-covered method of castration is preferred because inguinal/scrotal hernia is very common in the pig.

ANAESTHESIA

Local infiltration anaesthesia for small pigs. Large pigs that are difficult to control may be given general anaesthesia. Chloroform 1 to 1½ ounces or Nembutal 4% solution about 20 to 30 cc. I/V may be used as general anaesthetic.

Cryptorchid

In the cryptorchid condition the testicles fail to descend into the scrotum during embryonic life and they are retained in the abdomen or in the inguinal canal. The condition may be unilateral or bilateral. *Ectopia testis* is a condition wherein the testicle has come out of the inguinal canal but not come up to the scrotal sac. (It occupies a subcutaneous position along side the penis.) When a testicle is absent the condition is called anorchid.

Castration of the Cryptorchid Horse
(*Rig Castration*; *Castration of the Rig*; *Castration of the Rigling*)

A cryptorchid horse is called a rig or rigling. It is not advisable to operate on a rig until it is two years of age because before that the tissues of the abdominal wall are not strong enough and the operation might predispose to prolapse of the bowel. The inguinal canal also is too small in a young animal to allow the operator's hands to pass through.

PRE-OPERATIVE PREPARATION
The horse should be starved at least twenty four hours prior to the operation and enema should be given about half an hour before the operation. The operation is done under general anaesthesia.

TECHNIQUE
Any of the two methods (i.e., either the inguinal method or the flank method) may be adopted.

1. *Inguinal method*: The horse is secured in dorsal recumbency with the hind limbs drawn apart. An anteroposterior incision five inch long is made in level with external inguinal ring. The hand is introduced through the incision to search for the testicle. The testicle may be located in the inguinal canal or in the abdominal cavity. The recognition of the testicle in the abdominal cavity during the cryptorchid operation is facilitated by remembering the following features:

(i) The testicle has a characteristic feel and shape and is an isolated mass but for its attachment to the spermatic cord.

(ii) The epididymis can be palpated as an irregular or rough mass of tissue lying under a smooth surface; and after thus locating the epididymis the testicle can be traced and identified.

(iii) The vas deferens can sometimes be felt easily and is a wet, tubular or cord-like structure, and it can lead on to location of the testicle.

(iv) The peritoneal fold in the supero-lateral aspect of the pelvic inlet which forms a continuation of the suspensory ligament of the testicle and the gubernaculam testis, can be identified to locate the testicle.

(v) Palpate the uro-genital fold (Dougla's fold) on the upper surface of the bladder by introducing the hand. The vas deferens can be felt on either side of this fold and thereby the testicle can be located.

The testicle is removed by using an ecraseur, and the inguinal opening is packed with sterile gauze and retention sutures are placed on the skin. The gauze is removed fourteen to thirty six hours later. The wound is cleaned and dressed and light exercise is also given daily.

2. *Flank method*: The horse is secured in lateral recumbency. Laparotomy is performed either in the right or left flank, depending on which of the two testicles is to be removed. After locating the testicle through the laparotomy incision (following the guide lines already described), it is removed by an ecraseur, and the laparotomy wound is sutured as usual.

If both testicles are retained and are to be removed, the operation on the other flank is done after an interval of at least *three weeks*.

The flank method is preferred by many operators. The inguinal method is not practicable if the testicles to be removed are very large.

Vasectomy in the Bull

INDICATIONS

1. A vasectomised bull can be used to identify cows in heat.
2. To use as a teaser bull.

SITES

On the posterior aspect of the neck of the scrotum, a little lateral to the median line.

(*Note*: There are also other sites described for vasectomy. For example, on the anterior aspect of the neck of scrotum, on either side of median line; or on the lateral aspects of the neck of the scrotum.)

TECHNIQUE

Incise the skin and dartos and pull out portion of the spermatic cord enclosed in the tunica vaginalis, through the incision
using a blunt instrument. Incise the tunica vaginalis and identify
the vas deferens. Clamp the vas deferens with an artery forceps.
(You will notice that the vas deferens has its attachment to the
visceral layer of tunica vaginalis, but this is *not* to be separated
now.) Ligature the vas deferens on either side of the artery forceps and remove the piece after separating it from the attachment of the visceral layer of tunica vaginalis.

(*Note*: The portions of vas deferens left back are not
separated from their attachments to the visceral layer of tunica
vaginalis; and this is reported to be a safeguard against reunion
of the cut ends.)

The scrotal incision is sutured. Repeat on the other side.

Semen is collected and examined for spermatozoa once a week.
By the end of third week it is completely free of sperms.

Caudectomy of Epididymis in Bulls (*Epididymotomy*)

This operation is done as an alternative to vasectomy, and the
technique is very simple.

The tail of the epididymis at the bottom of the scrotum is
held tense against the skin and through a small incision through
skin, dartos and tunica vaginalis, the tail of the epididymis is
exposed and is snipped off close to the lower portion of the
testicle. When properly done the cut portions of the vas deferens
can be identified in the removed part of epididymis.

The skin incision need not be sutured, unless it is too large to
cause a prolapse.

The disadvantage of this technique is the tendency for the
epididymal ends to re-canalise, especially because they are without ligature. A modification of this technique is to expose the
tail of the epididymis a little more, and then ligature either
portion of its bend before snipping it off distal to the ligature.

The semen of an epididymotomised bull should be tested for
sperms at weekly intervals up to three weeks as in the case of a
vasectomised bull. Further, it should be re-tested every three
months to check possible re-canalisation of vas deferens and
presence of sperms in the ejaculate.

Spaying

See Operative Surgery. (Pages 493, 563, 566, 607).

CHAPTER 44

Urology

Urinary Calculi (*Uro-lithiasis*)

Calculi formation in the urinary tract is seen in all species of domestic animals. These calculi usually consist of the phosphates, oxalates and carbonates of Calcium, Magnesium and Ammonium. Calculi made up of phosphate, are seen in alkaline urine and those made up of oxalates and carbonates are seen in urine having an acidic reaction.

ETIO: OGY

The actual cause of formation of urinary calculi is not known. The following are some of the probable causes:

1. Decreased intake of water and consumption of hard water. Urinary calculi is common in places where the soil is of a chalky nature.

2. Mineral imbalance, imbalance in feed, especially with reference to Calcium and Phosphorus.

3. Chronic inflammatory condition of the urinary tract in which the epithelial casts may act as the nuclei over which deposition of minerals takes place to form calculi.

4. Vitamin A deficiency. Vitamin A is essential for the healthy condition of epithelial cells and therefore deficiency of Vitamin A may predispose to calculi formation.

The calculus in the urinary tract may be situated either in the kidney, ureters, urinary bladder or the urethra.

Renal Calculi and Ureteral Calculi

When calculi are situated in the kidneys or ureters no external symptoms may be observed. They are usually recognised post-mortem. Some cases may, however, exhibit haematuria and stiffness of loins and the presence of calculi may sometimes be diagnosed by rectal palpation in large animals or by radiography in small animals. Ureteral calculi may cause hydronephrosis.

Vesical Calculi (*Stones in the Urinary Bladder*)

Stones in the urinary bladder may or may not exhibit symptoms, depending on their position. Chronic haematuria, presence of casts in the urine, difficulty in micturition or complete blockage to the passage of urine, etc. are the usual symptoms. Complete obstructions may cause rupture of the bladder.

DIAGNOSIS

In Large Animals by rectal examination. In Small Animals by radiography.

TREATMENT

Cystotomy and removal of calculus. (Pages 500, 601).

Urethral Calculi in the Bull

The common seats of location of urethral calculi in the bovine are at the sigmoid flexure of the penis, or in level with the ischeal arch.

SYMPTOMS

(1) Uneasiness and restlessness. (2) Frequent attempts to urinate but only a few drops of urine are passed each time. The urine may be blood-tinged. (3) If the urethra is palpated at the ischeal arch while the animal attempts to pass urine, a characteristic pulsation of urethra can be felt because of the obstruction to the free flow of urine. (4) There is colic and the animal exhibits pain and restlessness by frequently lying down and getting up. (5) There is loss of appetite. (6) Anaemia is seen in chronic cases. (7) A certain degree of uraemia is present. (8) Frank mentions that a wiggling (=wave-like) sideward movement of the tail during urination is rather characteristic of urethral calculi in the bull. He also states that the animal may walk a few steps backwards because of the pain. (9) In some cases urine may contain precipitates which are seen adhering on to the prepucial hairs. (10) The distension of the urinary bladder

may be palpated per rectum. Due to accumulation of urine there may be rupture of bladder or urethra. If there is rupture of bladder urine escapes into the peritoneal cavity. In rupture of urethra urine collects subcutaneously and a swelling develops on the ventral aspect of the abdomen in the region of the sheath. If there is rupture of the bladder, there is bilateral distension of abdomen and symptoms of uraemia. In this case diagnosis can be confirmed by a paracentesis abdominis, using a small trocar and canula. If there is rupture of bladder, the fluid obtained from the peritoneal cavity will have the smell of urine when gently heated.

TREATMENT

1. If the calculus is located close to the distal extremity of the penis, its removal is easy. Expose the penis by giving 15 to 30 cc of 1% solution of Procaine hydrochloride epidurally. Locate the level of obstruction by passing a flexible probe or catheter. Incise the urethra longitudinally at this level and remove the calculus. The wound on urethra may be allowed to heal without suturing.

2. If the calculus is located at the sigmoid flexure, urethro-tomy may be performed through the post-scrotal site. (See pages 499, 558, 606).

3. If there is over-distentain of the bladder with urine it may be punctured through the pre-pubic site to remove the urine.

4. If there is rupture of the bladder destruction of the animal is advisable on economic grounds. If treatment is desired, laparotomy may be performed in the left or right flank and the fluid is syphoned out from the peritoneal cavity. The wound on the bladder and the abdominal wound are then sutured as for cystotomy. If the calculus is lodged in the urethra, urethrotomy also may have to be performed to prevent distension and rupture of the bladder.

Urethral Calculi in the Ram

In sheep calculi are sometimes seen located in the process urethra at the tip of the penis. Treatment in such cases is to amputate the urethral process where the calculi are lodged. This operation does not interfere with the breeding efficiency of the animal. Calculi in the form of sand-like particles are also of frequent occurrence in sheep. Successful treatment is difficult.

Urolithiasis in the Horse

Vesical and urethral calculi are commonly met with in the horse. Urethral calculi get lodged in level with the ischeal arch. The site for urethrotomy in the horse is in level with the ischeal arch. Because of the large calibre of the urethra in a horse, it is sometimes possible to remove small calculi from the bladder also by introducing a long "lithotomy forceps" through the urethrotomy incision.

Vesical Calculi in the Dog

Cystotomy may be performed to remove vesical calculi in the dog. The common site chosen is the pre-pubic site, along the linea alba. (In the male dog the skin incision is made lateral to the sheath.) The bladder is incised on its dorsal aspect close to its neck. After removing the calculus the bladder wound is sutured by inversion sutures (Cushing's suture; or, Lembert's suture; or, Connell's plus Lembert's), using 3/0 chromic catgut. The laparotomy wound is closed as usual.

Prognosis is "guarded", because recurrence is common.

Urethral Calculi in the Dog

The usual seat of urethral calculi in the dog is proximal to the os-penis. This can be removed by performing urethrotomy at this level. (See page 558).

Urethral Calculi in Male Cats

The calculi are usually in the form of sand-like particles. For removing urethral calculi in the male cat (tom cat), a cystotomy may be performed first and then the urethra is irrigated from the tip of the penis towards the bladder with normal saline solution, using a small size inoculation needle and 2 cc syringe.

In severe obstructions of the urethra, attempts have been made to connect the bladder directly to the outside and allow urine to flow out through a small opening in the abdomen in front of the pubis. This is called antepubic urethrotomy. The bladder is severed at the beginning of urethra and is fixed to the laparotomy wound. The laparotomy wound is then closed but for the small opening into the bladder.

Another method is to connect the bladder in a similar manner to the terminal portion of colon or the rectum. This is called urethrocolostomy. Urethrocolostomy and urethrotomy, however, have not been of much practical value.

Pyometra in the Bitch

Pyometra is a condition characterised by accumulation of pus in the uterus.

ETIOLOGY

Not known. Supposed to be due to some endocrine imbalance. There is hyperplasia of the endometrium and the proliferated cells of the endometrium degenerate and become necrotic. This necrotic material and discharges accumulate and cause the condition. The pus apparently is not due to any bacterial infection. Culture of pus do not reveal any specific causative organism.

INCIDENCE

Old bitches, six to seven years of age are usually affected.

SYMPTOMS

(1) There is history of irregular or abnormal heat periods. (2) The abdomen is greatly distended and is "pear-shaped". (3) Discharge through the vagina may or may not be present. The discharge is grey-yellow to brownish red and has a foul smell. (4) General depression. (5) Visible mucous membranes are injected due to toxaemia. (6) Frequent vomiting and thirst.

DIAGNOSIS

(1) From the symptoms. (2) Laboratory examination of blood may reveal marked leucocytosis and neutrophilia and left shift. The RBC count may be between 2 to 6 million. (3) A laboratory test, called "formol-gel test" is stated to be fairly diagnostic: Place 1 cc of the serum of the patient in a small test tube. Add 1 drop of 40% formaldehyde (i.e., formalin). Keep for one hour. A positive result is indicated by complete coagulation of the serum. If coagulation is complete serum will not move when the tube is inverted. (Details of the test, see book: *Clinical Laboratory Methods* by Gradwohl, Vol. II

1956 ed., page 1880). (4) Exploratory puncture using a thin inoculation needle and syringe. (5) Radiography.

TREATMENT

1. If the cervix is open temporary relief may be provided by evacuating the uterus by giving stilboestrol followed by pituitrin ½ to 1 cc S/C. (10 U. S.P. units), after twenty-four hours. 2. Surgical treatment is perferable. The uterus and ovaries may be removed. (Ovariohysterectomy or panhysterectomy.) If the condition of the patient is bad, blood transfusion or parenteral administration òf physiologic saline solutions are advisable before the operation. The patient is a bad surgical risk if the RBC count is 3 to 4 million or less. For details of operation see page 566.

Marsupial Operation for Pyometra in the Bitch

Marsupialisation is advocated in a case of pyometra if the patient is very weak and toxaemic that hysterectomy is not safe at that time. The purpose of the operation is to immediately drain the pus from the uterus. Under local infiltration or epidural anaesthesia a laparotomy is performed in the lower flank on the left or right side. The uterus is fixed to the laparotomy wound by sutures and is then incised to drain the pus. A fenestrated rubber tube is passed through the incision and is retained in position by one or two stitches, to facilitate good drainage. Draining of pus is complete within about three days and then the uterine and laparotomy wounds are sutured. Panhysterectomy may be done later, after the generual condition of the animal is good enough to withstand the operation. Usually an interval of three weeks is given between marsupialisation and panhysterectomy.

REFERENCE
William, R.E., *Vet. Rec.* May 10, 1967.

Caesarian Section in the Bitch (*Caesarotomy; Hysterotomy*).

INDICATIONS
(1) In dystocia as a life-saving measure especially in toy breeds. (2) Mummified foetus. (3) Pathological condition where

normal parturition is not possible. (4) Atony of the uterus. (5) Exhausted condition. (6) Where it is safer for the dam and/or litter than natural whelping. Twenty four to forty eight hours before parturition temperature drops to 100°F or below. Before attempting caesarian section in dystocia make an examination per vaginum to ascertain the position of the foetus and the condition of the cervix. A greenish black vaginal discharge indicates that the foetal membrane of at least one foetus is broken and that the foetus is dead because it cannot breathe without placenta. If the presentation is correct and if there is no other abnormality Pituitrin 1 cc (10 USP units) can be given. If there is no action after 30 minutes the injection can be repeated. Caesarian section may have to be done if there is no effect for the second injection. If the operation is performed within twelve hours after the onset of labour and if the foetal membranes were not broken the puppies are likely to be got alive. When the operation could be done only 24 hours after the onset of labour the chance of survival of the bitch is very little.

PRE-OPERATIVE PREPARATION

If the condition of the patient is bad, saline injections or blood transfusion may be necessary.

ANAESTHESIA

Any of the following may be adopted. (1) Morphine-Atropine plus ether. This is quite safe for the bitch and does not have any bad effects on the foetus. Morphine 1/8 to 1/2 grain; Atropine Sulphate 1/150 grain. (2) Nembutal is not recommended because it can pass through the placenta in quantities sufficient to weaken or kill the puppies. (3) Morphine-Atropine combined with local infiltration anaesthesia or with epidural anaesthesia may be resorted to in very debilitated patients.

TECHNIQUE

The mid-ventral site through the linea alba extending from in front of the pubis anteriorly is chosen. Avoid incising through the mammary glands. The uterus is incised on its dorsal aspect at its body. Usually the pup causing dystocia is located at this point. All pups (situated in either of the horns) may be removed through this incision. The pups are brought to the site, one after the other, by squeezing gently on the uterine horns. However, if there is difficulty in moving the foetuses in this manner, separate incisions may be put to remove each pup. The foetus can be removed enclosed in its placenta since the placenta is separate for each foetus. Remove the placental covering immediately. Clean the nose and pharynx of any adhering mucus and rub the pup vigorously in a clean, dry towel to stimulate respiration.

Before suturing the uterine incision make sure that there are no more pups left inside. Each horn should be searched up to its ovarian and cervical ends. Inversion sutures (Cushing's) using 3/0 chromic catgut and straight atraumatic needle are suitable for closing the uterine incision. The laparotomy wound is closed as usual. Pituitrin 2 cc S/C and calcium gluconas 5% solution 5 cc I/V may be given to affect uterine contraction and control bleeding. (See also page 565)

Prolapse of Vagina in the Bitch (*Eversion of Vagina*)

Eversion of the vagina is noticed in some bitches during oestrus. It is usually the floor of the vagina which prolapses. Some of these cases recover spontaneously after the oestrus is over. Some others respond to manual correction and treatment with mild antiseptic douches.

Surgical treatment consists of excising the prolapsed portion of vaginal wall by an elliptical incision at its base and then suturing the corresponding edges. Before doing this operation, an episiotomy may be performed to make sufficient room for manipulation. It is also advisable to retain a catheter in the urethra during surgery in order to identify it and thereby prevent accidental injury to it.

Fracture of Penis in the Dog

When the penis gets fractured in the dog, the fracture includes the os-penis also.

TREATMENT

Amputation of penis. (See page 559).

Caesarian Section in the Cow

See page 495.

Note: Many diseases pertaining to the genital system are either omitted or are referred to only briefly in this book because they are expected to be handled by the Department of Obstetries and Gynaecology.

Hydrocele

Collection of fluid between the layers of tunica vaginalis is called hydrocele. When the fluid collection is between the tunica vaginalis propria and the tunica albugenia of the testicle it may be called a spermatocele. The fluid is usually non-inflammatory and amber-coloured (=clear, light brownish yellow). If it is blood tinged the condition is called a haematocele.

PROGNOSIS

The fluid does not usually get reabsorbed but its presence does not cause much discomfort. In some cases, however, the pressure exerted by the fluid may cause atrophy of testicle.

SYMPTOMS

Non-inflammatory, soft, fluctuating swelling in the scrotum. Can be differentiated from scrotal hernia because here the swelling is confined mostly to the lower aspect of the scrotum where the fluid accumulates. Confirmation can be made by exploratory puncture.

TREATMENT

(1) Aspiration and injection of an irritant like Tinct. Iodine can be tried in order to produce adhesions and obliteration of the cavity where the fluid accumulates. (2) Surgical treatment is preferable. Prior treatment with irritant injections makes surgical treatment more difficult. Surgical treatment consists of incising the scrotum and removing as much of the tunica vaginalis as possible.

If the animal is not desired to be kept for breeding purpose, a better treatment is to castrate it by the open covered method, thus removing the tunica vaginalis along with testicle.

Acrobustitis and Balanoposthitis in Horse

Acrobustitis or Posthitis means inflammation of prepuce, (*acrobystia*: Gr=prepuce; *posthe*: Gr=prepuce).

Balanoposthitis is inflammation of the glans penis and prepuce. *Balanitis* is inflammation of glans penis. Acrobystitis and balanoposthitis are caused by accumulation of dirt; urine particles and smegma. Inflammatory swelling of the sheath is noticed. Urination into the sheath (because of some inability to expose the penis) may cause the condition. (*Note*: Urination without exposing the penis is normal in cattle but not in the horse.) Another cause is accumulation of smegma. Sometimes smegma accumulating in the urethral sinus may be as hard as a stone interfering with the flow of urine and causes symptoms of urethral obstruction by calculi. The *urethral sinus* which is the dorsal diverticulum of the fossa glandis of the penis, is an anatomical peculiarity in the horse. In all disease conditions wherein a horse exhibits difficulty in passing urine it is customary to examine the urethral sinus to rule out the possibility of urethral obstruction at this point.

TREATMFNT

On general principles. The penis is pulled out of the sheath and is washed with soap and warm water. Apply a lubricant protective antiseptic ointment (e.g., BIPP) and return the penis back to the sheath. This may be repeated daily for one to two days if necessary.

Balanoposthitis in the Ox (*Inflammation of Glans Penis and Prepuce*)

CAUSES

(1) Foreign particles gaining entrance into the sheath. (2) Accumulation or smegma. (3) Coital infection.

SYMPTOMS

(1) Swelling extending from preputial orifice along the entire length of sheath up to the level of scrotum. (2) Phymosis. (3) Dribbling of urine. (4) Palpation per rectum may show the bladder distended because of the obstruction to urine flow. (5) Subcutaneous tissues surrounding the sheath may later get infiltrated with urine and sloughing may follow.

TREATMENT

Puncture of the bladder per rectum to provide immediate

exit to urine. The long hair around the preputial orifice is clipped and a finger or curette is introduced into the sheath to remove the smegma. The sheath is then irrigated with warm soap water. If there is accumulation of urine which cannot be removed otherwise, the sheath may be incised on its ventral aspect for this purpose or, a V-shaped opening may be created on the ventral aspect of the sheath in level with the tip of the penis, to drain the urine.

Subsequent treatment is symptomatic as for balanoposthitis in horse.

Posthitis or Acrobustitis in the Pig

In the pig the *umbilical pouch* (preputial diverticulum) in the dorsal aspect of the sheath may get distended with urine or sebacious secretion. The swelling may resemble umbilical hernia. Difficulty in passing urine may be noticed.

TREATMENT

The umbilical pouch is squeezed with fingers to expel its contents. If there is difficulty in removing the contents, the preputial opening may be enlarged as follows. Remove a triangular piece of skin on the ventral aspect of the prepuce adjacent to the preputial orifice, the base of this triangle being along the junction of skin and mucous membrane. Incise the mucous membrane also antero-posteriorly from the base to the apex of the triangle. The corresponding mucous and skin edges on either side are united to provide an enlarged preputial orifice. After irrigating the prepuce and the umbilical pouch with warm soap water or a mild antiseptic lotion a lubricant antiseptic ointment may be applied.

Balanoposthitis in the Dog

The usual symptom noticed in the dog is the accumulation of a greenish purulent discharge at the preputial orifice. The dog frequently licks the part. If the penis is exposed granular eruptions or vegetations on the glans penis is visible.

TREATMENT

Mild cases recover without any treatment. Irrigation with antiseptic lotions like potassium permanganate (1 in 1000), zinc sulphate (1 to 2%) etc. and application of antiseptic ointments.

Phimosis

Phimosis is the inability to protrude the penis through the prepuce. It may be congenital. The urine is passed in a thin stream or in drops.

TREATMENT

The preputial opening is enlarged by cutting and removing a triangular piece of skin and mucous layers on its ventral aspect and suturing the corresponding skin and mucous edges of either side.

Paraphimosis

Paraphimosis is the inability to retract the penis into the sheath.

INCIDENCE

The condition is seen in all animals. Common in the dog after coitus. In bulls, another related condition is also seen, i.e., a portion of the mucous membrane of the sheath sometimes fail to return into the sheath and appears as a tumour-like mass.

ETIOLOGY

(1) In dogs the circular erectile swelling at the base of the penis resulting from the engorgement during copulation prevents its easy return to the prepuce. (2) Swelling due to injury or infection. (3) Paralysis involving retractor muscles of the penis.

TREATMENT

(1) Clean the exposed portion of penis with a mild antiseptic and astringent lotion. (2) Application of cold in the form of ice. (3) Application of a mild antiseptic or antibiotic lubricant ointment or liquid paraffin over the penis and pushing it back into the sheath, at the same time manually pulling the sheath over it with the other hand. (4) The preputial opening may be incised if necessary to facilitate return. (5) In cases which cannot be relieved otherwise, amputation of penis may have to be done. (6) In

bulls, if the protruding mucous membrane cannot be returned, it may be trimmed and sutured.

Prolapse of the Bladder

This is a condition met with in the sow and rarely in the cow and mare.

CAUSES

Due to rupture of floor of vagina, e.g., during parturition.

SYMPTOMS

The prolapse of the bladder can be recognised by its serus surface. The tear in the floor of the vagina can also be located. Urine accumulates in the bladder but it cannot drain because of the kinking of the urethra.

TREATMENT

Aspirate the urine and return the bladder to the normal position under epidural anaesthesia. Suture the tear in the vagina, if possible. In the sow recovery usually takes place even if the vaginal tear is not sutured.

Eversion of Bladder (*Inversion of Bladder: Invagination of Bladder*)

This is a condition met with in the mare. In the mare the urethra is relatively large and is easily dilatable and hence it predisposes to eversion of bladder.

CAUSES

Increase in the intra-abdominal pressure. May occur during parturition.

SYMPTOMS AND DIAGNOSIS

(1) Protrusion of the bladder through the vulva. The mucous membrane of the bladder can be identified. If the base of the protruding mass is examined it will be found to be at the usual place of the urethral opening. (2) Another feature which will assist diagnosis is the presence of the two small openings of the ureters through which there is more or less continuous dribbling of urine.

PROGNOSIS

Favourable in a recent case.

TREATMENT

The exposed tissues are cleaned with mild antiseptic solutions and the bladder is returned to the normal position through the urethral opening. If reduction is not possible or there is necrosis of the exposed portion, amputation is advisable. The fundus of the bladder is cut and removed after placing haemostatic mattress sutures. The ureters are identified by keeping two catheters in them so that they are excluded from the haemostatic sutures.

Questions

1. What are the indications for amputation of penis? Describe the operation in a case of cancer of penis.

2. Describe the indications and techniques of spaying.

3. Describe the etiology, symptoms and treatment of urethral calculi in the bull.

4. What are the indications for hysterectomy in the bitch? Describe the operation and its sequelae.

5. *Write short notes on*: (1) Egg bound, (2) Vasectomy, (3) Caponisation, (4) Scirrhous cord, (5) Pyometra, (6) Nymphomania, (7) Supernumerary teat, (8) Teat fistula, (9) Paraphimosis, (10) Phimosis.

6. What are the indications for ovariotomy in the cow? Describe the technique, complication and sequelae of the operation.

7. Describe the causes, symptoms and surgical treatment of "Scirrhous cord" in the horse.

8. Discuss briefly the etiology of urethral calculi in the bull and describe the symptoms and the line of treatment.

9. Describe in general the different techniques for sterilization of male bovine and canine, emphasising their merits and demerits.

10. Give a brief general account of uro-lithiasis in animals. How will you proceed to treat surgically a suspected case of urethral obstruction in the dog?

11. How will you differentiate between a prolapse and eversion of an organ or viscera? Indicate the normal channels through

which eversion may take place, name the structures and describe the treatment recommended.

12. What are the disease conditions causing an abnormally distended abdomen? How is distension in pyometra differentiated in bitches? Describe the blood picture and other clinical features presented which would determine the safety of an immediate surgical intervention as against a two-stage operation.

13. Give the indications for ovariotomy in animals and describe the procedure in full with reference to spaying of kittens.

14. Describe the incidence and treatment of pyometra in bitches.

15. Discuss the scope for and importance of exploratory laparotomy in cattle practice and describe the procedure adopted for cystotomy in mares.

16. Discuss the indications for ovariotomy in animals and describe the operation for spaying in cattle and cats.

17. Describe the incidence, symptoms diagnosis and treatment of prostate enlargement in the dog.

18. Describe the methods of castration commonly adopted in cattle and pigs with special reference to surgical anatomy, anaesthesia, control and post operative care.

19. Write briefly the etiology, diagnosis and treatment of empyaema of the uterus in canine practice.

20. Name the usual methods followed for castration of animals. Discuss the usefulness of each method with your reasons for choice made.

21. Discuss the importance of haematuria as a symptom of surgical disorder of the urinary system and explain in detail the procedure adopted for obtaining differential diagnosis by radiological technique with or without biochemical support.

22. Discuss briefly the etiology of cystic calculi in dogs and describe the symptoms and line of treatment.

23. What are the causes for retention of urine in animals? Describe the treatment adopted for surgical relief of high urethral obstruction in working cattle.

24. Write an essay on the incidence, symptoms and treatment of clinical condition commonly described as venereal granuloma in dogs (male and female).

25. Define paraphymosis and phymosis. How will you treat these conditions?

CHAPTER 45

Surgical Conditions Affecting the Teats and Mammary Glands

1. Stricture of Teat (See page 504)
2. Teat fistula (Milk fistula) (See pages 503, 504)
3. Amputation (Ablation) of Udder (See page 501)
4. **Fissured Teats (*Sore Teats: Chapped Teats*)**
   Wrinkles and fissures on the teats are common in the winter season.

TREATMENT
Clean and dry the teats after each milking and apply an antiseptic preparation like: 1) Tincture iodine one part plus Glycerine four parts. 2) Tannic acid in Glycerine, 20%, or, 3) Phenol in Glycerine, 5%.

5. **Necrosis of the Skin of Udder**
   Localised necrosis of skin on the udder with foetid purulent discharge. Dressing daily with equal parts Formalin and Tinct. Iodine is found effective in some cases. Surgical removal of the dead tissue may be necessary.

6. **Amputation of Teat**
   This is sometimes advisable in purulent mastitis to drain the pus and save the life of the animal. A local anaesthetic (2% procaine solution) is injected around the base of the teat and the teat is removed by an elliptical incision at this site. There is severe bleeding but this can be controlled by suturing the skin and mucous edges.

7. **Accessory Teat**
   Surgical removal of accessory teats can be done, if so desired.

Milk usually flows through the accessory teats also. Therefore the operation is postponed until the animal is dry. The operation is done under infiltration anaesthesia. An elliptical incision is made around the base of the teat and it is extirpated. The edges of the incision are sutured by simple apposition sutures.

8. Destruction of the Udder

Destruction of the udder is done when the gland tissue is damaged or inflammed to such an extent that it will not be capable of normal milk secretion. An irritant solution is injected through the teat canal for this purpose. The quantity injected will depend on the capacity of the udder. In a good Jersey cow about 200 to 300 cc of the following solution may be injected into a quarter. The solution is left in the quarter for one or two days after which the solution/exudates may be milked out. Solution for destruction of udder: 1 gramme of Silver Nitrate in one pint of water.

9. Milk Stones (*Lacteal Calculi*)

These calculi are formed of calcium salts contained in milk.

TREATMENT

Smaller stones can be broken by introducing a small forceps through the teat canal. To remove larger sized calculi the teat sphincter may be incised, if necessary.

10. Contracted Sphincter (*Hard Milker*)

If the constriction of the sphincter is at the terminal portion of the teat it can be incised using a Stinsen's teat director. (See Operative Surgery.) A constriction higher up in the teat canal is cut by using a teat bistoury or a concealed teat knife.

11. Imperforate teats

This is a congenital deformity wherein the teat canal has no external opening.

TREATMENT

The opening is made artificially, using an inoculation needle. After each milking a teat dilator plug is introduced through this opening until it becomes permanent.

12. Growths in Teat Canal

Small sized growths in the teat canal can be removed by manipulation with fingers or by using "Trump's Teat Rollers". When the growths are extensive and large they are difficult to remove and the udder ultimately becomes inactive.

13. Membranous Obstruction of the Teats (*Spider Teats*)

A partial or complete membranous obstruction develops at the base of the teat close to the milk cistern. In can be detected by palpation. The teat might have been normal during the previous lactation.

TREATMENT

1. If the membrane is very thick, it is advisable not to attempt treatment. The quarter may be allowed to become inactive.

2. If the membrane is thin, it may be divided into four by introducing a concealed knife through the teat canal. (The knife is to be introduced and withdrawn four times to cut the membrane in a crucial fashion.)

3. Successful removal of the membrane through a surgical incision through the base of teat ("Open Teat Surgery) is also possible in some cases.

Questions

1. Describe the operation for removal of mammary gland in the cow.

2. Describe the surgical treatment for gangrene of the right fore-quarter of the udder in a cow. Name the various structures you will encounter during the operation.

3. Describe how you will treat a lacerated wound in the teat of a milch cow.

4. What are the indications for the ablation of udder in a cow? Describe the operation.

5. Describe how you will treat a lacerated wound of the teat of a cow in lactation.

6. Name the different surgical affections of the udder of the cow. Give the symptoms and treatment of one such in detail.

Chapter 46

Surgical Conditions Affecting the Frontal and Maxillary Sinuses in Ox and Horse

Empyema of the Sinus

Causes

1. Traumatic injuries resulting in open wound and infection.
2. Diseased condition of a tooth rooted in the sinus. 3. Tumours involving the sinus. 4. Infection carried through the blood stream.

Symptoms

1. Mucopurulent nasal discharge which in later stages may have a foetid smell. When the discharge is tinged with blood it indicates ulceration of the bone. If only one side is affected the discharge is only from one of the nostrils.

2. Enlargement of the submaxillary lymph nodes. But the lymph nodes continue to fluctuate under the skin and have no tendency to adhere to the skin or subcutaneous tissues unlike in the case of nasal form of glanders.

3. An outside swelling due to the distension of the sinus with pus may or may not be noticed.

4. On percussion of the sinus, a dullness may be appreciated on the affected side.

5. Constitutional disturbances are usually absent.

6. The eye of the affected side may show lacrimation.

Diagnosis

From the symptoms. Should be differentiated from purulent inflammation of the nasal cavity which also causes noise during respiration due to inflammatory swelling of the lining mucous membrane. Glanders can be eliminated by mallein test. Diagnosis can be confirmed by exploration of the sinus using a gimlet or trephine.

PROGNOSIS

Guarded, because recurrence is common.

TREATMENT

The sinus is opened to drain the pus. (See trephining of sinuses in the Operative Surgery.) The cavity is then irrigated with warm sterile saline solution followed by a mild antiseptic lotion like potassium permanganate 1 in 1000 or hydrogen peroxide. The treatment is repeated daily or on alternate days. The trephine opening should be kept patent by plugging with gauze.

Tumours in the Sinus

Benign tumours can sometimes be removed after trephining the sinus.

Questions

1. Discuss the etiology and incidence of sinusitis in cattle. Describe the anatomical peculiarities of the sinuses in horse and cattle as well as the line of treatment and prognosis.

2. What are the symptoms of empyema of the sinuses in cattle and what is the prognosis? Describe the line of treatment recommended.

3. Describe the peculiarities of the facial sinuses of the horse and ox which influence the relative frequency of empyema of maxillary and frontal sinuses in these two animals. Discuss the prognosis in each case and indicate the line of treatment.

4. Write a short note on Empyema.

CHAPTER 47

Surgical Conditions Affecting Horns in Cattle

Anatomical Considerations

The horns are formed by the cornual processes of the frontal bones. The cavity of the horn core is continuous with the frontal sinus. The horn core is covered by the horn proper which is secreted by the corium at its base.

Avulsion of Horn (*Evulsion of Horn*)

Separation of the horny covering of the horn core sometimes happens due to traumatic injury. This is called avulsion of horn.

TREATMENT

See chapter on wounds. (See pages 42; 40)

Cancer of Horn

Cancer of the horn is a very common condition. The horn becomes shaky and falls off. A foul-smelling purulent discharge is noticed. Discharge may be seen from the nostrils. When the horn falls off or when it is amputated the typical cauliflower-like growths are seen.

There is no satisfactory treatment for this condition.

Fracture of Horn

Incomplete fracture of horn involving its distal portion may heal if properly immobilised. Immobilisation is difficult if the lower portions are involved.

Fracture of horn causes haemorrhage into the frontal sinus and bleeding from the nostrils is one of the symptoms noticed. A possible complication is accumulation of blood in the frontal sinus causing purulent sinusitis and empyema of the sinus.

TREATMENT

In fractures that are difficult to immobilise, amputation of the horn is advisable. (See page 470)

Disbudding of Calves

This operation is done to prevent the growth of horns in cattle, and such hornless cattle are referred to as *polled* cattle. The most suitable age for doing the operation is when the calf is five to ten days old.

METHODS

There are three methods used in calves.

1. *Application of caustics*: Caustic Potash (Potassium hydroxide) sticks are used to rub off the horn bud.

This method, although simple, is very painful to the animal. The pain persists sometime after the operation because of the continued action of the chemical locally.

2. *Use of a red-hot iron*: An ordinary bud-point firing iron can be used to destroy the horn bud. There is no haemorrhage. No pain after the operation. Healing is complete in ten to fourteen days. *Use of an electrically heated, Disbudding iron*: The principle is the same as in the case of using a red-hot iron. There are two types of instruments. Any one of them may be used. In one of these types, there is a spherical knob of about one inch diameter at the end of a rod-like handle. The knob is heated red-hot by means of electrical connections coming through the handle. The heated knob is pressed on to destroy the horn bud, after switching off the current.

The other pattern of Disbudding iron, which is perhaps more desirable, consists of a circular heating rim at the end of the rod-like handle (instead of the spherical knob in the other pattern). It looks like a circular rim of about one inch inner diameter fitted at the tip of a rod. The rim extends beyond the end of the rod by about ½ inch so that when seen from the tip, there appears a cylindrical cavity ½ inch deep. This is actually a safety device to prevent penetration of the heated rim too deep into the tissue. The heated circular rim destroys the corium surrounding the horn bud and thereby prevents growth of horn.

3. *Disbudding forceps*: If disbudding is to be done after the horn bud has started growing, it may not be practicable to

remove it by any of the above two methods. At this stage, a disbudding forceps (which works like a scissors), may be used to clip off the horn bud.

In *adult* cattle, de-horning can be done by using an amputation saw under cornual nerve block. It is necessary in that case to remove about ½ inch of skin around the base of horn so as to ensure removal of the corium and prevent the development of any stump or distorted horn.

Questions

1. What are the causes and symptoms of horn cancer in bullocks? What surgical treatment will you adopt?

2. Describe the causation, symptoms and treatment of cancer of horn.

3. Write a short note on avulsion of horn.

4. What are the indications for dehorning in cattle? Describe briefly the various methods adopted.

CHAPTER 48

Surgical Conditions Affecting the Ear

Foreign Bodies in the Ear

The animal constantly shakes the head due to the irritation when foreign bodies or inspissated cerumen (=ear wax) are lodged in the ear. The condition can be easily diagnosed on careful examination of the ear using an ear speculum if necessary.

TREATMENT

The foreign body can be removed by any of the following methods: (1) By injecting warm water with a syringe. (2) By using a forceps. Hartman's Ear Forceps with crocodile jaws is very much suitable for this purpose. (3) Hard ear wax can be softened by instilling glycerine or a mixture of Sodium Carbonate 1 part + Glycerine 20 parts + water 20 parts.

Parasites in the Ear

Parasitic otorrhoea (Otacariasis) in the dog and cat is caused by Symbiotes auriculatum and in the horse, sheep and goat by Psoroptes communis. Sometimes insects may accidently get into the ear.

TREATMENT

Insects getting into the ear can be expelled by injecting warm water, coconut oil or olive oil. For removing parasites an antiparasitic ointment like sulphur ointment or Lorexane cream may be used.

Haematoma of the Ear (Othaematoma)

Haematoma of the ear is very common in the dog especially in the long-eared breeds. The blood collects on the inner or the outer aspect of the ear flap, between the skin and cartilage.

TREATMENT

See Operative Surgery. (page 522)

Otorrhoea (*Ear Canker; Otitis of the External Ear, Inflammation of the External Ear*)

INCIDENCE

Common in the dog especially in the long-eared breeds. Very rarely met with in the horse. Uncommon in other animals.

ETIOLOGY

(1) Sometimes seen during an attack of distemper. (2) As a result of some unrecognised constitutional disorder (Eczematous otorrhoea). (3) Hypersecretion of the sebacious and ceruminous glands (Glandular otorrhoea). (4) Due to accumulation of cerumen.

SYMPTOMS

(1) Discharge from the ear which may be purulent having a bad smell. (2) The dog may feel uneasy, constantly shake the head and rub the ear with paws. (3) If only one ear is affected the head may be held towards the affected side. (4) In some chronic cases hypertrophic changes are noticed and vegetations are found occluding the ear canal causing deafness.

TREATMENT

(i) Clip the hair and clean with soap and water.

(ii) The ear may then be cleaned with any of the following. Hydrogen peroxide, methylated spirit, zinc sulphate lotion (1 to 2%), potassium permanganate lotion 1 in 1000.

(iii) An antiseptic powder or ointment is applied into the ear after cleaning. The powder is removed next day to repeat dressing. If there is much pain and irritation, an anodyne ointment containing Cocane or Anethaine is indicated. Iodoform has both anodyne and antiseptic properties. Some of the commonly used powders and ointments are:

1. Bismuth subnitras + starch + zinc oxide + Iodoform.

2. Zinc ointment.

3. Equal parts of Zinc ointment and Sulphur ointment is reported to be very effective against otitis in the horse.

4. Iodoform in ether (5 to 10%).

5. Cleaning only with Petrol once weekly has been reported to be effective in some cases.

(iv) Attention should also be paid to the general health of the patient. A laxative diet is prescribed. Administration of arsenical preparations (like Aricyl, Acetylarsan, etc.) have a beneficial effect.

(v) In chronic cases irritant solutions like Tinct, Iodine, Carbolic acid (2 to 5%), Carbolic acid in Glycerine (2½ to 5%), etc. may be applied to the inflammed area.

(vi) In cases with vegetative growth obstructing the ear canal and in which there is no proper drainage, *Zepps' operation* for chronic otorrhoea is advisable. (See Operative Surgery.) (page 524)

Questions

1 Describe the causes, symptoms and treatment of chronic otorrhoea in the dog.

2. What are the types of otorrhoea encountered in canine? How would you afford surgical drainage in such cases?

3. Describe the etiology of canker of the ear in dogs and value of therapeutic measures adopted for draining the external ear.

4. What are the different clinical forms of canker of the ear in dogs and what is the line of treatment recommended in the more chronic forms.

5. Illustrate the incidence of deafness due to disease in the different breeds of dogs and describe the treatment and prognosis in the productive forms of otorrhoea.

6. Describe the etiology, symptoms and treatment of haematoma of the dog's ear.

CHAPTER 49

Roaring

(Laryngeal hemiplegia; Paralysis of the Recurrent Laryngeal Nerve)

The recurrent laryngeal nerve supplies the intrinsic muscles of the larynx. The muscles are concerned with the outward movement of arytenoid cartilages and thus bring about dilatation of the larynx during inspiration. Therefore when there is paralysis of this nerve, the arytenoid cartilage of the affected side of the larynx fails to move outwards during inspiration. As a result of this the vocal cord and arytenoid cartilage partially obstruct the lumen of the larynx and produce an abnormal noise during inspiration. Depending on the nature of the noise, the condition is called *whistling* or *roaring*.

INCIDENCE

Roaring is met with in equines. The condition is usually unilateral affecting more commonly the left side.

ETIOLOGY

1. As an after effect of equine influenza. 2. Over-extension of the recurrent laryngeal nerve. 3. Plant poisoning. 4. Since the left recurrent laryngeal nerve is situated close to the oesophagus, careless and repeated use of the stomach tube may cause injury to the nerve.

DIAGNOSIS

If the roaring or whistling noise is not evident at rest, the animal may be trotted for sometime to make possible the diagnosis.

TREATMENT

Laryngotomy is performed and the mucous membrane lining the lateral ventricle of the affected side of larynx is removed so that when healing occurs the movement of the vocal cord and arytenoid cartilage will be restricted by the adhesions formed. The operation is done under local infiltration anaesthesia or general anaesthesia. The interior of the larynx may be anaesthetised by spraying or swabing a 20% solution of cocaine. (For details of "roaring operation" see Operative Surgery.) (page 594)

Questions

1. Discuss the causes of laryngeal hemiplegia in equiness and give the symptoms and line of treatment for the condition.

2. Name the indications for emergency tracheotomy in cattle as against horses and discuss the use of permanent tubing as a measure of treatment for roaring.

3. Describe the endoscopic and surgical treatment of roaring in horse.

4. What is roaring? Describe the incidence, symptoms and treatment in detail.

CHAPTER 50

Empyema of Guttural Pouch

The guttural pouches are seen only in equines. Empyema (collection of pus) in the guttural pouches occurs usually as a result of infection from the pharynx through the eustachean tube. It may also follow diseases like influenza or strangles. The pus in the guttural pouch may be partly inspissated. The empyema persists for want of complete drainage.

SYMPTOMS

1. There is usually an intermittent nasal discharge when the head is lowered during feeding or drinking. The discharge may be seen from both nostrils even if only one guttural pouch is affected. The discharge is thin and is not foul smelling.
2. The nasal discharge is also seen when the distended pouch is pressed with the hand.
3. If the distention is more there is difficulty in swallowing and breathing because of pressure on the pharynx and larynx.
4. Swelling of submaxillay (mandibular) lymph glands.
5. The horse may hold the head towards the sound side.
6. A rattling noise in the pouch may be heard during trotting due to agitation of the contents.

DIAGNOSIS

The diagnosis may be confirmed by passing a Gunther's catheter into the pouch. It is passed through the nostril into the pharynx and is carefully directed into the opening of the eustachean tube at the pharynx, to reach the guttural pouch of the affected side. (The pharyngeal entrance of the eustachean tube is roughly on an imaginary line connecting the temporal canthii of the eyes.)

PROGNOSIS

Prognosis is favourable if complete drainage is provided by a surgical operation. Sometimes there is symptomatic relief when the pus gets inspissated and the quantity of fluid is diminished. Rarely death takes place due to the inflammation persisting and causing ulceration of the mucous membrane. The ulceration causes injury to surrounding vessels and haemorrhage follows. Death may occur from severe haemorrhage, also from complications like pneumonia due to ingested food materials entering the lungs because of the difficulty in swallowing.

TREATMENT

1. In early stages of inflammation inhalations and antibiotic therapy may be helpful. But when pus is formed, drainage is to be effected surgically.

2. Effecting drainage by passing Gunther's catheter and irrigating with a mild antiseptic lotion. This provides only temporary relief and the inspissated pus in the cavity (called chondroids) cannot be completely removed through the catheter.

3. Providing drainage of pus surgically. There are two sites for this operation, viz., (i) by incising along the anterio-inferior border of the wing of atlas and doing what is called "hyovertebrotomy"*, and (ii) through the Viborg's triangle. Any of these two sites may be chosen. But for better drainage, sometimes it is necessary to open at both sites and pass a seton. (For details, see page 592).

Questions

1. Give a brief account of empyema of the guttural pouches. In what species is this condition met with? Describe the operation hyovertibrotomy.

---

*Dieterich's method of hyovertebrotomy.

CHAPTER 51

Ophthalmology

Ophthalmology is the science dealing with the structure, functions and diseases of the eye. Optometry deals with the powers of vision and the adaptation of lenses or prisms for the aid of vision, utilising means other than drugs. Orthoptics is the treatment of defective visual habits, defects of binocular vision, defects of ocular motivity, etc., by training.

Anatomical Considerations

The eyeball and its surroundings: The eyeball is situated within the bony cavity known as the orbit. The front portion of the eye is protected by the eyelids. Within the orbit it is surrounded by muscles and a thick padding of retrobulbar fat.

The bony orbital rim is complete in some species. It is incomplete in others. The term closed orbit is used when the bony orbital rim surrounding the eyeball is complete. Closed orbit is seen in man, horse, cattle and camel. An open orbit is an orbit with the bony rim incomplete so that part of it is made up of a fibrous ligament. Open orbit is seen in cat, elephant, pig, dog and birds.

The anterior segment of the eye is the portion of the eye consisting of the eyelids, conjunctiva, cornea, iris and pupil, and the anterior capsule of the lens. Posterior segment of the eye includes the remaining portions of the eye.

Eyelids: The front portion of eyeball is protected by the eyelids. The borders of the two eyelids contain the eye lashes. The third eyelid (membrana nictitans) is a piece of elastic cartilagenous structure situated at the inner canthus of the eye. The deep part of it is embedded in the retrobulbar fat. When the eyeball is forcefully retracted, the resulting pressure in the retrobulbar fat pushes the third eyelid forwards to cover the eye more or less completely, e.g., protrusion of membrana nictitans seen in tetanus due to the contraction of the Retractor oculi muscle.

Conjunctiva: The conjunctiva has two parts, the palpebral conjunctiva lining the inner surface of the eyelid and the bulbar conjunctiva attached to the eyeball. The epithelial lining of the conjucntiva is continuous with the epithelial lining of the cornea.

Lacrimal gland: The lacrimal gland secretes tears. It lies in a depression beneath the supra-orbital process. It opens into the conjunctival fornix by means of small openings. There are in addition numerous accessory lacrimal glands in the conjunctiva. The tears lubricate the epithelial surfaces of the cornea and conjunctiva. It has bactericidal properties and is also concerned with the nutrition of the cornea. The excess tears is drained through the two puncta lacrimalia situated at the inner canthus of the eye into the lacrimal sac and from the lacrimal sac to the nasal cavity through the lacrimal duct. The conjunctival epithelium is continuous with the epithelium of the lacrimal canal and epithelial lining of the cornea. The patency of the lacrimal canal can be tested by instilling a 2% solution of Fluorescein.

Harder's gland (Harderian gland): Resembles lacrimal gland. Situated on the inner surface of the third eyelid close to its outer border.

Tarsal glands: These are modified sebacious glands situated within the tarsal plate. The ducts of these glands open along the free border of the eyelid.

Refractive media of the eye: Cornea, aqueous humour, lens and vitreous humour.

Refractive surfaces of the eye: Anterior surface of the cornea, anterior surface of the lens and posterior surface of lens.

Tunics of the eye: There are three coats (tunics) of the eye: (1) the Tunica fibrosa (external fibrous tunic) comprising the cornea and sclera. (2) the Vascular tunic or Uvea, consisting of the choroid, ciliary body and iris which provides nourishment to the eyeball, and (3) the Tunica interna (inner layer) formed by expansion of the optic nerve. Also called the nervous tunic or *retina*.

Structure of the cornea: A section of the cornea reveals the following histological structure from before backwards: Anterior epithelium, Bowman's membrane, Corneal substance or substantia propria or stroma, Decemet's membrane, and Endothelium (ABCDE). The anterior epithelium of the cornea and of con-

ESSENTIALS OF VETERINARY SURGERY

382   ESSENTIALS OF VETERINARY SURGERY

junctiva are continuous with each other.

Muscles of the eyeball: There are five straight and two oblique muscles for the eyeball. They are: Superior rectus, Inferior rectus, External rectus, Internal rectus, Posterior rectus (Retractor oculi), Superior oblique and Inferior oblique muscles. All the straight muscles originate around the optic foramen and are inserted to the sclera immediately behind the attachment of the bulbar conjunctiva. (Posterior rectus or retractor oculi muscle is absent in man.)

Motor nerve supply to the muscles of the eyeball: All the muscles except three (the superior oblique, posterior rectus and external rectus), are supplied by the oculomotor nerve. The Superior Oblique muscle is supplied by the Fourth cranial or the Trochlear nerve, the Posterior and External recti muscles are supplied by the Abducent or Sixth cranial nerve (SOFT PEAS).

Sensory nerve supply to the eye: It is derived from the ophthalmic and nasociliary branches.

Blood supply: Blood supply to the eye is from the ophthalmic arteries and veins.

Iris: Iris is a muscular diaphragm between the cornea and the lens, with an opening in its centre. The opening is called the *pupil*. The pupils of horse, cattle and sheep are horizontally elliptical in shape. In the young horse below five years it is more roundish; in man, dog, monkey and most birds it is circular; and in cat and fox it is vertically elliptical.

The anterior surface of the iris as well as the posterior surface of the cornea are covered by endothelium. The posterior surface of the iris is continuous with the pigment layer of retina.

Corpora Nigra are small black bodies seen on the pupillary border.

Anterior chamber of the eye is the space situated between the iris and cornea.

Posterior chamber of the eye is the space situated between the iris and the lens.

Aqueous humour is the clear fluid filling the entire space between the cornea and lens, i.e., the anterior chamber and posterior chamber inclusive.

The *lens* has a vertical position. It is kept in position by the *suspensory ligament of the lens*. The suspensory ligament is attached along the *equator* of the lens. The lens has anterior and posterior *poles.*

Before reading this chapter, the student is expected to refresh his memory regarding the following parts and structures of the eye.

1. Cornea—The structure of the cornea comprising the Anterior epithelial covering, the Basement membrane, Corneal matrix, Decemet's membrane, and Endothelial lining on its posterior part. (The first letters of these give the formula ABCDE for purposes of memorising.)

2. Sclera.

3. The sclero-corneal junction or limbus.

4. Choroid—the vascular networks in it.

5. Supra-choroidal lymph space or peri-choroidal lymph space.

6. Ciliary body comprising the ciliary process and the ciliary muscles.

7. Retina—the three regions of the retina, namely, (i) Tapetum lucidum which has a combination of green, blue and yellow colour; (ii) Tapetum nigram which is black or chocolate colour, and (iii) the optic papilla.

8. The optic disc of the retina and the optic nerve.

9. The junction of the retinal periphery and the ciliary body called the Ora serrata retinae.

10. Suspensory ligament of the lens and Zonule of Zinn or Zonula ciliaris.

11. Entrance and distribution of ciliary nerve and posterior retinal artery and vein into the eyeball.

12. The Vorticose veins.

13. The pectinate ligaments or Ligamentum pectinatum iridis situated at the angle formed between the iris and the sclerocornea.

14. The spaces of Fontana, which are the open spaces between the pactinate ligaments and they communicate the anterior chamber of the eye to the canal of Schlem.

15. The Canal of Schlem.

16. Aqueous humour.

17. Vitreous humour.

18. Hyaloid membrane enclosing the Vitreous humour.

19. Hyaloid fossa or the depression in the hyaloid which

accommodates the posterior convex surface of the lens.

20. Anterior and posterior capsules of the lens, cortex of the lens and nucleus of the lens.

Tests for Visual Function (*Diagnosis of Blindness*)

1. A blind animal is nervous and is easily excitable.

2. It shows anxious movements of the ears in an attempt to grasp the environment.

3. It walks with the head held upwards and takes very cautious steps and has a "feeling gait".

4. During progression it stumbles on account of the inability to see obstacles on an uneven ground; and in order to avoid such obstacles it may lift the limbs unusually high ("high stepping").

5. When driven towards an object like a wall or a post, the animal may go and strike against the object because of the inability to see.

6. When light is suddenly flashed into a normal eye, immediate closure of the eyelids is noticed. This is a protective reflex known as *palpebral reflex*. Palpebral reflex is absent in a blind eye.

7. *Photomotor pupillary reflex* (*Photomotor pupillary reaction*): This is the ability of the pupil to react to changes in light. If the eyes are normal, the pupil contracts when exposed to bright light and dilates when there is shade or darkness. Absence of this reflex may indicate some abnormality.

8. *Crossed reflex* (*Consensual reflex*): If both eyes are normal the flashing of light into one eye constricts both the pupils. This is called crossed reflex or consensual reflex. If one eye is blind, flashing of light into the blind eye will not induce pupillary reflex of the normal eye.

Note: Crossed reflex is, however, not very marked in animals.

Clinical Examination of the Eye

1. *Naked eye examination*: Gross abnormalities of the anterior segment of the eye can be detected by naked eye examination, with the aid of artificial illumination if necessary.

2. *Using binocular loupe*: The binocular loupe consists of two magnifying lenses and its use is therefore preferable to naked eye examination.

3. *Catoptric test*: The word catoptric means relating to reflection. This test is useful for detecting opacities of the cornea and lens. The animal is taken to dark room or shade and a lighted candle is held in front of the eye about 6 inches from the eye. In the normal eye three distinct images can be observed respectively on the cornea, the anterior capsule of the lens and the posterior capsule of the lens. Of these three images, the first two are erect images and the third one is inverted. The first image is the biggest and the brightest and the third one is the smallest and the least bright. These images are called Purkinjee-Sanson's images. By moving the candle first in a horizontal and then in a vertical direction, opacities if any can be detected.

4. *By using ophthalmoscope (ophthalmoscopy)*: This is a better method of examining the eye than those mentioned above. In order to facilitate examination of the interior of the eye with the ophthalmoscope, it is necessary to dilate the pupil. This can be brought about by instilling a solution of homatropine (2%) into eye about fifteen to thirty minutes before.

The ophthalmoscope contains lenses of varying powers through which the examination can be conducted. The anterior segment of the eye can be examined by using a lens ranging from +12 to +20. For observing the lens +8 to +12, and for vitreous humour 0 to +8, are required. For the fundus of the eye (retina, optic disc) —3 or less, may be suitable.

5. *By using tonometer (tonometry)*: The *intraocular pressure* (IOP) can be measured by using an instrument called tonometer and the increase or decrease in the intraocular pressure can be found out. The normal intraocular pressure in the dog ranges from 16 to 30 mm of mercury. The normal IOP in man is 15 to 20 mm of mercury.

DIRECTIONS FOR USE OF THE SCHIOETZ TONOMETER
Familiarise with the following parts of the Tonometer:
(a) Test block.
(b) The outer cylinder with *handle*, which slides over the inner cylinder above the level of the *foot plate* of the inner cylinder.
(c) The *handle* of the tonometer which is attached to the outer cylinder.
(d) The *inner cylinder* which rests on the test block by a *foot plate* and which has an *inner lumen* through which the lower

portion of the *plunger* slides.

(e) Plunger, which has an upper or top portion to carry the adjustible weights and a lower portion which runs through the inner cylinder mentioned above. The uppermost tip of the *plunger* touches the base of the *pointer*.

(f) The *pointer* which slides on a graduated scale.

Before use, the tonometer is placed upon the convex side of *test block* and the *pointer* is adjusted to zero. If the pointer has another position, the instrument requires readjustment. The weight marked 5.5 grammes always remains on the plunger so that the other weights must be added supplementarily to the weight 5.5 grammes. For measuring the tension, the patient is laid in the recumbent position and the cornea anaesthetised with two or three drops of 2% Holocain or ½% Pontocain. While the patient is made to look straight upwards; the eyelids are retracted gently with one hand without exerting pressure on the eyeball. An eye speculam may be used, if necessary. The other hand seizes the handle and the tonometer is placed in a vertical position on the centre of the cornea. The handle of the tonometer is lowered to a position midway between the top and the foot plate of the inner cylinder, thereby the instrument will act independently by its own weight. Add additional weight, if necessary, on the plunger. Now the position of the pointer on the scale can be read. The tension in mm/Hg may be determined from the following table.

The average normal intraocular tension in man is 15 to 20 mm of mercury. A tension more than 20 mm is considered high, while tension above 25 mm is suspicious of a pathological condition.

After use, the plunger should be removed from the cylinder. This is done after unscrewing the weight 5.5 gramme. The plunger, the groove and the foot plate should be cleaned with ether and rubbed dry in order to avoid corrosion.

Illustration: If the, scale reading is 4.5 and the plunger load is 7.5 grammes, the intraocular pressure is 28 mm of Hg.

6. *Digital palpation of eyeball to assess intraocular pressure*: During clinical examination, a rough idea of intraocular tension can be obtained by this method. The cornea is gently pressed by the index finger kept over the closed upper eyelid while the thumb is placed below the lower eyelid to support the eyeball

Table indicating the intraocular pressure, based on scale reading of the pointer and the plunger load (weight on the plunger).

Scale reading	5.5 g.	7.5 g.	10.0 g.	15.0 g.
0.0	41.5	59.1	81.7	127.5
0.5	37.8	54.2	75.1	117.9
1.0	34.5	49.8	69.3	109.3
1.5	31.6	45.8	64.0	101.4
2.0	29.0	42.1	59.1	94.3
2.5	26.6	38.8	54.7	88.0
3.0	24.4	35.8	50.6	81.8
3.5	22.4	33.0	46.9	76.2
4.0	20.6	30.4	43.4	71.0
4.5	18.9	28.0	40.2	66.2
5.0	17.3	25.8	37.2	61.8
5.5	15.9	23.8	34.4	57.6
6.0	14.6	21.9	31.8	53.6
6.5	13.4	20.1	29.4	49.9
7.0	12.2	18.5	27.2	46.5
7.5	11.2	17.0	25.1	43.2
8.0	10.2	15.6	23.1	40.2
8.5	9.4	14.3	21.3	38.1
9.0	8.5	13.1	19.6	34.6
9.5	7.8	12.0	18.0	32 0
10.0	7.1	10.9	16.5	29.6
10.5	6.5	10.0	15.1	27.4
11.0	5.9	9.0	13.8	25.3
11.5	5.3	8.3	12.6	23.3
12.0	4.9	7.5	11.5	21.4
12.5	4.4	6.8	10.5	19.7
13.0	4.0	6.2	9.5	18.1
13.5	—	5.6	8.6	16.5
14.0	—	5.0	7.8	15.1
14.5	—	4.5	7.1	13.7
15.0	—	4.0	6.4	12.6
15.5	—	—	5.8	11.4
16.0	—	—	5.2	10.4
16.5	—	—	4.7	9.4
17.0	—	—	4.2	8.5
17.5	—	—	—	7.7
18.0	—	—	—	6.9
18.5	—	—	—	6.2
19.0	—	—	—	5.6
19.5	—	—	—	4.9
20.0	—	—	—	4.5

from below. By this method a relative idea of intraocular tension can be obtained by comparison with the normal eye.

Other Specialised Procedures for Examination of the Interior of the Eye

Electroretinography (ERG): All nervous tissues generate electric current. The principle underlying electroretinography is the fact that the retina generates electrical current and that it can be recorded by using the electrodes of a specialised Electroencephalograph. One of the two electrodes is placed on the cornea and the other is placed in an area over the skin adjacent to the eye. Electroretinography is particularly useful to assess the condition of the retina when ophthalmoscopic examination is not possible, as in cataract. It is also helpful in arriving at the prognosis in glaucoma and also to arrive at the cause of partial or complete blindness.

Ultrasonography: This is carried out by an ultrasound machine with a transducer attached to it. The transducer is taken along various positions over the corneal surface in the process of examination. Ultrasonography *helps* in the diagnosis of luxation of lens and retinal detachments.

Fluorescein angiography: This is taking photograph of the fundus of the eye as the injected dye (Fluorescein) circulates through the retinal vessels.

REFERENCE

Magrane, William G. (1977). *Canine ophthalmology*, 3rd ed. Lea & Febiger, Philadelphia.

SURGICAL CONDITIONS AFFECTING THE EYELIDS

Chalazion *(Tarsal Cyst)*

This is a cyst caused by the distension of a tarsal gland with secretion. The size of the cyst may be about the size of a pea or more. It contains cheesy material.

TREATMENT

Incise and remove the contents of the cyst.

Hordeolum or Stye

It is a localised inflammation of the hair follicles of the eyelashes. In the beginning stage there is inflammatory swelling of the eyelid which later points to a small abscess. The condition is due to staphylococcal infection.

TREATMENT

One or two neighbouring eyelashes are plucked with forceps so as to open the abscess and drain the pus. After draining the pus sulphacetamide eye ointment is indicated.

Dacryo-adenitis

Inflammation of lacrimal gland.

TREATMENT

Fomentations, antibiotics, etc. Do not open before it is mature. Spontaneous rupture and healing usually happens.

Blepharitis

Blepharitis or inflammation of eyelids, causes ulceration of the palpebral borders. The ulcers contain a yellowish or greyish sticky discharge. The eyelids may stick together.

TREATMENT

Symptomatic. Antibiotics may be used to control infection.

Ectropion and Entropion

See Operative Surgery. (See pages 466 and 465).

Trichiasis and Districhiasis

In trichiasis the eyelashes are directed slightly inwards so that they irritate the cornea and conjunctiva.Districhiasis is a congenital condition in which two rows of eyelashes are noticed on each lid and the inner row causes irritation of the conjunctiva. Districhiasis is supposed to be hereditary.

TREATMENT

1. Epilation or plucking of the eyelashes. 2. Destroying he hair roots by electrocautery. 3. Complete removal of the ιair roots by snipping the inner border of the lid. 4. Opera-

tion for entropion may prevent the eyelashes irritating the cornea.

Ptosis *(Blepharo ptosis)*

Dropping of the upper eyelid, due to inability to raise it, may be congenital. It may be due to paralysis of the seventh cranial nerve.

TREATMENT

The condition may be temporary and may become normal without treatment. Surgical correction when necessary can be done as for entropion, for symptomatic relief.

Lagophthalmos

A condition in which the eye cannot be completely closed. (*Lagos* = hare).

CAUSES

1. Paralysis of the orbicularis oculi muscle resulting from injury to the seventh cranial nerve.
2. Prolapse of Harderian gland.
3. Inflammed lacrimal gland.
4. Growth on the cornea.
5. Staphyloma.
6. Granulations on the edges of the eyelids.

Lagophthalmos causes drying of the cornea and conjunctiva (as the eyelids do not move over the cornea and smear it with the lacrimal secretion).

TREATMENT

Remove the cause. Normal saline or liquid paraffin may be instilled at frequent intervals to moisten the cornea and conjunctiva. The lids may be kept closed by means of one or two skin sutures over the closed lids.

Blepharospasm

It is a state of partial or complete closure of eyelids. It may be due to foreign particles irritating the cornea, early keratitis and conjunctivitis, photophobia, etc.

TREATMENT
Blepharospasm is only a symptom and treatment depends on the cause.

Parasites in the Conjunctival Cul-de-sac
Thelazia rhodesii in cattle.

Prolapse of Harderian Gland
(Luxation of the superficial gland of the third eyelid.) Prolapse of the Harder's gland is common in the dog due to inflammatory swelling or hypertrophy. The gland protrudes outwards.

TREATMENT
Surgical removal. 1 in 50,000 adrenalin may be applied locally to control haemorrhage.

Removal of Membrana Nictitans
(Third eyelid).

INDICATIONS
Hypertrophy. Neoplasm. Carcinoma.

ANAESTHESIA
1% solution of Novocaine injected under conjunctival lining, along base of the third eyelid.

TECHNIQUE
Haemostatic matress sutures are put along the base of the third eyelid to control haemorrhage and afterwards it is cut distal to the sutures.

SURGICAL CONDITIONS AFFECTING THE EYEBALL

Exophthalmos (Proptosis)
It is an abnormal protrusion of the eyeball. It may be a congenital condition or may be due to retrobulbar abscess, haematoma, or inflammation. It may be seen as a symptom of diseases like hydrophthalmos and glaucoma. Exophthalmos may also be due to goitre resulting from iodine deficiency but this is rare in animals.

Enophthalmos (*Pig Eye*)

Enophthalmos is an abnormal retraction of the eyeball into the orbit. May be congenital or sometimes due to debility or exhaustion.

Hyphema

Haemorrhage into the anterior chamber.

Hydrophthalmos

It is an enlargement of the eyeball associated with increase in the quantity of aqueous humour. When hydrophthalmos is congenital it is called megalophthalmos or megalophthalmos congenitus.

Hydrophthalmos is usually the result of interference with the drainage of aqueous humour and may be due to the adhesion of iris to the cornea at the filtration angle. The tunics of the eyeball, especially the selera and cornea, become thin and weak. This weakening is supposed to be due to a deficiency of Calcium and Vitamin D. Rickets may predispose to hydrophthalmos.

SYMPTOMS

Due to the general increase in the fluid contents the eyeball bulges forward causing exophthalmos and lagophthalmos. This causes drying or desiccation and interference with the nourishment of the cornea. The cornea becomes opaque, the vessels from the limbus penetrate into the cornea radiating towards its centre. The lens is detached and usually floats in the aqueous humour and may become adherent to the cornea or vitreous humour. Keratoglobus (protrusion of cornea into a globular enlargement) or Keratoconus (conical enlargement of the cornea) may be observed. In very advanced cases the eyeball may burst.

PROGNOSIS

Guarded.

TREATMENT

1. Dropping pilocarpine ($\frac{1}{2}$%) into the eye to constrict the pupil and reduce intraocular tension.

2. Keratocentesis, to let out the excess of aqueous humour.

3. Diuretics.
4. Salt-free diet.
5. Limited water intake.
6. Laxative diet.
7. If hydrophthalmos is due to adhesion of the iris to the cornea or other structural deformities, treatment is useless and removal of eyeball is indicated.

Excision (*Removal*) *of the Eye*
See Operative Surgery.

Strabismus (*Squint*)
It is a condition where there is abnormal deviation in the position of the eyeball.
Varieties of squint are:
1. Horizontal squint when the deviation is along a horizontal plane. Horizontal squint may again be classified as Lateral (divergent) squint and Medial (convergent) squint.
2. Vertical squint when the deviation is in the vertical plane. Vertical squint may be in the form of an upward deviation of the eyeball or a downward deviation of eyeball.
3. Oblique squint when the deviation is in a direction other than the horizontal or vertical plane.

CAUSES
1. Squint may be a congenital condition without any apparent cause.
2. Middle ear infections, brain tumours, etc. are sometimes responsible for squint.

TREATMENT
If squint is not due to any apparent disease condition like meningitis, surgical treatment may be adopted. The object of the operation is to correct the position of the eyeball by cutting the particular eye muscle which is causing undue tension on the eyeball.

TECHNIQUE
With proper aseptic precaution, the eyelids are kept well dilated with a speculum. The conjunctiva in level with the

muscle to be divided is held with a conjunctival forceps and is incised. Through this incision a strbismus hook is introduced to locate the muscle to be divided. The muscle is then cut close to its scleral attachment with a narrow, thin bladed knife introduced through the conjunctival wound. The eyeball may rotate to the normal position as soon as the muscle is cut. The eye speculum is released. A suitable antibiotic eye ointment is applied to the eye daily and a bandage is put. Care is necessary to prevent the animal interfering with the eye post-operatively. Operation for squint is only very rarely successful in animals because of the difficulty in preventing post-operative interference.

Glaucoma

Glaucoma is a disease condition of the eye characterised by marked rise in the intraocular pressure.

Glaucoma is sometimes seen in dogs, it is very rare in other animals.

There is increased intraocular pressure due to excessive quantity of aqueous humour. It may result from increased production or decreased drainage of aqueous humour. (Glaucoma is different from hydrophthalmos. In hydrophthalmos there is enlargement of the eyeball due to weakening of its tunics, in addition to increased retention of aqueous humour.)

SYMPTOMS

1. There is severe pain. 2. Vision is greatly reduced. 3. The pupil is dilated. 4. Thère is increased tension in the eyeball. 5. The cornea is sensitive to touch. 6. There is lacrimation. 7. If the interior of the eye is examined with an ophthalmoscope the optic disc appears to be concave ("cupping of the optic disc"). 8. The retinal arteries appear constricted because of the pressure, and retinal veins are engorged with blood due to the compression at the optic disc. 9. Pressure atrophy of the choroid and retina is evident by greyish patches.

TREATMENT

Palliative treatment consists of instilling pilocarpine ($\frac{1}{4}\%$), diuretics, laxatives, salt-free diet, restricted water intake, etc. Surgical treatment is not of much curative value but may provide temporary relief. The following operations may be tried.

1. *Scleral puncture*: Site—On the sclera, immediately behind the limbus and in front of iris, near the temporal canthus of the eye. Before operation, sterilize the conjunctival cul-de-sac by instilling antibiotic eye drops and flush with sterile normal saline. Four per cent cocaine is used as anaesthetic. The puncture is made through the bulbar conjunctiva and sclera to let out the aqueous humour.

2. *Iridectomy*: Eye is prepared by frequent instillation of antibiotic eye drops about twenty-four hours prior to the operation and is flushed with sterile normal saline immediately before the operation. Four per cent cocaine solution is used as a surface anaesthetic. Eye is kept open with speculum. Using a Keratome the cornea is incised close to the limbus and in front of the iris, taking care not to injure the iris. When the knife is withdrawn, portion of aqueous humour escapes through this incision. A portion of iris also protrudes and this is held with iris forceps or iris hook and is drawn out of the wound as much as required. Then it is swabbed with 1 in 2,000 adrenaline. After a few seconds the protruding portion of iris is incised with a fine iris scissors. An iris probe is then introduced to push the remaining portion of iris back into position. Eye is again washed with normal saline.

Another method of doing iridectomy is by performing keratectomy, using a corneal trephine. A portion of cornea $\frac{1}{2}$ cm in diameter is cut and removed close to the limbus using a Walker's trephine. Through this opening iridectomy is conducted as in the previous case. This opening is covered with a conjunctival keratoplasty.

Parasites in the Anterior Chamber (*Worm in the Eye*)

The worm causes keratitis and opacity of the cornea. Setaria equi is seen in cattle and Setaria cervi in the horse.

DIAGNOSIS

The presence of worm can be recognised on careful examination.

TREATMENT

Operation for "worm in the eye" is recommended. An incision is made on the upper half of the cornea close to and parallel to the corneoscleral junction. near the outer canthus. When the incision is made, the aqueous humour escapes through it. A portion of the worm also may protrude through the wound and it can be removed with a forceps. If the worm does not protrude through the incision, inject a small quantity of warm normal saline solution into the anterior chamber to make it appear close to the wound and facilitate removal.

SURGICAL CONDITIONS AFFECTING THE CONJUNCTIVA

Conjunctiva has two parts namely, lining the inner surface of eyelids, called *palpebral conjunctiva* and the *bulbar conjunctiva* lining the sclera and the cornea. Over the cornea, however, only the epithelial layer of conjunctiva is present (Magrane, 1971).

Normal appearance of the conjunctiva is rosy pink and it is soft, smooth and moist. The appearance of conjunctiva is altered in various systemic diseases e.g., in gastrointestinal disorders it is congested, in jaundice it is yellow or icteric; shows petichae (pinpoint heamorrhages) in toxaemia and septicaemic conditions.

Echymosis of conjunctiva is noticed in protozoan diseases like surra. It is dry and pale in shock, pale and watery in anaemia, ulcerated in riboflavin deficiency, and thickened in Vitamin A deficiency (Xerophthalmia).

Conjunctivitis

Conjunctivitis or inflammation of the conjunctiva is one of the most common eye diseases.

CAUSES

1. Bacterial or virus infection, sometimes primary virus infection followed by secondary bacterial infection. 2. Irritation caused by chemical substances. 3. Presence of foreign bodies. 4. Trauma. 5. Allergy. 6. Nutritional deficiencies.

CLASSIFICATION

Based on etiology, conjunctivitis may be classified as Specific conjunctivitis (e.g., seen in pink eye in horses, distemper in dogs), and Non-specific conjunctivitis.

Clinically conjunctivitis is classified into three types, viz., acute, subacute and chronic conjunctivitis.

According to the nature of inflammation the following vari-

eties of conjunctivitis are also recognised.
1. Catarrhal conjunctivitis, e.g., conjunctivitis due to mild
bacterial infection or trauma.
2. Purulent (suppurative) conjunctivitis, e.g., conjunctivitis
seen in pink eye of horses, distemper of dogs, etc.
3. Croupous or Diphtheritic conjunctivitis, e.g., croupous con-
juctivitis seen in birds. Diphtheritic conjunctivitis seen in calves
due to infection by Fusiformis necroforus.
4. Granular or follicular conjunctivitis, causing small follicular
enlargements on the conjunctiva known as *trachoma*.

SYMPTOMS
1. Lacrimation: In the beginning stages of conjunctivitis
lacrimation is thin and watery. Later it becomes thicker and
has a tendency to stick on to the edges of lids and cheek. There
is tendency for the lids to stick together.
2. Photophobia and blepharospasm are not marked in simple
conjunctivitis. If these symptoms are present extension of inflammation to the cornea should be suspected.
3. Pain is not much. There is more of a discomfort than
actual pain.
4. Chemosis (protrusion of the swollen conjunctiva through
the palpebral fissure).

DIAGNOSIS
Diagnosis is easily made from the symptoms.

TREATMENT
The conjunctival sac is irrigated at frequent intervals with
warm saline solution or a mild antiseptic lotion. The eye lotions
commonly used are: ZAB lotion (zinc sulphate ½%, alum 1%,
boric acid 2%), Perchloride of mercury lotion (1 in 30,000 to 1
in 10,000), Argyrol (5%) and Boric lotion (2 to 3%). "Chloro
mycetin applicaps" are found effective in many cases of conjunctivitis due to bacterial infection. Other antibiotic eye ointments
like "Teramycin eye ointment" are also effective. In allergic conjunctivitis Hydrocortisone eye ointments are indicated (See p. 655).

Epiphora
Epiphora is a symptom characterised by excessive flow of

tears. It may be due to conjunctivitis, or due to stricture, atresia or obstruction of the lacrimal passages. If due to conjunctivitis it passes off when the inflammation subsides. Irrigation of the lacrimal passage or exploration with a flexible probe is necessary if the condition is due to obstruction or atresia.

Symblepharon

Symblepharon is a condition wherein the bulbar conjunctiva is adherent to the palpebral conjunctiva. This may be congenital or may result from blepharitis.

Ankyloblepharon

It is adhesion of the eyelids.

Pterygium

Pterygium is a condition where there is growth of conjunctiva extending towards the cornea. It can be removed surgically after ligation.

Dermoid (*Dermoid Cyst*; *Teratoma*)

Dermoid is a misplaced embryonic cutaneous tissue. It is sometimes seen in the eye. Dermoid cyst usually contains hairs growing on it and causes irritation of the conjunctiva and cornea. There is lacrimation. Dermoids may be cauterised by using silver nitrate sticks. The eye is irrigated with normal saline solution immediately after the application of silver nitrate to neutralise the effect of the caustic. Large sized dermoids may be removed surgically.

Keratitis

Keratitis means inflammation of cornea.

CAUSES

1. Infections due to bacteria, virus, richetssia, etc.
2. Trauma (including irritation caused by eyelashes, in entropion, trichiasis, distichiasis, etc.).
3. Chemical irritants.
4. Parasites in the eye.
5. Allergy.
6. Deficiency diseases (Vitamin A, Riboflavin, etc.).

7. Senility (due to old age).
8. Neoplastic conditions as dermoids.
9. Toxaemia
10. Diabetes.

CLASSIFICATION

Keratitis may be classified as follows.
1. Superficial keratitis, 2. Interstitial keratitis (parenchymatous keratitis), 3. Vascular keratitis, 4. Ulcerative keratitis, 5. Suppurative keratitis, and 6. Non-suppurative keratitis. The normal, clear, transparent, moist and glistening appearance of cornea is altered.

SYMPTOMS

Unlike conjunctivitis keratitis is a painful condition. Photophobia and blepharospasm are seen. There is loss of lusture (the shining appearance) of the cornea. The transparency of the cornea is altered and cloudiness or opacity is evident. Vascularisation of the cornea (pannus) may be noticed in severe cases.

The vessels invading the cornea may originate either from the superficial vessels of the conjunctiva or from the deeper ciliary vessels, situated at the limbus. Vessels originating from the conjunctiva are *bright red, wavy and superficial* whereas the ciliary vessels appear pale or bluish grey and have a more or less straight course. In chronic cases these vessels are arranged in a birch-broom fashion. In suppurative keratitis there is collection of pus in the anterior chamber of the eye. This is called *hypopyon*. The pus appears in the form of cloudy precipitates deposited at the bottom of the anterior chamber. When the inflammation subsides these precipitates usually get absorbed. But rarely they may remain permanently.

TREATMENT

1. Remove the cause.
2. Dionine (Merck) 5% solution is instilled into the eye to relieve pain.
3. Irrigating with antiseptic solutions like Perchoride of mercury lotion (1 in 30,000 to 1 in 10,000), ZAB lotion (zinc sulphate ½%, alum 1%, boric acid 2%), boric acid lotion (2 to 3%) etc.

4. Adequate intake of vitamin A, D and B-complex.

5. Instilling emollients like cod liver oil, milk, penicillin in oil, etc.

6. Hydrocortisone eye ointment.

7. Hydrocortisone injection subconjunctivally. Dose for dog: 0.1 to 0.3 cc of a 25 mg per cc solution.

8. Placental extract intramuscularly or subcutaneously: 1 to 4 cc for dog, cattle 5 to 20 cc. The injections are to be given daily for 30 days. This treatment is effective but costly.

9. Milk injections: Sterilized milk I/M or S/C: Cattle 5 to 25 cc. Dog 0.5 to 1 cc. To be repeated at intervals of 1 to 5 days.

Corneal Ulcer (*Ulcerative Keratitis*)

Ulcerative Keratitis is frequently met with in animals.

ETIOLOGY

The causes may be trauma, infections (like distemper in dogs), or nutritional deficiencies (like riboflavin deficiency).

Note. "Injections of live hepatitis vaccines are reported to cause occasionally allergic corneal and iridal reactions (corneal opacity and congestion of iris), one to three weeks after their injection. No treatment is necessary for this as the reactions subside spontaneously. Corticosteroids are contraindicated as corneal scarring and blindness have been reported with their use".*

SYMPTOMS

The ulcer on the cornea is easily recognised. If necessary, a 2% fluorescein solution may be used to aid diagnosis. The solution is instilled into the eye so as to stain the ulcer and make it visible.

PROGNOSIS

Guarded. When the ulcer heals a localised opacity of cornea results, because of the scar tissue.

COMPLICATIONS

1. *Keratocele*: Protrusion of an intact Decemet's membrane through the ulcer is called Keratocele. Keratocele may rupture.

---

*Smithcors, J.F. and Catcott, E.J. (Editors) (1968). Progress in Veterinary Practice. Book No. 7. American Veterinary Publications, Inc., California p. 475.

The rupture might help correction of the Keratocele and the ulcer might heal up, if small. Rupture may predispose to prolapse of iris if the wound on the cornea is sufficiently large. So it is better to make a small puncture of the Keratocele artificially to let out the aqueous humour and facilitate collapse of the protruded portion. The Keratocentesis may be repeated, if necessary.

2. *Staphyloma*: It is a protrusion of iris through a wound or ulcer on the cornea. There is leakage of aqueous humour and there is also chance of infection being carried through the perforation of the cornea. If the opening is large the lens may also prolapse. A small staphyloma resulting from a narrow opening in the cornea may slough off during the healing of the corneal wound.

TREATMENT OF CORNEAL ULCERS
1. Remove the cause.
2. Instilling Dionine 5% solution to relieve pain.
3. Administration of Vitamin A, C, D and B-complex.
For example, for dog: Vitamin C. 500 to 1000 mg daily orally.
Vitamin A. 5000 Units orally.
Niacin 100 to 150 mg. I/V every third or fourth day.
4. Antibiotic ointments and administration of antibiotics in case of infection.
5. Touching the ulcer carefully with carbolic acid is recommended if there is infection. A small match stick dipped in carbolic acid may be used for this purpose.
6. In Keratocele, Keratocentesis may be performed.
7. In staphyloma, snipping the iris in level with the corneal surface may be helpful.

Opacity of Cornea
Opacity of cornea is one of the symptoms of chronic Keratitis. In milder forms there is only cloudiness which clears up after the inflammation subsides. In chronic cases there is invasion of the corneal tissue by fibrous tissue and therefore the opacity becomes permanent.

CLASSIFICATION

According to the degree of opacity, opacities of the cornea may be classified as: (1) Nebula (light cloudiness), (2) Macula (moderate opacity), and (3) Leucoma (well-marked, dense, milky white opacity).

TREATMENT

1. Mildly irritant antiseptics like: Yellow eye ointment of mercury (Oculentum Hydrargyri Oxidi Flavum. 1 to 2%); Calomel powder; Mixture of Calomel plus Quinine sulphate plus Sugar in equal parts, etc. These are applied into the eye to stimulate re-absorption of the opacity.

2. Subconjunctival injection of 5 cc (in cattle) of normal saline solution, or normal saline with sodium iodide $\frac{1}{2}$%, is found to be effective in some cases.

3. Hydrocortisone injection subconjunctivally. Dose for dog is 0.1 to 0.3 cc of a 25 mg per cc solution.

4. Placental extract, milk injections, etc. as mentioned under treatment of Keratitis.

Luxation of the Lens

Displacement of the lens from its normal position is called "luxation of the lens". The lens may get displaced into the posterior chamber or into the anterior chamber. If associated with liquefaction of vitreous humour, it may get displaced backwards sinking into the liquefied vitreous humour.

CAUSES

1. Trauma. 2. As a complication of hydrophthalmos, iridocyclitis, etc. 3. Disease conditions causing wide variations in the aqueous humour causes softening of the lens, especially at the equator of lens and this facilitates loosening of its attachments to the suspensory ligament and luxation of the lens.

SYMPTOMS

1. *Irido donesis* or vibration of the iris when the head is moved.

2. *Aphakia*, i.e., the appearance of a portion of the suspensory ligament of the lens in the form of a shining cresent at pupillary margin.

3. Hydrophthalmos and opacity of cornea may be caused.

TREATMENT

Sometimes the displaced lens may atrophy and may get absorbed. Removal of the displaced lens may be advised in certain cases.

TECHNIQUE

Dilate the pupil with atropine or homatropine (2%). Puncture the cornea with the keratotomy knife (Graefe's knife) at 3-o clock position on the cornea and by using iris scissors make a semicircular incision on the upper half of cornea about 1 mm from the limbus. A small glass rod or a clinical thermometer may be used to gently press over the cornea so as to push the displaced lens towards the corneal wound. The lens is then removed with a forceps. The corneal wound is sutured with a size 6/0 eye silk. Conjunctival keratoplasty may also be done.

Cataract

Opacity of the lens is known as *cataract*. It is a degenerative lesion of the lens.

CLASSIFICATION

1. Congenital cataract—Cataract present at birth. (*Note*: In foetal life the lens receives its nutrition through vascular channels. After birth the lens is entirely dependent on the aqueous humour for its nutrition. In puppies and kittens it is normal for the vascular covering of the foetal lens to persist for a few days after the eyes have opened. This should not be mistaken for congenital cataract.)

2. Acquired cataract—Cataract developing later in life.

3. Complete cataract, involving the lens completely.

4. Partial cataract.

5. Progressive cataract.

6. Stationary cataract.

7. Senile cataract—Cataract developing due to old age.

8. Diabetic cataract—This also is not seen in Veterinary practice. Diabetic cataract is characterised by minute opacities developing on the superficial cortex of the lens due to turgidity

of cells in the superficial cortex of the lens. The turgidity of cells is apparently associated with the sugar content of aqueous humour.

9. Toxic cataract—Cataract caused by the circulation of toxins or poisons in the body, e.g., cataract due to equine influenza, periodic ophthalmia, distemper, chronic nephritis, ergot poisoning in cattle and pigs, experimental feeding of naphthalene, etc.

10. Capsular cataract—(Anterior capsular cataract and posterior capsular cataract). This is not common.

11. Cortical cataract—(Anterior cortical and posterior cortical cataracts). Majority of cortical cataracts are stellate cataracts, i.e., spreading from the centre of the lens to its periphery. Cortical cataract sometimes develops as a complication of a perforating corneal ulcer.

12. Pyramidal cataract—A localised opacity of the lens.

13. Lamellar cataract—The opacity is seen in the area between the lens nucleus and cortex.

14. Perinuclear cataract—This is lamellar cataract seen in horses.

15. Nuclear cataract—Confined to the central portion (nucleus) of the lens.

16. Diffuse cataract—Spreading evenly through the entire lens substance.

17. Calcareous cataract—Cataract in which the lens substance is partly converted into chalky materials.

18. At the *immature* (unripe) stage, when the cataract has not fully developed, it has a cloudy appearance. When *mature* (ripe) the colour is grey-white, amber, or, rarely, blackish. In the *hypermature* stage the lens is milky-white and there is partial liquification and calcification; the nucleus may actually sink down into the liquified lens substance. Surgical removal and replacement of the lens by an intraocular artificial lens, is possible at the right stage of maturity of the cataract; surgery is not likely to be successful at the hypermature stage.

ETIOLOGY
1. There might be a hereditory predisposition.
2. Toxins.
3. Senile changes attended with old age.
4. As a sequela of diseases of the eye like iridocyclitis or systemic diseases like diabetes.
5. Prolonged use of corticosteroids, locally or systemically.

PROGNOSIS
For juvenile cataract seen in young animals, the prognosis is good.

DIAGNOSIS
The pupil is dilated by instilling atropine or homatropine (2%) into the eye, in order to facilitate examination of the lens. The diagnosis can be made by using an ophthalmoscope or by the catoptric test.

TREATMENT
1. *Discission* or *Needling*: The anterior capsule of the lens is incised in a cruciate fashion, using a cataract needle so that the aqueous humour will come in contact with the lens substance and will facilitate re-absorption of the opacity. Discission will have to be repeated periodically to obtain the desired effect. It may not be effective in all cases.
2. *Couching of the lens*: The lens is pushed downwards and backwards by introducing a proper instrument through an incision in the cornea. Couching of the lens is not a practicable treatment in Veterinary practice because the suspensory ligament of the lens in animals is very strong.
3. In man, dissolution of the opaque lens by using 0.02% trypsine has been reported.
4. *Removal of the lens*: This operation is not usually done in Veterinary practice. It is occasionally done in the dog. The removal of the lens in the dog is more difficult than in man because the lens of the dog is proportionately much larger, and the suspensory ligament of the lens is tougher.
    Removal of the lens will not serve any purpose if there are degenerative changes in the retina associated with cataract. In estimating the prospects of the operation the existence of pupillary reflex is of some help.

There are two methods for removal of the lens, viz., the intracapsular extraction, and the extracapsular extraction.

Intracapsular extraction is the extraction of the lens *with its capsule.* This is difficult in animals because of the tough suspensory ligament.

Extracapsular extraction is the extraction of the lens without its capsule. The anterior capsule of the lens is incised and through that the lens substance is removed. Extracapsular extraction is successful only if the cataract is ripe (mature). At this stage the endothelial cells of the capsule that are left behind are incapable of proliferating. Whereas, if the operation is done before fully ripe, the proliferation of the endothelial cells after surgery may once again create opacity and this will interfere with vision. Extracapsular extraction of the lens is difficult if the cataract is hyper-mature because of the partial liquefaction or softening of the lens substance.

TECHNIQUE FOR REMOVAL OF LENS

The operation is done under general anaesthesia.

The eyeball is fixed during the operation by one or more stay sutures passed through the sclera. *Temporary canthotomy* may be done, if necessary to get more space for manipulation. (Canthotomy is the opening out of the lateral cathus of the eye by incising the skin. After completion of the operation the skin incision is sutured.)

The cornea is punctured above the 3-O-clock point, about 0.1 cm away from the limbus. By using a small scissors or the Graefes' knife the incision is extended upwards along the cornea parallel to the limbus, to the 9-O-clock point.

In intracapsular extraction, the lens is held close to its equator with a special forceps (Duthies' forceps or Arrugas' forceps) and then it is gently moved and detached from its suspensory ligament.

If extracapsular extraction is desired, the anterior capsule of the lens is incised in the form of a T and a cataract scoop is used to remove the lens substance.

After removal of the lens the corneal wound is sutured. *Conjunctival keratoplasty* is advisable. Postoperative interference by patient should be guarded against. For this it is desirable to administer sedatives for at least two or three days.

SURGICAL CONDITIONS AFFECTING THE UVEA

Coloboma of iris

Coloboma is a congenital condition in which portion of the iris is absent. This may give the pupil an irregular shape. When coloboma is situated away from the pupillary margin, more than one pupil may become apparent.

Aniridia

Aniridia is a condition in which iris is completely absent.

Iritis

Inflammation of the iris.

Cyclitis

Inflammation of the ciliary body.

Iridocyclitis

Iridocyclitis is inflammation of the iris and the ciliary body. A very characteristic symptom of this condition is flushing (engorgement) of vessels at the sclerocorneal junction. This type of persistent flushing of vessels at the limbus is stated to be one of the symptoms of tuberculosis of the eye in man.

Choroiditis

Inflammation of the choroid.

Uveitis .

Inflammation of the iris, ciliary body and choroid.

Hyalitis

Inflammation of the vitreous body (vitreous humour).

Retinitis

Inflammation of retina.

Anterior Synechia

Attachment of the iris to the cornea is called anterior synechia. This is sometimes seen as a sequela of staphyloma.

Posterior Synechia

Attachment of the iris to the lens is called posterior synechia. Sometimes seen as a sequela of periodic ophthalmia in the horse.

Periodic Ophthalmia of Horses (*Moon Blindness*; *Recurrent Opthalmia*)

Periodic ophthalmia of horses is characterised initially by repeated attacks of iridocyclitis. After repeated attacks of the disease there is atrophy of the eyeball. The retrobulbar fat gets absorbed and consequently the eyeball sinks into the orbit. The eyelids become greatly wrinkled and shrunken.

ETIOLOGY

The cause of the disease is not definitely known. The disease appears to be contagious but attempts to transmit the disease artificially have not been successful. The disease occurs in places where a number of horses are housed together, as in the army.

SYMPTOMS

The disease usually affects only one eye in the beginning. Photophobia, blepharospasm and lacrimation are present. The tears are sticky and become adherent to the eyelids and cheek. Conjunctivitis and engorgement of blood vessels around the sclero-corneal junction are seen. The consistency of the aqueous humour is altered, there is accumulation of whitish or yellowish precipitates in the anterior chamber (hypopyon) and due to this the cornea may appear completely opaque. Pupil is constricted. Recovery takes place in about 3 weeks, the precipitates get absorbed and the pupil dilates to the normal size.

After seven to ten days the symptoms recur either in the same eye or in the other eye. During this second attack symptoms are more severe. Thus the same eye may become affected repeatedly. Due to these recurrent attacks the eye is permanently damaged. The cornea and lens show opacity; posterior synechia is a constant sequela of the disease: the retina atrophies; and the vitreous humour undergoes liquefaction.

The vitreous humour when examined through an ophthalmoscope presents a characteristic appearance with star-like floating bodies described as *synchysis scintillans*. The aqueous humour gets partially absorbed and the eyeball shrinks. The fat in the orbit gets absorbed, the eyeball sinks into the orbit and the eyelids get wrinkled. Permanent blindness is caused.

DIAGNOSIS

The disease is characterised by its sudden onset without any apparent cause. The pupil is constricted and fails to dilate with atropine. Pressure on the supraorbital fossa evinces pain. Posterior synechia may be noticed.

TREATMENT

There is no curative treatment. Symptomatic treatment may be tried.

Amaurosis

Amaurosis is blindness without any apparent lesion in the eye. It may be temporary or permanent. Possible causes are toxaemia, lesions in the brain, etc.

(*Note*: A temporary form of amaurosis is sometimes seen in cattle due to deficiency of Vitamin A which can be corrected by administration of Vitamin A.)

Refraction of the Eye

Parallel rays: The amount of divergence of light rays falling on a given area is inversely proportionate to the distance from the source of light. When the distance is 20 feet or *more*, the divergence is so slight that the rays can be considered as parallel.

Emmetropia (*Normal sight*): When the refraction of the eye is normal, parallel rays coming into the eye in a condition of rest, are focussed exactly on the retina. The normal reading range in a man of 38 to 45 years is 50 cm.

Ametropia: Ametropia is a term used to denote a condition of abnormal refraction of the eye due to hypermetropia, myopia, or astigmatism, in which parallel rays are focussed either in front or behind the retina.

Hypermetropia (*Hyperopia*; *Long sight*; *Far sight*): Hypermetropia is a condition of abnormal refraction of the eye in which parallel rays come to a focus behind the retina. This type of ametropia is caused if the axis of the eyeball is too short or if the refractive power of the eye is too weak.

Myopia (*Short sight*; *Near sight*): Myopia is a condition of abnormal refraction of the eye in which parallel rays get focussed in front of the retina. This may happen either due to the axis of the eyeball being too long or due to the refractive power of the eye being too strong. (In this condition the eye is able to see clearly only objects very close to it.)

Astigmatism: When the refraction through several meridians of the eye is different, the condition is called astigmatism. Astigmatism may be caused by irregularities in the cornea or the lens. Astigmatism causes blurred vision.

(*Note*: A certain degree of astigmatism is normally present in the horse.)

Prisms and Lenses

Refraction by a prism: Light rays passing through a prism are bent toward its base; an object seen through a prism appears displaced towards its apex.

Formation of lenses by prisms: See figures in textbooks on ophthalmology.

Numbering of Prisms

There are three methods for expressing the strength of a prism.

1. *Prism diopters* ($\triangle$): The prism diopter is a deviation, the tangent of which is 1/100 of the radius, and is expressed as 1$\triangle$, 2$\triangle$, 3$\triangle$, etc.

2. *Degrees*: In this method the strength of the prism is equal to the refracting angle (geometrical angle), e.g., Prism 1°, 2°, 3°, etc.

3. *Centrad* ($\triangle$): A centrad corresponds to a deviation the arc of which is 1/100 of the radius, and is expressed 1$\triangledown$, 2$\triangledown$, 3$\triangledown$, etc.

(*Note*: For practical purposes, the three scales (diopters, degrees and centrad) can be considered almost alike.)

Varieties of Lenses

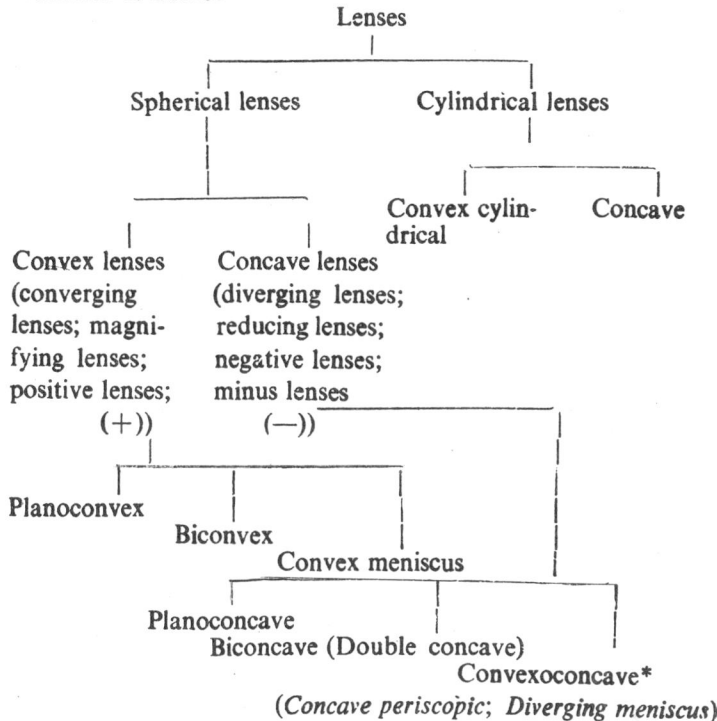

```
                              Lenses
                                |
          ┌─────────────────────┴──────────────────────┐
   Spherical lenses                          Cylindrical lenses
          |                                             |
          |                               ┌─────────────┴──────┐
   ┌──────┴──────┐                  Convex cylin-        Concave
   |             |                    drical
Convex lenses  Concave lenses
(converging    (diverging lenses;
lenses; magni- reducing lenses;
fying lenses;  negative lenses;
positive lenses;  minus lenses
   (+))           (—))
```

Planoconvex
Biconvex
Convex meniscus
Planoconcave
Biconcave (Double concave)
Convexoconcave*
(*Concave periscopic; Diverging meniscus*)

Numbering of Lenses

The strength (refractive power) of the lens is indicated by its principal focal distance. The principal focal distance is the distance between optical centre (c) and principal focus (Pf); i.e., the distance between Pf and c.

The shorter this distance the stronger is the lens, and the longer the distance, the weaker is the lens. The strength of a lens is the inverse of its focal distance.

The strength or refractive power of a lens is commonly expressed in the Metric or *dioptric system*.

The lens which has a principal focal distance of 1 metre (about 40 inches) is taken as the standard (unit) and is known as 1 diopter (1 D). A lens which has twice this strength is known as

---

*(*Note*: In the convexo-concave lens, the concave side has the shorter radius of curvature.)

2D and its principal focal distance will be 0.5 metre.

A lens half as strong as the standard lens is referred to as 0.50 D and its principal focal distance is 2 metres. The principal focal distance is obtained by dividing 100 by the number of the lens.

Example:

Number of the lens = 4.00 D

$$\text{Principal focal distance} = \frac{100}{4.00} \text{ Cm.}$$

$$= 25 \text{ Cm. } (0.25 \text{ metre})$$

Questions

1. What are the symptoms of intraocular filariasis in horses? What complications are likely to result from a keratocentesis?

2. Give an account of corneal ulceration with special reference to its etiology, complications and treatment.

3. Give the etiology, symptoms and treatment of moon blindness in horse.

4. Give an account of keratitis in cattle, its complications and methods of treatment.

5. Describe the condition popularly called "worm in the eye". How will you treat it? What is the prognosis?

6. Write short notes on:

(a) Entropion, (b) Pannus, (c) Staphyloma, (d) Cataract, (e) Glaucoma, (f) Corneal ulcer, (g) Corneal opacity, (h) Cupping of the optic disc.

7. Describe the tests used for determining visual function in domestic animals.

8. Discuss the incidence of cataract in animals and describe the treatment advised.

9. Enumerate the common causes of blindness in horse and dog. Describe how visual function may be tested and state how defective vision due to organic changes in the lens may be rectified.

10. What is a teratoma? Write briefly on its incidence, with special reference to dogs and calves and give an outline of the treatment advised.

11. Describe briefly the procedures for examination of vision. State the conditions that cause defective vision in cattle.

CHAPTER 52

Surgical Conditions Affecting Birds

The reproductive system of the *male* fowl consists of two testes and the vasa deferentia (one from each testes) leading to the cloaca.

The reproductive system of the *female* fowl normally consists of only *one* ovary (the left) and the oviduct; because out of the two ovaries seen in early embryonic life, only the left ovary develops and the other one remains undeveloped. In cases where the right ovary is recognised in adult life, it can usually be seen only as a non-functioning rudiment. However, there are reported extraordinary cases wherein both ovaries are present and functioning.

General Anaesthesia

Sl. No.	Kind of animal	Drug	Route	Time taken to set in	Duration	Supplementary dose for extended duration	Remark
1.	Fowl	Nembutal solution 0.5 to 0.75 ml of a 5% solution.	I/V slowly into wing vein.	Immediate	2 hours	Up to 0.25 ml.	The duration is extended to several hours if a supplementary dose is given.

		Nembutal 5% solution				
2.	Turkey	1 to 2ml. per pound body weight.	-do-	Immediate	2 hours	— —

			By mouth 1 to 2% solution			
3.	Fowl	Chloral Hydras.	at the rate of 0.2g per kg body weight.	25 to 30 minutes	4 hours	— —

(*Note*: Even though ether and chloroform can be used as general anaesthetic for the fowl, the use of these drugs is frequently followed by fatal results. The use of Nembutal (Pentobarbital Sodium) is comparatively safe.)

Caponization
Castration of male fowls is called *caponizing*.

INDICATION
For fattening broiler cockerels, for improving quality and quantity of meat.

The recommended age for caponization is ten weeks or about six to eight weeks prior to slaughter for meat.

PRE-OPERATIVE
No feed should be given eighteen to twenty-four hours prior to the operation. Better to withold water also twelve hours before operation because this minimises bleeding.

ANAESTHESIA
Local infiltration anaesthesia.

SITE
The last intercostal space of either side, close to the anterior border of the last rib to avoid the major intercostal vessels along posterior border of the rib.

CONTROL

It is desirable to secure the bird on a sloping board so that the operator can see the testicle from the ventral aspect of the bird.

The legs are stretched and tied together in the extended position and secured to the upper portion of the sloping board, and the wings together are secured in the opposite direction. It might be advantageous to have holes made in the board for purposes of securing; otherwise an assistant may hold the wings and head with one hand and the legs with the other hand. The head is held by putting a finger around the base of the neck.

Proper stretching of the legs is very important to keep away the thigh muscle (tensor facia lata) from the site.

TECHNIQUE

The lower testicle should be removed first, if both testicles are to be removed through a single incision.

The skin is incised half to one inch at the site and the Tensor facia lata is pushed backwards to make visible the intercostal muscles.

Incise also the intercostal muscles, introduce a rib-retractor and dilate the wound. The parietal peritoneum is seen which is torn with the peritoneum tearing hook. The testicle will be seen as a maggot-like body anterior to the kindney. (In older birds the testis is much larger than the size of a maggot, with very prominent vessels.) Hold the testis with the jaws of a caponizing forceps, give a gentle twisting motion combined with traction and remove it. Damage to the posterior vena cava should be avoided. Remove the retractor and release the bird. No suture necessary.

The testicle and connecting portion of spermatic duct should be removed to ensure complete success for the operation. If a portion of testis is left back, the desired result may not be obtained and the bird is called a "*slip*".

The operation is repeated on the other side, if both testes are not removed through the same side.

POST-OPERATIVE CARE

Confine the bird in a small enclosure to avoid flying or running about and secondary haemorrhage. Usually no complications, and the bird is ready to take feed and water immediately after the operation.

Sub-cutaneous emphysema or "wing-puffs" rarely form due to entrance of air through the wound. This is not of much significance and can be easily relieved by puncturing the skin if necessary.

The incision heals completely in about two to three weeks. (See also page 626.).

Eye Worms

INDICATION
Removal of eyeworm (Oxyspirum mansoni) found under the nictitating membrane of the fowl, causing scratching with resultant inflammation and swelling of eye.

ANAESTHESIA
Instil into the eye a few drops of a suitable local anaesthetic. (e.g., Anethane (Glaxo); Butyn).

TECHNIQUE
After lifting the third eyelid with fingers or a blunt instrument, instil one or two drops of a 5% solution of Creolin on the worms and immediately thereafter, irrigate the eye with clean water. The worms are killed in this manner and can then be removed with a forceps.

Laparotomy
The common sites for laparotomy in the fowl are: Between the last two ribs. It is suitable for caponization, caecal ligation, etc.

Parallel to the left pubic bone. Also suitable for ligation of caecum.

Caecal Abligation (*Ligation of Caecum*)

INDICATION
Done in turkeys to control *black head*.

SITE
(1) Between the last two ribs, as described above for caponization. (2) Parallel to the left pubic bone.

TECHNIQUE

If approached through the last intercostal site (site No. 1), the junction of the two caeca to the main gut can be located almost opposite the site. Each caecum is ligated separately close to its junction with the main gut. The functional communication is thus severed and within a few days after the operation the caecum atrophies. It does not, however, undergo necrosis because the blood supply through its mesenteric attachment is retained.

Ascitis

Tapping the abdomen with a small trocar and canula or needle and syringe is recommended.

Up to about 12 ml may be removed daily. There might be tendency to refill.

Eggs in the Abdomen

Eggs or parts of eggs accumulated in the abdominal cavity may be removed surgically.

It is advisable during the operation to remove the larger egg yolks also from the ovary so that there may not be any laying of new eggs before healing is complete.

Deutectomy

Surgical removal of the yolk sac from newly hatched out chicks for experimental purposes when certain nutritional studies are conducted. Removal of the yolk sac ensures a uniform sample of chicks for the experiment that have derived little initial supply of vitamins and minerals from the yolk sac.

TECHNIQUE

Incise the abdomen through any of the sites described above and expel the yolk sac, and touch the yolk stalk with a small heated blunt instrument. Suture the abdominal wound. (Sloan, 1936; Harvey, Parrish and Sandford, 1955.)

Gizzardectomy

Removal of the gizzard is done for experimental studies relating to function of the gizzard, by comparing gizzardectomised and normal birds (Burrows, 1936).

Rectostomy

Connecting the rectum to an artificial anus, so that the urine and faeces can be collected separately (Rothchild, 1947).

Resection of Oviduct

For making studies of eggs produced by hens in which various sections of the oviduct have been surgically removed, and comparing with unoperated hens (Barger., Card. and Pomery, 1958).

Bumble Foot

Bumble foot is an abscess on the foot.

CAUSES

1. Traumatic injuries like contusion or small wounds with secondary infection. 2. Deficiency of Vitamin-A (Nutritional bumble foot).

SYMPTOMS

Lameness.

PROGNOSIS

Usually favourable.

TREATMENT

The scab or thick skin covering the abscess may be removed and the pus expelled. Clean and apply an antiseptic solution and put on a bandage. Repeat cleaning and dressing at intervals of two to three days. Administer Vitamin A (Barger., Card. and Pomery, 1958).

Ingluviotomy

Ingluviotomy or opening of the crop is done in severe impaction of the crop. The site of operation is over the distended crop which can be felt at the base of the neck towards the right side. The skin and the wall of the crop are incised to remove the contents. For closure, the edges of the incision on the crop are sutured by simple interrupted sutures; and the skin edges are sutured separately.

Cropectomy

Similar to ingluviotomy, but a large portion of the crop is removed before suturing.

Amputation of Comb (Dubbing) and Amputation of the Wattles (Cropping)

INDICATIONS
1. Abnormally large size of the comb/wattles interfering with feeding.
2. Oedema of the wattles, injury and necrosis, etc.

TECHNIQUE
After cutting away the excess portion with a scalpel or scissors, the bleeding can be controlled in a simple manner by placing a clean feather over the cut surface.

Or, the cutting away of the excess portion can be done distal to a line of haemostatic sutures to control bleeding.

Trimming the Spurs

INDICATIONS
The male birds are de-spurred to prevent injury to the female.

TECHNIQUE
1. Using a sharp knife of rasp, the spur is trimmed or rasped to a smooth, blunt end.
2. It is possible to prevent the growth of spurs by cutting off the spur cap at a very young age and touching it off with a caustic potash stick (as in the case of de-horning cattle). This is better done when the bird is about *ten to twelve weeks* old, or when the spur cap is not more than about ¼ inch long.

Pinioning
(See page 650).

De-beaking

In this operation, about one-third the length of the *upper* beak at its tip is cut and removed. The operation can be repeated once in forty days, if necessary, as the beak grows.

INDICATION

1. To enable the bird to feed better; otherwise it may have a tendency to feed selectively on grit/grains instead of consuming the mash as a whole.

2. To prevent the birds pecking at each other and causing injury. (Cannibalism).

TECHNIQUE

A special instrument called "De-beaking Forceps" is used. Alternatively, it can also be done with a suitable knife or scissors, but care is necessary to avoid splitting the beak.

De-beaking may be done even when chicks are ten-day old.

Part III

Operative Surgery

CHAPTER 53

Anaesthesia and Analgesia

Anaesthesia is a term used to indicate production of insensitivity. *Anaesthetics* are substances used for inducing anaesthesia. Anaesthesia is classified into four main types, viz.,

1. Local anaesthesia (analgesia) e.g., by surface application, by local infiltration S/C or intradermally.

2. Regional anaesthesia (analgesia) e.g., nerve blocks, epidural injection into the subarachnoid space.

3. Sedation and narcosis. Used usually before the administration of local or general anaesthesia and hence the drugs used for this purpose are generally termed preanaesthetics. Narcotics depress the activity of the central nervous system. Drugs which cause sedation without drowsiness are called *ataractics* or *tranquilizers*. A *hypnotic* is a drug used to induce sleep.

4. General anaesthesia.

Local Analgesia

For local anaesthesia drugs are applied about nerve terminals or injected around nerve fibres to prevent conduction of nerve impulses by the nerve tissue. According to modern terminology drugs used for this purpose are called local *analgesics* and not local *anaesthetics*. Therefore the term local analgesia has been preferred to the term local anaesthesia by certain authors.

The desensitisation of an area by injecting analgesics around its borders is called *field anaesthesia* or *field block*.

The local analgesics commonly used are as follows.

1. *Procaine (Novocaine) hydrochloride*: Commonly used as 2% to 2.5% solutions for local infiltration and nerve block and as 1 to 2.5 % solutions for epidural analgesia, perferably combined with adrenaline 1 in 100,000. Anaesthesia develops in about five minutes and lasts for about one hour. When combined

with adrenaline, procaine is ten times less toxic than cocaine. It is quickly detoxicated by the liver. Non-irritating. Can be sterilised by boiling but is decomposed in alkaline solutions.

2. *Amethocaine hpdrochloride (Anethaine)*: This is five to ten times more powerful than procaine, used as 1% solution for local infiltration and 2% solution for surface application. More toxic than procaine but the quantity required is less. Commonly used for surface anaesthesia.

3. *Lignocaine hydrochloride*: Effective both for surface application (4%) and for local infiltration (2%). Solutions are very stable and are not decomposed by boiling, strong alkalies or acids.

4. *Cocaine*: For surface anaesthesia on mucous membranes. Four per cent solution for eye and 10 % to 20% solution for nasal and laryngeal mucous membranes. Can be used for local infiltration (2% to 4%) but being very toxic other drugs are perferable. Convulsions, loss of consciousness and respiratory depression due to paralysis of medullary centres are likely to be caused by toxic doses exceeding 15 mg for cat, 45 mg for small dog, 120 mg for large dog, and 780 mg for horse.

Regional Analgesia

In regional analgesia the analgesic is injected over the main nerve trunk (e.g., nerve block) supplying a given area or region. *Epidural anaesthesia* also comes under regional analgesia because the effect is brought about by the analgesic solution coming in contact with the spinal nerves at their origin in the vertebral canal.

The details regarding various nerve blocks and epidural anaesthesia in different species may be obtained elsewhere from this book.

Pre-anaesthetic Medication (*Pre-medication*)

Pre-anaesthetic medication includes administration of sedatives, narcotics, tranquilizers, etc., with a view to minimise excitement and struggling during induction of and recovery from anaesthesia. They also make, anaesthesia safer and more comfortable for the patient by dercreasing irritability of the central nervous system and by enhancing the effects of the anaesthetic. Most sedatives are respiratory depressants.

DRUGS USED FOR PRE-MEDICATION

1. *Atropine*: Atropine is given S/C to the horse, pig, dog and cat, thirty to forty minutes before the administration of the anaesthetic to reduce mucous and salivary secretions. It should not be given to ruminents for this purpose because in these animals atropine makes secretions much thicker.

Dose: *Pig* and *Dog* 1/50 to 1/200 grain S/C; *Cat* 1/200 grain S/C; *Horse* up to 1 grain S/C. For quicker effect atropine can be given I/M or I/V. (See also page-652).

2. *Morphine*: Morphine is given S/C to the dog thirty to forty minutes before the administration of anaesthesia usually in combination with atropine, for sedative effect. It induces vomiting within about fifteen minutes due to stimulation of vomiting centre but since this is followed by depression of the vomiting centre, there is no danger of its causing vomiting during anaesthesia. Morphine causes respiratory depression. It may cause death of foetus if given to pregnant animals by passing through the placenta.

Dose: 1/4 grain S/C is sufficient even for the large sized *Dog*. Higher doses are unnecessary and may produce undesirable respiratory depression.

Morphine is not recommended for other species.

3. *Pethidine* (Burroughs Wellcome & Co.) is a drug whose action is similar to morphine but unlike morphine it can be prescribed for all species. It is given with atropine. Pethidine is quite safe for cats also. Available in 2cc ampoules containing 100 mg.

Dose: *Cat* 10 mg S/C; *Dog* 100 mg S/C; *Horse, Cattle* and *Pig* up to 1 gramme S/C.

4. *Largactyl* (M & B) (Chlor promazine hydrochloride) is a tranquilizing agent. It is also antiemetic, antiadrenaline and vagolytic.

Dose: *Horse* maximum dose 0.4 mg per kg body weight I/M 60 to 90 minutes before induction of anaesthesia. *Pig* 1.0 mg per kg body weight I/M 40 to 60 minutes prior to anaesthesia. *Dog* maximum dose 1 mg per kg I/M 60 to 90 minutes before anaesthesia (If I/V 10 to 15 minutes before). *Cat* 1 mg per kg body weight I/M 40 to 60 minutes before anaesthesia.

5. *Siquil* (squibb) available in rubber-capped vials of 5 ml containing 20 mg per ml.

When given before anaesthesia, reduces the dose of barbiturates required to one-half for general anaesthesia.

Should be given five to fifteen minutes before the anaesthetic drug, if intravenously; ten to thirty minutes if intramuscularly; forty to forty five minutes if orally.

Species	Intravenous	Intramuscular
Dog	0.5 to 1 mg per pound body weight.	1 to 2 mg/lb.
Cat	—	2 to 4 mg/lb.
Cattle	5 to 8 mg per 100 lb.	10 to 15 mg. per 100 lb.
Horse	10 to 15 mg per 100 lb. (Max. 100 mg)	As for I/V.
Pig	40 mg/100 lb.	60 mg per 100 lb.
Sheep	1 mg/2 lb (Max. 40 mg)	—

(*Note*: The intra-peritoneal dose is same as intravenous dose. The oral dose is approximately double the parenteral dose.)

Basal Narcosis

Basal narcosis is a stage of narcosis at which the animal is unconscious but still is capable of responding to painful stimuli. In *light narcosis* the animal may be able to keep standing but its responses to external stimuli are reduced. In *medium narcosis* the animal is unable to stand but in the recumbent position it may struggle and try to get up unless properly restrained. In *deep narcosis* which is very close to the stage of anaesthesia, there is muscular relaxation and responses to external stimuli are very sluggish though not absent.

Medium narcosis is sufficient to perform operations combined with local and regional anaesthesia.

Inducing basal narcosis before administration of general anaesthesia is desirable because it reduces the quantity of anaesthetic required and thus increases the safety margin. The involuntary excitement during induction is minimised, the onset becomes smooth and regular and a uniform depth of anaesthesia is more easily maintained. Drugs commonly used for basal narcosis are Chloral hydras and Pentobarbitone Sodium (Nembutal).

1. *Chloral hydras*: Freely soluble in water but chemically incompatible with alkalies. The drug can be used as a general anaesthetic also by increasing beyond th narcotic dose. Toxic doses cause death by respiratory failure and circulatory depre-

ssion. The drug can be administrated by stomach tube, by enema, by intraperitoneal or I/V injections. However, the rectal route is unreliable in bringing about proper effect and the intraperitonal route is not very desirable due to the irritant nature of the drug. Chloral hydras is the *best basal narcotic for horse and adult* cattle. Can be used in pigs also.

Dose: The general dose for horse and cattle is 5 to 6 grammes per 50 kg body weight. Accordingly a horse can be given (by stomach tube), 1¼ to 1¾ ounces for light narcosis, 1¾ to 2½ ounces for medium narcosis and 2¼ to 3 ounces for deep narcosis. The stomach should be kept empty by withholding feed for 24 hours. Narcosis commences from 5 to 10 minutes and maximum depth is obtained in 10 to 20 minutes. The duration in deep narcosis is about 1 hour.

For intravenous administration in the horse quantities up to the above dosage limits can be given but if the desired depth of narcosis is obtained before the calculated dose has been administered, the injection is discontinued. The strength of solution for I/V is 10%.

For cattle 1 to 2 ounces are given as a drench for light to medium narcosis. Maximum depth of narcosis is obtained in 10 to 20 minutes. To induce deep narcosis or light general anaesthesia the drug is better given intravenously as a 10 to 12% solution in the calculated dose of 5 to 6 grammes per 50 kg body weight.

2. *Pentobarbitone sodium (Nembutal)*: Nembutal is a good basal narcotic for small animals, calves and foals. In horse and adult cattle it can be used I/V as a 6.5% solution 15 to 20 cc, to prolong the basal narcosis induced by chloral hydras. Nembutal is not generally used alone in large animals because of its cost, prolonged action and due to the excitement and struggling produced during the stage of recovery. For calves and foals it can be used as a 6.5% solution I/V for basal narcosis or anaesthesia. For dogs and cats it is given I/V as a 3 to 6% solution up to a calculated dose of 1/5 grain per lb body weight, the injection discontained when the desired stage of narcosis or anaesthesia is obtained.

General Anaesthesia

General anaesthesia is a state of unconsciousness combined with loss of sensitivity and reduced motor response to stimuli, produced in a controlled manner by a process of reversible intoxication of the central nervous system.

General anaesthesia may be grouped into the following two types.

1. *Intravenous anaesthesia*: The anaesthetic drug chosen is administered I/V, e.g., Chloral hydras, Pentobarbitone Sodium (Nembutal), Thiopentone Sodium (Intraval Sodium), Thialbarbitone Sodium, Thiamylal, Methohexital Sodium, etc.

2. *Inhalation anaesthesia*: For this volatile drugs are administered by inhalation, e.g., Chloroform, Ether (Diethyl Ether), Ethyl chloride, Trichloroethylene, Halothane (Fluothane), Methoxyflurane, Nitrous oxide, Cyclopropane, etc.

MODE OF ACTION OF GENERAL ANAESTHETICS

There are several theories about the action of anaesthetics, but none of these have been accepted as completely satisfactory.

1. *The colloid theory*: According to this theory, anaesthesia is brought about by the reversible aggregation of cell colloids. Aggregation of colloids in the cell is brought about with the onset of anaesthesia and this is reversed with the recovery from anaesthesia.

Although this theory may to some extent explain changes brought about in the cells of lower forms of life like amoeba, by the anaesthetic drugs, the action produced in higher species of animals appears to be not so simple.

2. *Lipoid (lipid) solubility theory*: Mayer (1899) brought out a theory that: "All chemical substances which are soluble in fats or fatty substances, must exert a narcotic action on living protoplasm, in so long as they become distributed in it." In other words, the capacity of an anaesthetic drug to act depends on its solubility in fats (lipoids).

It has been observed, however, that certain drugs soluble in fats cause convulsions and not depression or anaesthesia and this questions the lipoid theory. Further, it is argued, that even through the fat solubility may throw some light on how the drug is brought to the central nervous system, it does not satisfactorily explain the mode of action of the drug. It is also worthwhile to note that certain drugs like morphine which are insoluble in fats are still capable of bringing about narcosis.

3. *Cell permeability theory*: This theory assumes that anaes-

thesia is produced because of the capacity of the drug to affect the permeability of the cell membrane, thereby altering the cellular constitution; but it also is not satisfacto.y because drugs like digitalis which affect cell permeability do not cause anaesthesia.

4. *Biochemical theory*: It has been proved experimentally that there is decreased oxygen consumption during anaesthesia and, therefore, decreased oxygen consumption brought about in the brain tissue by certain biochemical changes was proposed as the cause of anaesthesia.

The decrease in oxygen consumption might be only a reflection of the decreased metabolic activity resulting from anaesthesia, rather than the causing of anaesthesia. Hence this theory only indicates a phenomenon resu'ting from anaesthesia and does not explain the mechanism of production of anaesthesia.

5. *Neuro-physiological theories*: The impulses to the brain normally travel through two pathways, namely, (1) the relatively rapid lemniscal pathway through thalamus to sensory cortex, and (2) the more slow extra-lemniscal pathway. It is believed that consciousness of the individual is maintained by the constant travelling of impulses through the extra-lemniscal pathway.

The neuro-physical theroy is based on the demonstration in 1952 of Larrabee (quoted by Soma, 1971) that anaesthetics *selectively* inhibit transmission of impulses through synapses and proposes that anaesthesia is brought about by the blocking of the extra-lemniscal pathway (which is responsible for normal consciousness), without blocking the lemniscal pathway.

It is, however, noted that the theory does not explain the mechanism as to how exactly this selective blocking is brought about. Hence some authors have rather humourously commented that this theory "simply says that anaesthetics act by causing anaesthesia".

6. *Physical theories*: Many investigators have tried to correlate the action of anaesthetic drugs to the physical properties like solubility in fat/protein/water, and the thermodynamic activity exhibited by vapour pressure/surface tension/ intermolecular attraction/molecular volume. But no satisfactory explanation is forthcoming regarding the actual mechanism of production of anaesthesia, for which considerably ɔre work seems necessary.

STAGES OF GENERAL ANAESTHESIA

The development of complete general anaesthesia has been described in 4 stages.

Stage 1: This is called the stage of induction or the stage of voluntary excitement. The animal is fully conscious and is excited. The pulse and respiration rates are accelerated. Breath-holding may be noticed. Faeces and urine may be passed.

Stage 2: Stage of *involuntary excitement*. Consciousness is lost, respirations are regular and breath-holding also may occur. Exaggerated response to stimuli, violent limb movements or muscular rigidity may be noticed. This is followed by a gradual relaxation of muscles when the animal enters the next stage.

The stages 1 and 2 can be shortened and made to pass off smoothly by the use of pre-anaesthetics.

Stage 3: This is the stage of *surgical anaesthesia* and is further subdivided into 3 planes. In the *first plane* of surgical anaesthesia (*light anaesthesia*) breathing becomes regular and the limb movements stop. The eyeballs may be moving from side to side but they soon get fixed when the second plane of anaesthesia is entered. The palpebral, cojunctival and corneal reflexes become sluggish or almost absent. In dogs and cats the *pedal reflex* is present. (The pedal reflex is the pulling away of the limb when the web of the foot is pinched.) Minor operations like openings of abscesses can be done under light anaesthesia.

In the *second plane* of surgical anaesthesia (*medium anaesthesia*) the respirations are more or less same as in the first plane but the pedal reflex becomes sluggish and muscular relaxation becomes progressively more pronounced. In cattle, horse, pig and sheep the eyeball is fixed and central but in the dog it may rotate downwards. Most operations, except laparotomy and thoracotomy, can be performed under medium anaesthesia.

In the *third plane* of surgical anaesthesia (*deep anaesthesia*) respiration rate is increased but the depth of respiration is decreased. A pause between inspiration and expiration may also be evident. The pedal reflex disappears. In the dog and cat the eyeball may once again become central because of loss of tone of its muscles. There is generalised muscular relaxation.

(*Note*:—Some authors describe a *fourth plane* of surgical anaesthesia, but actually it is nothing but the stage-4 of general anaesthesia, described above.

Stage 4: Anaesthesia develops to this stage when there is *overdosage* and the administration should be stopped immediately. The pulse becomes rapid. The eyeballs appear dry and the pupil is dilated. The thoracic muscles are paralysed and during inspiration the movements of the diaphragm causes bulging of the abdomen and inward movement of the thorax. Since the movements of the diaphragm are jerky the respiration is gasping in character. If proper counter measures are not taken at this stage the respiration ceases and mucous membranes become cyanotic. Soon heart failure follows and this is indicated by an ash-grey colour of the mucous membranes.

INTRAVENOUS ANAESTHESIA
Horse: 1. A freshly prepared solution containing Chloral hydras. (28 grammes)+Magnesium sulphate (14 grammes) + Nembutal (100 grains)+Distilled water (1000 cc) is stated to be the best intravenous anaesthetic for the horse. The injection is given slowly "to effect", until the animal comes under anaesthesia. Approximately 670 cc is required for a 1000 lb (450 kg) horse. The chief indication of anaesthesia is slowing of the nystagmus (=oscillatory movement of eyeball) and the disappearance of corneal reflex.
2. A solution of Chloral hydras plus Magnesium sulphas (10% of each) also can be used.
3. 10% solution of Chloral hydras alone can be used but is not as good as the other 2 solutions mentioned.
Bovine: The bovine is not a good subject for general anaesthesia. Probably the safest is to use I/V a combination of Chloral hydras (12%) +Magnesium sulphas (6%). The flacidity of tail is a good indication of surgical anaesthesia in this species (besides the slowing of nystagmus and disappearance of corneal reflex). The injection should stop when the tail just becomes completely flacid. About 10 grammes of Chloralhydras per 100 kg body weight is the average dose required. Food should be withheld for at least 24 hours before anaesthesia. Many major operations in the bovine are however done under sedation with Chloral hydras plus local anaesthesia, because of the difficulties and complications associated with general anaesthesia.
Porcine: 1. Chloral hydras (12%)+ Magnesium sulphate (6%) solution, 1/V. Approximate dosage required is equivalent to 2

grains of Chloral hydras per lb body weight. Anaesthesia lasts for one-and-a-half to four hours.

2. Nembutal l/V is a very good general anaesthetic for the pig but for its cost. Anaesthesia lasts for one-and-a-half to four hours.

Ovine: Nembutal may be used for basal narcosis and Chloral hydras is administered I/V as a 7% solution. About 5 to 10 gramme of chloral hydras may be required.

Dog: Nembutal may be given I/V, after preanaesthetic medication of Morphine-Atropine. Approximately 1/5 grain per lb body weight is the quantity of Nembutal required. The strength of the solution recommended is 3 to 6%. Usually a 4% solution is used. The injection is given slowly "to effect", until the animal comes under anaesthesia.

Cat: Similar to the dog but do not use Morphine. Pethidine may be used instead of morphine.

The sign of surgical anaesthesia in the cat is the disappearance of the following reflexes in stages: (i) digital reflex, (ii) palpebral reflex, (iii) corneal reflex, and (iv) ear-wisker reflex.

The pedal reflex may vanish in the hind limbs first in some individuals, while in fore limbs first in certain others. The forelimb reflexes are generally more reliable in cats than hind limb reflexes. The ear-wisker reflex is manifested by movement of wiskers and/or extension of tongue and/or movement of head when the ear is pinched.

Inhalation Anaesthesia

Equine: Excellent surgical anaesthesia can be obtained in the horse with chloroform. 1 to 2 ounces may be required. If Chloral hydras is given by stomach tube for basal narcosis, the excitement stage during induction can be shortened or abolished. A mask can be used for inhalation; or the direct "drop method" of putting it over the nostril can be adopted. For the latter method the animal is cast and secured in lateral recumbency, the lower nostril is closed with towel and chloroform is periodically dropped over a sponge or piece of cotton wool placed over the other nostril according to requirement.

Cattle, Pig, Sheep and Goats: There is no satisfactory inhalation anaesthesia practicable under ordinary field conditions for cattle, pig, sheep and goats. Chloroform is sometimes used in cattle and pig but is not very safe.

Inhalation Anaesthesia in the Dog

Inhalation anaesthesia can be practised safely in the dog. Some of the methods and drugs used are described below. The administration can be done using a mask or by passing an endotracheal tube. A special apparatus like the Boyle's Anaesthesia Apparatus may be used.

METHODS

There are four methods:

1. Open method
2. Semi-open method
3. Closed method with carbon dioxide absorption by:
   (a) the "to-and-fro" system
   (b) the "circle" system
4. Semi-closed method

1. *Open method*: In this method the volatile anaesthetic agent like chloroform or ether is dropped on a gauze held over the nostrils of the animal; or a mask is used.

2. *Semi-open method*: In this method the inspired air is made to pass through the mask in which the anaesthetic agent is allowed to vapourise.

3. *Closed method using carbon dioxide absorption*: When an anaesthetic vapour is inhaled by the animal only a part of it is consumed by the animal; the majority of it is exhaled. This exhaled vapour in addition contains a larger quantity of carbon dioxide and proportionately less of oxygen. Therefore, if this carbon dioxide is regularly absorbed (and a little of oxygen added to it if necessary) the same vapour can be used over and over again. This is the principle of the closed method. The carbon dioxide is absorbed by using soda lime. So the animal breathes and rebreathes from a closed system containing a rebreathing bag, soda lime canister, and an inlet for fresh mixture of oxygen and the anaesthetic gas. There are two types of apparatus available for this method either of which may be used. They are: (1) the "to-and-fro" system which consists of a rebreathing bag connected to the animal through a soda lime canister. A side tube situated between the animal and the canister feeds into the system fresh gases. This system is simple to operate and is widely used in veterinary practice. But some of the disadvantages are: (a) the particles inhaled from the canister may be irritating to the

animal and may cause bronchitis, (b) the gases may become very hot after sometime because of the chemical action of the canister, and (c) the size and shape of the apparatus is rather inconvenient to handle and it is difficult to keep it air-tight. (2) the "circle" system also consists of canister and rebreathing bag but it also contains two separate tubes fitted with valves, one for expiration and the other for inspiration. These tubes are connected to the mask or endotracheal tube. The canister is situated between these tubes, at the other end. The carbon dioxide absorption is more efficient in this system but a disadvantage is that the valves and tubing offer some resistance to breathing. For this reason they are unsuitable for small dogs and cats.

4. *Semi-closed method*: In this method the anaesthetic gases flow into a reservoir bag. The animal inhales from this bag but the expired air is permitted to escape more or less completely through an expiratory valve.

Muscle Relaxants

Muscle relaxants commonly used in veterinary practice are: *Flaxedil* (Gallamine Triethiodide).

Horse: 0.5 to 1.5 mg per kg body weight I/V. Apnoea (cessation of breathing) and complete paralysis lasting for 10 to 20 minutes is produced.

Calf and Lamb: 0.4 mg/kg, I/V. Apnoea is prolonged.

Pig: Effect unreliable.

Dog: 1.0 mg/kg, I/V. Within two minutes complete paralysis. Apnoea lasts for 15 to 20 minutes.

Cat: 1.0 mg/kg, I/V. Apnoea lasts for ten to twenty minutes. A temporary hypotension lasting for short period also is produced.

Brevedil (Scoline) i.e., Suxamethonium/(Suxethonium): This drug may be used in the dog, cattle and sheep but the horse, cat and pig are somewhat resistant.

Horse: 0.12 to 0.15 mg/kg I/V.

Cattle and Sheep: 0.02 mg/kg I/V.

Dog: 0.3 mg/kg I/V.

Pig: 2.2 mg/kg I/V.

Questions

1. Write short notes on: (i) Epidural anaesthesia, (ii) Nerve blocking, (iii) Pudental nerve block.

2. Name the different anaesthetics used in dogs. How will you proceed to induce Nembutal anaesthesia in a dog? What measures will you adopt in a case of collapse?

3. Define a major operation. Describe briefly the techniques of anaesthesia required for the following operations: (i) Rumenotomy, (ii) Extraction of molar in a dog, (iii) Median neurectomy in a horse.

4. Define the different sites for epidural anaesthesia for animals of the bovine and ovine species. Name the anaesthetic used and the specific purpose for which it is used describing the depth and area of anaesthesia in each case.

5. Write an essay on the choice of anaesthetics and nature of anaesthesia to be induced for surgical interference in the different animal patients.

6. Describe the procedure followed for inducing epidural anaesthesia at different levels, for performing pelvic and abdominal surgery, giving also details of choice of anaesthetic and site for administration.

7. Describe briefly the indications for general anaesthesia in animal surgery and illustrate your answer with suitable examples from the full range of anaesthetics available indicating their suitability or otherwise for use in the different species of animals.

CHAPTER 54

Control of Haemorrhage

Haemorrhage

Haemorrhage (bleeding) may be arterial haemorrhage, venous haemorrhage, or capillary haemorrhage. The usual cause of haemorrhage is trauma. It may also be due to congenital diseases like haemophilia or due to diseases of blood vessels.

CLASSIFICATION

Haemorrhage is classified as external haemorrhage and internal haemorrhage. External haemorrhage occurs from open wounds or through one of the natural orifices of the body, e.g., epistaxis (bleeding from nose), haemoptysis (from lungs or respiratory passages), haematemesis (vomiting blood), meloena (blood passed through faeces), haematuria (through urine). The blood in epistaxis and haemoptysis is bright red and frothy being recently oxygenated and mixed with air. The blood in haematemesis may have been swallowed from nasopharynx. Its colour depends on the duration of contact with gastric juice which gives it a dark brown colour. Bleeding from colon and small intestines has blackish colour due to partial digestion of blood.

In internal haemorrhage bleeding takes place within the body and blood collects in any of the natural body cavities or in a newly formed cavity. When blood collects in a newly formed cavity it is called a haematoma. Examples of internal haemorrhage are: haemopleura (haemorrhage into pleural cavity), haemoperitoneum (into the peritoneal cavity), haematocele (into the tunica vaginalis), haemarthrosis (into a joint), haematosalpinx (into the fallopian tube), haemometra (into the uterus), haematocolpos (into the extradural portion of spinal cord), haematomyelia (into the spinal cord), apoplexy (into the brain substance), petechiae (pin-point haemorrhages on skin and subcutis), ecchymosis (haemorrhagic spots on skin and subcutis).

Haemorrhage is also classified as primary, reactionary and secondary haemorrhages. *Primary haemorrhage* occurs immediately after the injury. *Reactionary haemorrhage* (intermediate or recurrent haemorrhage) is haemorrhage occurring within about 24 hours after the primary bleeding has been controlled. Reactionary haemorrhage is due to mechanical disturbance of clot in the vessel or due to slipping of the ligature. *Secondary haemorrhage* takes place after 14 days or more due to septic disintegration of the clot or due to sloughing of portion of vessel because of a septic or gangrenous lesion.

Haemorrhage may be : Arterial, Venous, or Capillary.

PROGNOSIS

Prognosis depends on the amount of blood loss. Shock may develop if large quantity of blood is lost.

TREATMENT

Control bleeding. Measures to prevent shock are also necessary.

General Methods for Controlling Haemorrhage

1. *By using a tourniquet*: A tourniquet is a cord tied around an extremity (like limb, tail, penis) so as to control bleeding. A tourniquet is applied proximal to the bleeding point. A tourniquet should not be applied very tightly because it may completely arrest blood supply to the part and cause tissue damage. It should not be kept continuously for more than 15 minutes.

2. *By the use of Esmarch's bandage*: This method may be employed while doing operations on the limb or tail so as to minimise bleeding during the course of the operation. A tight bandage is applied completely covering the distal part of the extremity up to a point above the seat of operation so as to compress the vessels and drive away blood from the area. Afterwards a tourniquet is applied close to the upper limit of the bandage to prevent return of blood and then the bandage is removed. After the operation is completed the tourniquet also is removed.

3. *Thermocautery*: A red-hot iron applied to a bleeding point usually causes arrest of haemorrhage unless the vessel is very large. This method is very useful for small vessels which are difficult to hold with artery forceps. Thermocautery may be

practised with an electro-cautery apparatus.

4. *Crushing*: When a vessel is crushed the inner coats of the vessel (viz., the endothelial and muscular coats) rupture first and they retract slightly into the lumen of the vessel and the tough areolar coat forms a cap over this. A clot is soon formed inside the vessel adjoining the ruptured ends of the inner coats. Crushing small vessels can be done by using artery forceps; crushing of large vessels can be done by using ecraseur.

5. Applying *artery forceps* (Haemostatic forceps or Haemostats)for a few minutes stops bleeding from small vessels.

6. *Torsion* or twisting a vessel on its long axis also prevents bleeding in the same way as crushing of the vessel. Torsion is commonly employed in castration. Torsion of the spermatic vessels in castration of large animals is done by using castration calm and torsion forceps. In small animals torsion of spermatic vessels can be done using 2 artery forceps instead.

7. *Ligation* is the best method of stopping bleeding from a vessel. The vessel is first grasped with an artery forceps and the ligature is then tied on the vessel.

8. Control of bleeding from a large wound cavity wherein the bleeding points cannot be identified, is achieved by plugging *or packing the cavity* with sterilised gauze pieces called tampon. Tamponing (tamponade or tamponment) mechanically prevents bleeding by exerting pressure and it also favours coagulation of blood.

9. *Adrenalin* when applied to a small bleeding vessel constricts the vessel and thus controls bleeding.

10. Application of Liq. Ferri Perchlor, Tincture Benzoin, collodion, ice, cold water, etc. is also helpful to arrest bleeding from small vessels.

11. *Gell-foam* (a patent product made of fibrin available in small pieces of $\frac{1}{4}'' \times 4'' \times 2''$) when applied directly on to a bleeding point favours immediate coagulation of blood. "Gelatin sponges" also have the same effect.

12. Injection of coagulen-ciba. Coagulen-ciba is a physiological haemostatic derived from unclotted bovine blood. Manufactured by Messers Ciba pharmaceuticals and is supplied in ampoules of 5 cc. It contains *prothrombin* and *thrombokinase*. *Dose*: *Dog*: 5 to 20 cc I/V; *Horse* and *Cattle*: 50 cc I/V every 12 hours.

13. Administration of Vitamin K. eg., Kapilin (Glaxo) 10 mg per cc solution, supplied in ampoules of 1 cc. *Dose*: *Dog*: ½ to 1 cc; *Cattle*: 10 to 20 cc.

14. *Calcium* has remarkable effect in bringing about coagulation of blood. Calcium borogluconas 10 to 25% may be given S/C or I/V. *Dog*: 5 to 10 cc; *Cattle*: 100 to 300 cc.

15. *Congo-red* (a dye substance) when injected as a 1% solution seems to favour coagulation of blood. *Dose*: *Dog*: 15 to 20 cc I/V: *Cattle*: 100 to 200 cc I/V.

16. Solutions of *sodium citrate*, sodium iodide, formalin and gelatin when injected intravenously in the following doses are found useful to control bleeding in cattle and horse; Sodium citrate 20% solution up to 1 pint I/V, Sodium iodide 1 ounce dissolved in 1 pint of water I/V. Formalin (i.e., 38% Formaldehyde) 10 cc in 100 cc of distilled water I/V. Gelatin 5% I/V about 500 cc.

During surgery, mopping, digital pressure, use of thermo-cautery/haemostat/crushing/torsion/ligation can be employed depending on size, loation and accessibility of vessel. Cutting tissues under traction empties veins causing their accidental section, especially during extirpations. Some veins (e.g. Jugular) cannot collapse when cut on account of deep facial attachment, hence risk of air getting aspirated to the heart (The characteristic sound may be audible). Avoid these happenings, by prior ligation before cutting.

Questions

1. Classify haemorrhage. What are its causes? State briefly the different methods of haemostasis in practice.

2. Write short notes on: (i) Haemostatic methods, (ii) Internal haemorrhage. (iii) Venous haemorrhage.

3. Define haemorrhage. Describe the methods of haemostasis adopted in Surgery.

CHAPTER 55

Pre-operative Preparations

1. The patient should be examined to decide whether it will be safe to operate. Very young and very old animals are poor risks for anaesthesia and surgery. Cardiovascular diseases, pneumonia, uraemia, renal inefficiency, pregnancy, etc. complicate surgery. So adequate precautions are necessary when surgery is undertaken in such cases.

2. The operation is conducted preferably in the morning so that time is available for post-operative observation.

3. Before major surgery and general anaesthesia the patient is to be starved for twelve to eighteen hours or more. A mild purgative may be administered on the previous day to reduce the volume of abdominal contents. An enema is given half to one hour before the administration of preanaesthetic.

4. Do not administer general anaesthetic to an animal in shock. When surgery is undertaken immediately after automobile accidents, fractures, etc., make sure that there is no internal haemorrhage, rupture of bladder, etc.

5. Postpone cosmetic surgery if the animal is undernourished and debilitated, anaemic or is heavily infested with parasites.

6. Enquire into the history as to whether the animal had been under general anaesthesia at any time previously, whether it has any idiosyncracy or hypersensitivity to any drug, etc.

7. Auscultation of heart and lungs, laboratory tests for urine and blood including PCV, may be conducted.

8. If there is protein deficiency or loss of electrolytes (due to vomiting, diarrhoea, etc.), protein hydrolysates and isotonic saline solutions may be administered before the operation.

9. If there has been heavy blood loss, blood transfusion or saline injections should be given.

Operation Room (*Operation Theatre*)

The operating room should be clean and airy and should have adequate light. The flooring, walls, desks, etc. should be clean. The instrument table and the operation table should be simple in order to ensure rapid and thorough cleaning. Wash basins with hot and cold water connections should be provided. A wall-clock and x-ray viewing box (x-ray illuminator) are useful additional equipments.

Conducting the Operation

Asep.ic technique (Sterile technique) should be followed as far as possible.

1. All the equipments used (instruments, gowns, towles, gloves, etc.) should be sterilised.

2. The skin at the operative area should be clipped or shaved and smeared with an effective antiseptic.

3. The hands of the surgeon should be cleaned and sterile gloves should be worn. If available, caps, gown and masks also may be worn.

4. All chances of contamination of the surgical wound should be prevented.

5. The wound should be protected until healing is complete.

Sterilisation of instruments

METHODS

    (1) Chemical sterilisation.

    (2) By heat: (a) Dry heat.

                (b) Moist heat.

    (3) By U-V rays.

1. *Chemical sterilisation*: By immersing in antiseptic chemical solutions. Chemical sterilisation is not as good as heat sterilisation. But for sharp cutting instruments, gum elastic articles, etc. that are likely to be spoiled by heat, chemical sterilisation is advocated (e.g., 10% formalin). Sharp cutting instruments may be sterilised by keeping them immersed in 1 to 5% carbolic acid and afterwards washing in sterile distilled water.

2. *Dry heat*: By placing in hot air oven at 350°F for three hours.

3. *Moist heat*: (i) By boiling in water for 15 minutes.

Two per cent Sod. Carb. may be added to the water to prevent corrosion of metallic instruments.

(ii) By autoclaving at 250°F and 15 lb pressure per sq inch, for fifteen minutes. This is one of the best methods of sterilisation. The articles to be sterilised for an operation are kept in a bundle and the bundle is placed in the autoclave. The autoclave is closed and steam is allowed into it. The valve is kept open until all the air is let out and then closed, and the pressure is gradually raised to 15 lb and maintained for 15 minutes. After 15 minutes the valve is opened to let out the steam and sometime later the autoclave is opened. Before removing the "sterile pack" the door of the autoclave is kept open for sometime.

Preparation of a "General Surgery Pack"

The instruments, towels, etc. are usually bundled in cloth towels and autoclaved for sterilisation. A *General Surgery Pack* is a bundle of this type, containing sterilized equipments commonly required for most of the major surgical operations. Any special instrument required for particular operation and which is not available in the general pack will be taken in an additional bundle called a Special Pack or "Special Surgery Pack".

The contents of General Surgery Pack are preferably taken in the following four separate subsidiary bundles within the main bundle.

Bundle No. 1: Containing: Scalpel-1; Tissue forceps, toothed-1; Allis tissue forceps-2; Spencerwell's artery forceps-6; Scissors, straight, blunt pointed-1; Scissors, blunt-pointed, curved-1 Wound retractors-1 pair; Grooved director-1; Spaying hook-1; Bowel forceps-1; Suture needles, straight, cutting-2; Suture needles, curved, round-tipped-1; Vetafil or other non-absorbable suture; Needle holder-1; Gauze sponges for mopping-10; Laparotomy sheet-1; Towel clamps-4; Towels-4; Gowns-1 pair; Hand towels-2.

Bundle No. 2: Containing: Gloves-2 pairs; Talcum powder 2 pkt.

Bundle No. 3: Containing: syringes and Inoculation needles-5 cc, and 10 cc, one each.

Bundle No. 4: Containing: Masks-1 pair; Caps-1 pair.

Preparing the Site of Operation (*Sterilisation of Skin in and around the Site of Operation*)

The hair should be closely clipped or shaved. Then the area is washed with plenty of soap and water, scrubbing with a brush. Dry with a towel and wash again with a fat solvent like turpentine or ether to remove grease from the skin. Repeat washing with soap and water. Dry with ethyl alcohol (70% alcohol, by weight). Apply an effective antiseptic like Tincture iodine. The iodine is then washed off with alcohol. (Instead of Tincture iodine any other of the effective antiseptic solutions like: 5% Mercurochrome, 2% Picric acid, 1 to 2% Acriflavin in spirit, 5% Carbolic acid, etc. may be used).

In birds the operation site is prepared by plucking the feathers, cleaning the skin with soap and water and drying. Antiseptics are not generally used because the skin is very delicate.

Routine Steps before Starting an Aseptic Operation

1. Put on the cap and mask. The cap is intended to prevent loose hair, sweat, etc. falling on the wound. The mask prevents, to a certain extent, bacterial contamination of the wound while talking, sneezing, coughing, etc.

2. The hands of the surgeon and his assistant should be washed very well with soap and water, scrubbing with a brush. (It is stated that the skin should be scrubbed about ten times and nails twenty times while cleaning.) Rinse with water and then with a suitable non-irritant antiseptic lotion like savlon. The hand is then held lifted a little with elbow half-flexed.

3. Open the Sterile Pack and pick up the hand towel to dry the hands.

4. Put on the *gown*.

5. Put on the *gloves*.

Draping the Patient

Covering the skin of the patient with sterilised towels excluding the actual site of operation, is called draping the patient. There are two methods of draping: (1) Four-towel draping, and (2) Double-thickness draping.

(1) *Four-towel draping*: In this method four towels are spread and clipped around the operative area.

(2) *Double-thickness draping*: After the preliminary four-towel draping the skin is incised for the operation. Double thickness draping is done at this stage by clamping two more towels to the edges of the incision. The clamping to edges is done in such a way that the skin edge gets everted and covered by the towel.

Laparotomy sheet: This is an additional piece of towel used in operations like gastrotomy, enterotomy, hysterotomy, etc. wherein lot of contamination with foreign matter is possible. The laparotomy sheet has a central opening corresponding to the incision. It is spread over the other drapes and is changed whenever required during the course of operation.

Sizes

Laparotomy sheet (Surgical shroud):
For large animals: 60 cm. × 100 cm., with a central slit of 18 cm. × 3 cm.
For Small animals: 50 cm. × 50 cm., with a central slit of 10 cm. × 2 cm.
Towels: 40 cm. × 40 cm.

Note: Chalk powder can be used for preserving rubber articles like gloves; but talcum powders are not desirable because they contain Magnesium silicate which has a tendency to stimulate granulomas in wounds.

CHAPTER 56

Post-operative Care of Patient

1. After the operation keep the animal in a comfortable position. Never in dorsal recumbency.
2. The tongue should be placed out to avoid breathing difficulties, if the animal has not completely recovered from general anaesthesia.
3. If the weather is cold preserve the body temperature by covering the body.
4. While recovering from anaesthesia, most animals struggle and if this is severe a tranquilizer may be administered, if necessary.
5. Do not give water to an animal recovering from anaesthesia because aspiration pneumonia might be caused due to difficulty in swallowing.
6. Check the temperature, pulse, respiration, etc. periodically.
7. Change the position of the animal every 30 minutes to avoid hypostatic congestion.

Post-operative Complications

1. *Pneumonia* may develop due to inhalation of foreign bodies, secretions, vomitus, etc. To avoid this do not anaesthetise when the stomach is full; administer drugs like atropine to reduce secretions; administer antiemetics.
2. *Hypostatic congestion.* This can be prevented by periodically changing the position of the animal.
3. *Wound* infection and formation of stitch abscesses.
4. *Wound* dehiscence due to improper sutures, infection or suppuration.
5. *Evisceration* (Protrusion of viscera through the incision). The intestines or other viscera may protrude, and because of the damage caused to it by drying, soiling, infection, injury, etc. the animal may die.

6. *Herniation.* Herniation of viscera is more common than evisceration. Improper suture technique is one of the common causes. External violence may also cause it.

7. *Peritonitis.* Peritonitis may be caused due to rough handling of viscera,. due to the escape of contents from stomach, intestine, uterus, bladder, etc. Acute peritonitis causes sudden death.

Questions

1. What is meant by aseptic surgery? Describe the general principles and steps to be taken in the conduct of aseptic surgery.

2. Write short notes on: (a) Post-operative care, (b) General Surgery Pack.

CHAPTER 57

Surgical Instruments

A few of the commonly used instruments and some of the special instruments are listed below. For convenience they are arranged under the following headings:

1. Cutting instruments (scalpels, scissors).
2. Forceps.
3. Retractors.
4. Towel clips (Drape clips).
5. Gloves, drapes, etc.
6. Inoculation syringes. .
7. Inoculation needles.
8. Catheters.
9. Other general instruments.
10. Suturing instruments and materials.
11. Mouth gags.
12. Stomach tubes.
13. Tooth instruments.
14. Orthopaedic instruments.
15. Teat instruments.
16. Eye instruments.
17. Ear instruments.
18. Nasal instruments.
19. Roaring set.
20. Rumenotomy set.
21. Castration instruments.
22. Anaesthetic apparatus.
23. Miscellaneous instruments.
24. Special equipments.

1. Cutting Instruments

The two most important cutting instruments used in surgery are the scalpel and the scissors.

1. (a) Scalpels

1. *Ordinary scalpel*: Made up of a single piece of metal comprising a blade and a handle. Several varieties are available, depending essentially on the shape and size of the blade. To put an incision, the scalpel is to be held like a pen with the thumb and middle finger, with the index finger supporting the back of the blade.

2. *Scalpel with separate blade and handle*: Two common varieties available are: (i) Bard-Parker handle and blades and (ii) Swann-Morton handle and blades.

Each of these varieties have different sizes of handles numbered as 1, 2, 3, 4, etc., and also blades to suit each variety. The blades may be broad or narrow, pointed, curved, etc., of different lengths and shape. They are chosen according to the need for a particular operation.

3. *Electroscalpel*: Electroscalpels are designed to provide passage of electrical current through a small point of contact with the tissue to be incised. The incision actually is brought about by coagulation of tissue proteins. It is necessary to see that the earth connection (grounding) of the instrument from the animal is provided close to the point of incision, as otherwise the electric current will be spread over a wider area. The contact area of the scalpel is reduced to the minimum to minimise the tissue damage.

The advantage of the electroscalpel is that the bleeding is greatly reduced. But it has been reported that the healing after use of electroscalpel takes about 3 days longer than with the use of ordinary scalpel, because of the additional tissue damage resulting from electrocautery.

4. *Cryo-surgery*: This is described in a separate chapter. (p. 456).

1. (b) Scissors

The four common varieties of scissors are:

    (i) Operating scissors,

    (ii) Suture scissors,

    (iii) Suture removal scissors, and

    (iv) Bandage scissors.

The recommended method for holding a scissors during surgery is as follows:

The thumb and ring finger should be in the 2 rings of the

scissors. (Some persons use the index finger or the middle finger instead of the ring finger, which is not correct.) The index finger should be used only to guide the scissors by placing on the shaft of the scissors. The middle finger gently holds or rests outside the ring in which the ring finger is placed.

(i) *Operating scissors*: Operating scissors are available in two major styles, namely, (a) the Metzenbaum style, and (b) the Mayo style. The Metzenbaum scissors are thinner with narrow blades and they have comparatively shorter blades and longer handles. The Mayo scissors are more popular and are better for the cutting of dense tissue.

Many va ieties of operating scissors are available, depending on the type of their points, shape of blades, type of cutting edge, etc.

Type of points: (1) Blunt-blunt (or, Blunt-pointed), if both blades have blunt points.

(2) Sharp-sharp, if both blades have sharp points.

(3) Sharp-blunt, when one blade has sharp point and the other blade has blunt point.

Shape of blades: (1) Straight, (2) Curved.

Type of cutting edges: (1) Plain, (2) Serrated.

Example of describing a scissors: Scissors, straight, broad blade, blunt-pointed, plain, 10 inches, stainless steel.

(ii) *Suture scissors*: Used to cut suture materials. May have either ordinary or serrated edges.

(iii) *Scissors for suture removal*: One of the blades is shaped at the tip in the form of a blunt hook.

(iv) *Bandage scissors*: The lower blade of this scissors has a blunt. flattened tip which can be introduced under the bandage.

2 Forceps

(1) Tissue forceps, plain. (2) Tissue forceps, toothed. (3) Allis tissue forceps. (4) Dressing forceps. (5) Tongue holding forceps. (6) Lung-grasping forceps (having hollow, broad, triangular, opposing surfaces as jaws). (7) Artery forceps (Haemostats). Many varieties are available. The commonly used variety is the Spencerwell's Artery Forceps. They may be (a) straight, or (b) curved. The curved type is also called a mosquito forceps. Available in different sizes: 6″, 10″, 12″, etc. (8) Alligator forceps. Having long handle which is bent at an obtuse angle, with small

jaws opening and closing at the tip. The jaws may be either serrated or rat-teethed. (9) Bull-dog forceps or Bull-dog clamps (Serrefine forceps), useful for temporarily clamping blood vessles during surgery, e.g., during vascular anastomosis. (10) Needle-holding forceps (Needle holder). (11) Cheetle's forceps.

3. Retractors

These are useful to retract wound edges during surgery. Those having flat, curved ends, or having hook-like ends are available. The hooks may be sharp or blunt. Examples: Durham's retractor, Czerney retractor.

Special type self-retaining retractors having two pieces joined together and provided with hachet are available with specific indications for their use. Examples: Laparotomy retractors, Balfour retractors, Laryngotomy retractors.

4. Towel Clips (*Drape Clips*)

The two common types are the following: (1) Towel clips, Schaedel type (the rear portion of this looks like that of a bull-dog-clamp). (2) Towel clips, Backhaus type (the rear portion of this resembles the handles of a scissors).

5. Gloves, Drapes, etc.

(1) Surgical gloves. Available in different sizes to suit different individuals. Examples: Size No. 9, 8, $7\frac{1}{2}$. (2) Obstetric sleeve with attached glove. (3) Surgical drapes, size 3 ft × 3ft. (4) Surgical drapes, 4 ft × $1\frac{1}{2}$ ft. (5) Surgical drapes, 4 ft × 2 ft. (6) Laparotomy sheet, 3ft × 3 ft. (7) Hand towels. (8) Surgical gowns. (9) Caps. (10) Masks.

6. Inoculation Syringes

There are two types of syringes, namely, (1) the all glass syringes, and (2) the syringes which have a metallic nozzle, popularly called the "record type" syringes. The typical "record-syringe" has a glass barrel with metallic protections at both ends (the metallic protection at one end having the metal nozzle), and a metal piston. Various modifications of this are also available with patent names. Example: "Arthro-veterinary" record syringes.

Syringes made of nylon with either glass type or record type

nozzles are available.
The common sizes of syringes are: 20 ml, 10 ml, 5 ml, 2 ml, 1 ml, etc.
Example of description of a syringe: Syringe, all glass, 10 ml.

7. Inoculation Needles

According to the type of syringe to which they are suitable, inoculation needles may be either: (1) the variety to suit glass syringes, or (2) the variety to suit record syringes. Various sizes are available, based on external diameter and length. The diameter is expressed in standard numbers of British Wire Gauge. (Examples: 16 BWG, 18 BWG, 21 BWG, etc.)
Example of describing a needle: Inoculation needle, record type, 21 BWG, 2 inches.

8. Catheters

(1) Dawson's cow catheter, single channel. (2) Cow catheter, double channel. (3) Flexible metal catheter, ox. (4) Mare catheter, metal. (5) Mare catheter, gum elastic. (6) Horse catheter, gum elastic. (7) Bitch catheter, gum elastic. (8) Bitch catheter, metal. (9) Dog catheter, gum elastic. (10) Flexible metal catheter, dog. (11) Uterine catheter, Bane's pattern, double channel, with tap adjustment.

9. Other General Instruments

(1) Grooved director: A simple rod-like instrument with a longitudinal groove and handle, which is useful for directing a cutting instrument like scissors or scalpel along its groove. (2) Probe: A blunt-pointed, rod-like instrument which may be flexible to some extent. (3) Director, probe-pointed (Director and probe combined). (4) Tenaculum. (5) Tenotome (Tenotomy knife), sharp-pointed, folding type. (6) Exploring needle. (7) Syme's abscess knife. (8) Seton needle with handle. (9) Volkmann's scoop. (10) Gimlet. (11) Izuka's needle.

10. Suturing Instruments and Materials

1. Needle holder (Needle holding forceps).
2. Suture needles, assorted. Examples: Suture needle, straight tapering 2 inches; Suture needle, half circle, tapering 1½ inches.
3. Suture materials: Examples: Catgut, medium chromic,

boilable, size 2/0; Catgut, plain, non-boilable, size No. 2; Surgical silk; Horse hair; Nylon; Catgut, size 2/0, with atraumatic needle.

4. Michel wound clips.
5. Michel wound clip applying forceps.
6. Michel wound clip extracting forceps.

11. Mouth Gags

(1) Wooden gag for cattle, with leather straps. (2) Drinkwater's mouth gag for cattle. (3) Varnell's mouth gag for horse. (4) Gray's mouth gag for dog (Spring gag).

12. Stomach Tubes

(1) Stomach tube for horse. (2) Probang for cattle. (3) Probang for dog, for removal of foreign bodies from oesophagus.

13. Tooth Instruments

(1) Dental scalers for dog. (2) Dental forceps for dog. (3) Pritchard's incisor tooth forceps for equine. (4) Gunther's tooth forceps for large animals. (5) Tooth chisel, English pattern. Use: To remove "hooks" on teeth. While using the chisel, it should be struck with caution, as otherwise the tooth may break in an oblique fashion cutting deeper down into the crown or the root. (6) Molar cutter, Danish pattern, with adjustable screw handle. (7) Thompson's heavy tooth shears. (8) Tooth rasp. Available with long or short handles. The short-handled rasp with blade set at an angle is specially useful for a prominent hook on the first molar.

14. Orthopaedic Instruments

(1) Bone cutting forceps. (The jaws are chisel-like intended for cutting, unlike in the case of Rongeurs.) (2) Rongeurs: For cutting and removing small bits of bone. The jaws are cupped and the remaining part of the instrument similar to bone cutting forceps. (3) Trephine: To cut and remove a circular (cylindrical) piece of bone. (4) Bone chisel: Note the sharp bevelled tip which is straight on one surface unlike an osteotome. (5) Osteotome: Similar to bone chisel, except that the tip is double-bevelled. (6) Amputation saw. (7) Wire saw. (8) Bone holding forceps. (9) Bone pinning chuck and key. (10) Bone pin. (11) Trephine.

(12) Plaster shears. (13) Plaster saw, Engel. (14) Ferguson's bone holding forceps. (15) Pollock's rib shears. (16) Vitellium plate and screws. (17) Amputation saw.

15. Teat Instruments

(1) Columbus teat plugs. (2) Bengen's self-expanding teat dilators. (3) Hudson's teat probe. (4) Hudson's teat dilater. (5) Mc'Lean's teat knife, for cutting the constricted sphincter at tip of teat. (6) Trifin teat knife; Use similar. (7) Stinson's teat director. (8) Milking tube (teat syphon), self-retaining. (9) Teat bistoury, probe-pointed. (10) Teat slitter, with adjustable blade. (11) Barrett's papilotome, for removal of growths from teat canal. (12) Milk fever outfit for infusing air into the udder.

16. Eye Instruments

(1) Binocular loupe. (2) Eye speculum, Graefe's. (3) Undyne, for eye irrigation. (4) Eyelid retractor, Desmarr's. (5) Lachrimal probe, Bowman's. (6) Iris forceps, straight. (7) Cataract knife, Graefe's, straight. (8) Cataract needle, straight. (9) Cataract needle, curved on flat. (10) Spoon (Scoop). (11) Spatula. (12) Sharp hook, Graefe's. (13) Refraction ophthalmoscope, plain.

17. Ear Instruments

(1) Ear scoop. (2) Ear speculum (can also be used as a nasal speculum)

18. Nasal Instruments

(1) Bull rings, self-piercing. (2) Forceps for applying bull rings. (3) Bull nose punch.

19. Roaring Set

(1) Hobday's automatic laryngeal retractor (laryngeal dilator). (2) Hobday's forceps cum dilator for lateral ventricles. (3) Knife for roaring operation. (4) Hobday's burr for roaring operation. (5) Blattenburg's burr (Modified Hobday's burr).

20. Rumenotomy Sets

(1) Mc'Lintock's rumenotomy set consisting of: Rubber drape with linear opening in the centre; Rubber covered hooks; Rubber tube with flexible rim; Rubber drape with circular

opening for rubber tube; Rubber-shod clamps for clamping rumen while suturing. (2) Weingart's rumenotomy set, consisting of: Fixation frame; Vulsellum forceps-2; Fixation tenacula-8.

21. Castration Instruments

(1) Burdizoo forceps, with cord stop jaws, 19 inches, for cattle. (2) "Elastrator" with rubber rings. (3) Castration knife for horse, folding type. (4) Castration clamp for holding spermatic cord for torsion (Vide Dollar, Fig. 145, p. 367). (5) Robertson's forceps for torsion of the spermatic cord, as advocated by Moller (Dollar, Fig. 145, p. 367). (6) Emasculator, Hausemann and Dunn's pattern. (7) Castration clam, wooden. (8) Ecraseur. (9) Dovault ovariectomy hook (Spaying hook). (10) Caponising set, Collingnon's pattern, consisting of: Scalpel (Caponising knife); Wound retractor; Peritoneum tearing hook and probe, combined; Caponising forceps (Testis removing forceps). (11) Pellet injector, for implanting "Stilkap" pellets.

22. Anaesthesia Equipments

(1) Cox's chloroform muzzle for horse (Dollar, Fig. 43). (2) Reynold's anaesthetic apparatus for cattle. (3) Hobday's chloroform apparatus for dog (Dollar, Fig. 47). (4) Boyle's anaesthetic apparatus. (5) Magill cuffed endotracheal tube. (6) Brook's eqidural needle. (7) Cat anaesthesia box.

23. Miscellaneous Instruments

(1) Flutter valve intravenous apparatus. (2) Bleeding fleam (phlebotomy knife). (3) Field's tracheotomy tube. (4) Pape's tracheotomy tube. (5) Tongue depressor for dogs. (6) Tongue forceps with rubber-shod jaws. (7) Throat forceps, long curved, for dogs. (8) Trocar and canula, assorted sizes. (9) Trocar and canula, large size for rumen puncture. (10) Wooden clamp for hernia. (11) Umbilical hernia clamps with leather straps. (12) Vaginal speculum, cow. (13) Coldlite bovine vaginoscope. (14) Firing irons for: Line firing; Bud-point firing; and Needle-point firing. (15) Sandcrack forceps. (16) Leather cow-boot. (17) Dog brush. (18) Hair clipper. (19) Claw cutter for dogs. (20) Docking scissors for puppies. (21) Hoffmann's docking machine for horse (or, Guillotine). (22) Wound irrigation syringe. (23) Enema can. (24) Percussion hammer.

24. Special Equipments

(1) Ultraviolet and infra red lamps. (2) Operation theatre lamp (Shadowless lamp). (3) X-ray machine (X-ray plant; X-ray equipment). (4) Fluorescent screen. (5) X-ray cassette. (6) X-ray exposure holder. (7) Intensifying screens. (8) X-ray protective apron. (9) X-ray protective gloves. (10) Beehive safe light. (11) X-ray film processing tanks. (12) X-ray illuminator (Viewing screen). (13) Pneumothorax apparatus. (14) Professor Wright's diagnostic instrument set. (15) Respiration pump. (16) Vacuum suction apparatus. (17) Satinsky clamp for ventriculotomy (of heart). (18) Furnis clamp.

CHAPTER 58

Cryosurgery (Cryogenic Technique)

Cryogenic technique is used to freeze and cause necrosis and sloughing of localised areas of living tissues of the body.

A *cryoprobe* which is in the form of a hollow metal rod is used for this purpose. It has an external diameter of about 1 cm and length of about 25 to 35 cm. The distal end is in the form of a probe. The proximal end has insulated handle and can be connected to the apparatus supplying the cooling agent. Liquid or *gaseous nitrous oxide,* or *liquid nitrogen* is circulated in it as the cooling agent. The cooling effect produced by gaseous nitrous oxide is $-70°C$, by liquid nitrous oxide $-80°C$ and by liquid nitrogen $-180°C$. The apparatus using liquid nitrogen is much more expensive (about 20 times) than the equipment using nitrous oxide.

Although the principle in cryosurgery is comparable to diathermy/thermocautery, there are some essential differences as noted below.

	Diathermy/ Thermocatery	*Cryogenic technique*
1. Action produced in the tissue	Localised destruction and necrosis of the tissue due to the coagulation of cell protein due to heat	Localised freezing, thrombosis of the microcirculation in the frozen tissue and gradual necrosis
2. Line of demarcation from surrounding healthy tissue	Not so sharp	Sharply well-demarcated
3. Pain during application	Painful	No pain, since the freezing itself has a local anaesthetic effect

4. Reactionary and secondary haemorrhage	Possible	Chances are less than in diathermy/ thermocautery
5. Inflammatory response to the necrosed tissue	More as compared to freezing	Negligible
6. Scar formation after healing	Scars are formed	Only little or negligible scarring
7. Time taken for separation and shedding of necrosed tissue	Three to five weeks	Three to five weeks

USES

To destroy tumours of the skin, mouth, pharynx, cauterisation of cervix, treatment of prostatic enlargement, destruction of haemorrhoids, etc.

Reference
Goligher, J.C, Duthie, H. L., and Nixon, H. H. (1975). *Surgery of the anus, rectum and colon.* 3rd ed. London: Baillere Tindall, pp. 1143-1145.

CHAPTER 59

Cornual Nerve Block

A. In Bovine

INDICATIONS

Analgesia of the horn core and the skin around the base of horn.

ANATOMY

The cornual nerve is the sensory nerve supplying the horn core and skin around its base. Cornual nerve is a branch of the Lachrymal nerve which is a branch of the ophthalmic branch of the Trigeminal nerve (fifth cranial or trifacial nerve). Remember this by remembering the letters CLOT.

The cornual nerve emerges behind the orbit and ascends (head vertical) behind the lateral ridge of frontal bone. The nerve is placed relatively superficial in the upper third, covered by skin and a thin layer of frontalis muscle only. The nerve in this region is in close association with the superficial temporal artery supplying the horn core and the vein from the horn core. The order, therefore, from before backwards is vein, nerve artery.

SITE

Close to and behind the lateral border of frontal bone, about one inch below the base of the horn (assuming the vertical position of head.)

TECHNIQUE

The needle is introduced through the site until its tip reaches a depth of ½ to 1 cm. The quantity of solution injected is 5 cc to 10 cc in a concentration of 2.5% to 5% of the local analgesic (usually Novocaine). Analgesia takes effect in about five to fifteen minutes and lasts for half to one hour or longer.

B. Cornual Nerve Block in Goat

In the goat, the lacrimal nerve as well as the infratrochlear nerve are to be blocked, and there are anatomical differences. The cornual branch of lacrymal nerve comes out of the orbit behind the root of the supra-orbital process where it is covered by the thin frontalis muscle. For blocking this nerve the needle is introduced close to the upper border of the supraorbital process about 1 cm above the lateral canthus of the eye described in the vertical position of head, for a depth of 1.0 to 1.5 cm.

The *infratrochlear nerve* after emerging from the antero-medial aspect of the orbit, divides into the dorsal (cornual) branch and the medial (frontal) branch. The cornual branch of the nerve should be blocked at the supero-medial margin of the orbit, i.e., at a point about 1 cm medial to and above the inner canthus of the eye (Ref.: Hall, L.W., 1966 for details).

CHAPTER 60

Ligation of Stenson's Duct in Bovine

INDICATIONS

In persistent salivary fistula. Ligation of the duct brings about atrophy of the gland.

ANAESTHESIA AND CONTROL

Local infiltration, controlled in the standing or recumbent state.

ANATOMY

The duct of the parotid salivary gland (Stenson's duct) arises from the ventro-medial aspect of the gland and proceeds along the ventral and anterior borders of the masseter muscle to open into the mouth in level with the fifth upper cheek tooth. At the anterior site described below, the duct is seen close to the masseter muscle, with the facial Artery and Vein, in the order: Artery anterior, then Vein and afterwards Duct. (AVD).

SITE

1. *Anterior or Distal Site*: Immediately in front of the anterior border of the masseter muscle and about ½ to 1 inch above the inferior border of the horizontal ramus of the mandible, where the duct can be *palpated*. (Palpate before incising skin).

2. *Posterior or Proximal Site*: In the Viborg's Triangle which is outlined by the posterior border of the vertical ramus in front, tendon of sternomaxillaris above and the submaxillary vein below.

TECHNIQUE

A ½ to 1 inch long skin incision along the course of the duct is made at the site. The head is held well extended if the posterior site is chosen. Identification of the duct is easy after cutting through the subcutaneous facia, by its pink colour and anatomical relationship.

In the *anterior site,* try to locate the anterior border of masseter muscle and pick out the duct carefully be pasing a blunt instrument like Tenaculum or closed Artery forceps underneath it.

In the *posterior site,* the neck should be well-extended as otherwise the sterno-maxillaris muscle will hide the duct and accompanying structures. The duct is not very deep and it is likely to be confused with the inferior buccal nerve accompanying it. Besides the nerve, the duct is also accompanied by the submaxillary artery and vein.

Whichever site is chosen, injury to the associated vessels is avoided; and after exposing the duct it is ligated with a broad, non-absorbable suture material like silk. Suture the skin with interrupted apposition sutures.

CHAPTER 61

Trephining of the Frontal Sinus in Bovine

INDICATIONS

Empyema; tumour or cyst; depressed fractures and removal of isolated fragments of bone; exploratory.

ANAESTHESIA AND CONTROL

Local infiltration anaesthesia. The animal may be controlled in the standing or cast position.

ANATOMY

The frontal sinus in the bovine may be outlined as follows:

Lower limit: A horizontal line connecting the inner canthi of the eyes.

Upper limit: Frontal crest and into horn cores.

Lateral limit: Frontal ridge (temporal or lateral ridge of frontal bone).

The frontal sinus of each side is separated by the *median septum*.

Each sinus is divided into a number of incomplete compartments by ridges of bone.

The sinuses drain into the nasal fossa directly through cribriform plate of the Ethomoids (and not via the maxillary sinus as in horse).

The three major compartments of the frontal sinus of each side consist of the three diverticuli, viz. the nuchal diverticulum, the post-orbital diverticulum behind the orbit, and the cornual diverticulum which occupies the horn core.

The frontalis muscle and its fascia (cutaneous muscle) covers the fore-head, and its thickness is very variable depending on the breed of catttle.

BLOOD SUPPLY

The frontal branch of the external ophthalmic artery enters the supra-orbital canal and ramifies chiefly in the frontal sinus.

SITES

1. To obtain complete drainage from the post-orbital diverticulum, about 1 to $1\frac{1}{2}$ inches above (head vertical) the upper border of orbit and medial and close to the temporal ridge.

2. Above a horizontal line connecting the supra-orbital processes and at a point between the midline and the supraorbital fissure which accommodates the frontal vein and artery. This site is not satisfactory due to the risk of puncturing the cranium.

3. Below the base of the horn.

4. Amputation of horn or trephining into horn core will also open the frontal sinus.

TECHNIQUE

Make an outline of the circumference of the trephine by direct pressure on skin with the trephine. Remove a circular piece of skin by making a crucial incision of a slightly larger diameter and by cutting along the outer aspect of the outline made. Scrape and remove the facia to expose the bone. If the frontalis muscle is thick and is interfering with the approach it will have to be cut and retracted. Fix the centre of the trephine head on the bone and by applying pressure, work in a to and fro semirotary fashion till the thickness of the plate of bone is gone through to enter the sinus.

CHAPTER 62

Trephining the Maxillary Sinus In Bovine

INDICATIONS

Usually for removal of a diseased upper molar tooth chiefly the fourth; empyema; exploratory purpose.

ANAESTHESIA AND CONTROL

Local infiltration analgesia. Controlled in the standing or cast position.

ANATOMY

In the bovine the maxillary sinus is not divided into superior and inferior compartments.

It communicates with the middle nasal meatus by a slit-like opening. The fourth and fifth cheek teeth are rooted in the sinus. The third cheek tooth is partly rooted in it.

SITE

Above the facial tuberosity (head horizontal position) and a variable point behind it according to the tooth to be removed.

TECHNIQUE

Similar to trephining of frontal sinus.

Removal of molar tooth, (See page 472).

CHAPTER 63

Operation for Entropion
(Surgical Correction of Entropion)

INDICATIONS

Inward deviation of the palpebral border, Trichiasis, Districhiasis, etc.

ANAESTHESIA AND CONTROL

Block the facial nerve as it emerges on to the cheek, below the temporo-maxillary articulation (motor). Block supra-orbital nerve as it comes out of supra-orbital foramen (sensory to upper lid) or by field block. The animal is controlled in standing or recumbent state.

TECHNIQUE

A fold of skin parallel to the affected palpebral border is held by a forceps, enough to cause the correction of the abnormality, and is severed and removed. The wound is sutured by ordinary apposition sutures.

Anatomy, Blood supply, Nerve supply: See under Ectropion.

CHAPTER 64

Operation for Ectropion
(Surgical Correction of Ectropion)

INDICATIONS

Outward deviation of the palpebral border resulting in an abnormal exposure of the conjunctiva.

ANAESTHESIA

Local infiltration.

SITE

It is $\frac{1}{2}$ to 1 cm away from the free border of the eyelid.

TECHNIQUE

A V-shaped cutaneous incision is put with the base of the "V" close to the affected border of the lid. The triangular flap of skin outlined is worked loose from its apex by undercutting to effect correction of palpebral border. The gap thus caused at the apex is closed by suturing the sides of the "V" incision to form a "Y".

Blood supply to the eyelids: Branches of the ophthalmic and facial arteries; the blood is drained by the corresponding veins.

·· *Nerve supply*: Sensory nerves are derived from the ophthalmic and maxillary branches of the fifth cranial nerve (trigeminal). The facial nerve supplies motor fibres to the muscles: Orbicularis oculi, Corrugator supercili, and Malaris. Oculo-motor nerve supplies the levator muscle of the eyelid.

CHAPTER 65

Removal of the Eye

INDICATIONS
Irreparable injury; orbital abscesses; malignant disease,

ANAESTHESIA AND CONTROL
General anaesthesia, controlled in lateral recumbent state.

ANATOMY
The eyeball is situated in the bony cavity of the orbit formed
by the frontal, lachrymal and malar bones. The conjunctiva lines
the inner surface of eyelids and is then reflected on to the scleral
surface (as palpebral and bulbar conjunctivae).

There are five straight and two oblique muscles of the eyeball: (1) Superior rectus, (2) Inferior rectus, (3) External rectus,
(4) Internal rectus, (5) Posterior rectus, (6) Superior oblique, and
(7) Inferior oblique. These muscles originate around the optic
foramen and are inserted on the sclera behind the attachment
of conjunctiva. The muscles are enclosed by a fibrous covering
called *Tenon's capsule.*

Blood supply: External and internal ophthalmic arteries and
veins. The external ophthalmic artery is a branch of the internal
maxillary and the internal ophthalmic is a branch of the internal
carotid artery. The orbital and periorbital veins form a venous
plexus between the periorbit and muscles of the eyeball. It
communicates with the carvernous sinus and dorsal cerebral veins
on the one side and frontal and facial veins on the other.

Nerve supply: Motor nerve supply—Superior Oblique muscle
by the Fourth cranial or the Trochlear nerve; Posterior and
External rectus by the Abducent or Sixth cranial nerve; and the
other muscles by the oculo-motor or third cranial. Sensory
supply is by the ophthalmic nerve and naso-ciliary nerves. (For

remembering motor nerve supply, the words SOFT PEAS formed by the beginning letters of important words is useful.)

TECHNIQUE

Method (1): Enucleation of eye—The conjunctiva is held by forceps and is divided around the eyeball exposing the scleral inser· tions of the muscles of eyeball. These are divided one by one so that it will be possible to turn the eyeball and sever the rest of the attachments. The eyeball is removed and the orbit is plugged to arrest haemorrhage. If tarsorrhaphy is to be performed, the edges of the lid are trimmed and sutured.

Method (2): Extirpation of eye (Eviseration of orbit)—The palpebral borders of the eyelids are temporarily sutured together. An elliptical cutaneous incision enclosing this suture line is made without opening into the conjunctival sac. Retracting the skin edges, the eyeball along with its muscles is detached from the bony orbit by blunt dissection between the Tenon's capsule and bony orbit. After division of the attachments close to the base of the orbit and removal of the eyeball the orbital cavity is packed with gauze to control bleeding. The skin edges are united by apposition sutures leaving a small gap at the inner commissure for removal of the gauze packing next day.

CHAPTER 66

Evisceration of the Eyeball

INDICATIONS

This operation is of very little application in bovine. When an artificial eye is desired to be introduced, this method is suitable.

ANAESTHESIA AND CONTROL

General anaesthesia; recumbent state.

TECHNIQUE

The cornea is dissected out and the contents of the eyeball are removed leaving the outer tunics intact.

CHAPTER 67

De-horning
(Amputation of Horn)

INDICATIONS

Irreparable injury or malignant disease. For making management and control easier.

ANAESTHESIA AND CONTROL

Cornual nerve block. Hold the animal in the standing or in the recumbent position.

ANATOMY

The horn core is a part of the frontal bone.

Blood supply: Cornual branch of superficial temporal artery and corresponding veins.

Nerve supply: Cornual nerve, which is a branch of the Lachyrmal which is a branch of the ophthalmic branch of the Trigemal (fifth cranial or Trifacial). (To remember this, remember the word CLOT formed with the beginning letters of important words.)

SITE

(1) Below the base of horn after "flapping" the skin; or (2) any level above the base of horn but below the seat of damage.

TECHNIQUE

Method (*1*): (The *Flap Method*)—The amputation is carried out through the frontal bone below the base of horn after flapping the skin forwards and backwards in two halves by a long elliptical incision around the base of horn, extending from the nuchal crest to the frontal ridge, long enough to expose the site of amputation. The bleeding is controlled and the operation is completed by suturing the skin flaps in apposition by interrupted sutures, after trimming the flaps as required. *Method* (*2*): Amputation at the desired level is carried out by the direct method using a saw. The bleeding in method (1) is arrested by ligature or torsion of the superficial temporary artery lying lateral to the base of the horn, behind the frontal ridge (i.e., the cornual artery). Thermocautery may also be used. In method (2) wherein amputation is done above the base of horn, bleeding is controlled by thermocautery. *Method* (*3*): By using de-horning shears. This is feasible only if the horn is small. *Method* (*4*): Destruction of the horn buds by applying potassium hydroxide sticks, so that the horn growth is completely suppressed. Can be done in young calves when they are five to ten days old. *Method* (*5*): Dishorning calves by electric dishorner.

Dishorning Calves Using Electric Dishorner

INDICATIONS

(1) For more safety in restraining the animals. (2) To save accommodation space in stalls. (3) Avoid risk to other animals and the farmer. (4) To increase the aesthetic value of the animal. (5) For safety of transport.

Optium age: Before the calves are one month old, preferably when they are five to ten days old.

PROCEDURE

The equipment consists of a circular tip which can be applied around the horn bud, and having a long handle with necessary electrical connections. It usually operates on 220 volts AC. The connections are plugged to the electrical supply for five minutes till the circular tip gets sufficiently hot. The current supply is then cut off and the circular tip applied slowly and steadily encircling the horn-bud, for about half a minute, thereby destroying the horny tissue.

We have been using the "Raico Electric Dishorner" (manufactured by Messrs. Raico Industries, Puttur, South Canara District, Karnataka State). The equipment is also provided with different accessories which can be fixed on to the tip for other purposes of thermo cauterisation, like point-firing, pin-point firing, branding, etc.

CHAPTER 68

Removal of Molars in Bovine

INDICATIONS

In cases such as ossifying alveolar periostitis, odontoma and in extensive caries.

ANAESTHESIA AND CONTROL

General anaesthesia or maxillary nerve block or local infiltra·tion anaesthesia. The animal is secured in lateral recumbent position.

ANATOMY

The roots of the first three cheek teeth are directed slightly forward and are not in the maxillary sinus. The other cheek teeth, particularly the fourth and fifth, have their roots in the floor of the maxillary sinus and are directed backwards.

Blood supply: Infra-orbital and alveolar branches of the internal maxillary artery.

Nerve supply: Branches of the maxillary nerve along its course in the superior dental canal before its exit through the infra-orbital foramen, supplies the upper cheek teeth. Similarly the mandibular nerve supplies the lower cheek teeth.

TECHNIQUE

Methods: (1) Simple extraction by using tooth forceps is possible in some cases when the tooth is diseased. (2) Repulsion through maxillary sinus after trephining the maxillary sinus and removal of the external alveolar plate in case of teeth with roots embedded in the sinus. (3) Repulsion through the trephine openings made on inferior border of the rami of mandible for the lower cheek teeth. *Technique for Method 2*: Trephine the maxillary sinus in level with the root of the affec-ted tooth. The mouth is kept open by using a mouth gag. The root of the tooth is identified by breaking the alveolar plate using chisel and mallet, through the trephine opening made. The crown of the tooth is held by a hand in the mouth. Through the trephined opening, a punch is applied against the root at an angle corresponding to the direction of the tooth and the assistant strikes the punch with a mallet repeatedly till the tooth could be safely extracted by the hand in the mouth. Occasionally it may become necessary to break the root from the crown and remove them separately.

The technique for trephining the maxillary sinus for removal of a molar tooth, is given on (page 464).

CHAPTER 69

Emergency Tracheotomy

INDICATIONS

(1) Threatened respiratory failure on account of allergic or other obstruction of the upper respiratory tract like oedema of the larynx, oedema of the upper lip and nostrils. For example in calf diphtheria. (2) Persistent epistaxis. (3) To prevent persistent straining in prolapse of rectum, eversion of uterus.

ANAESTHESIA AND CONTROL

Standing position with local analgesia.

ANATOMY

The trachea is a cartilaginous tube composed in cattle of a number of incomplete annular cartilages, covered by the two sterno-thyro-hyoid muscles on the ventral face.

Blood supply: The blood supply to the trachea is chiefly derived from branches of the common carotid arteries. The veins go mainly to the jugular veins.

Nerve supply: The nerve supply is from the vagosympathetic trunk.

SITE

1 to 2 inches longitudinally along the ventral aspect of neck, preferably at the junction of its upper and middle third.

TECHNIQUE

An incision about 2 inches long is made through the skin and subcutis on the mid-ventral line of the neck. After retracting apart sterno-hyoideus muscles, an incision is made between two tracheal rings. The opening is widened to suit the dimension of

Operation for "Tumour Neck" (Chronic Yoke Abscess) in Cattle

ANAESTHESIA AND CONTROL

Local infiltration around the base of the tumour. Controlled in standing or lateral recumbency.

TECHNIQUE

An elliptical incision enclosing the necrotic areas of the skin over the swelling is made parallel to or slightly oblique the long axis of the neck. By blunt dissection, reach base of the swelling and enucleate the mass. The wound is closed by interrupted apposition ·sutures after assuring ıthat the bleeding points are arrested. The length and shape of the incision is adjusted for proper closure without pouch formation and the skin is trimm-ed, if necessary, before suturing. (See also page 114)

Note: If possible, the direction of the skin incision may be so modified as to correspond to one of the natural skin creases of the neck, as it will minimise scarring. The skin creases, which are vertical or slightly oblique in the neck region, represent the natural clevage of collagen fibres of dermis.

CHAPTER 70

Oesophagotomy

INDICATIONS
Oesophageal obstructions.

ANAESTHESIA AND CONTROL
Local infiltration; standing or recumbent state.

ANATOMY
Lateral to the oesophagus are the carotid sheath containing the internal jugular vein; carotid artery and the common trunk of vago-sympathetic and the sternosuboccipitalis part of sterno-cephalicus muscle.

Ventro-medially the oesophagus is related to the trachea and the recurrent laryngeal nerve.

Dorsally the oesophagus is related to the Longus colli muscle.

Blood supply to the oesophagus: Branches of the carotid and brancheo-oesophageal arteries for cervical segment. Short branches of the gastric artery toward the terminal segment. Delicate branches from intercostal arteries in the thoracic segment run circumferentially to supply the oesophagus.

SITE
On the left side of the neck, along the superior border of jugular furro, close to the level of obstruction.

TECHNIQUE
An incision about 2 inches long is made along the superior border of jugular furrow cutting through the skin and cervical cutaneous facia. The jugular vein is retracted by separating it from the brancheo-cephalicus muscle; to encounter the sterno-sub-occipitalis muscle which is pushed downwards; and by blunt dissection the oesophagus lying adjacent to the trachea can be

located. The oesophagus is recognised by its characteristic pink colour. It is exposed by a tenaculum. The wall of the oesophagus is incised longitudinally over the desired length to get into the lumen and the obstruction is relieved. The mucous membrane is sutured by interrupted apposition sutures and the outer coat is sutured by interrupted or continuous apposition sutures with ¼ to ½ of an inch spacing. The overlying muscles and skin are sutured only if conditions are suitable for primary healing.

*Note: Some surgeons prefer inversion sutures for the mucous membrane, in which case care is taken to avoid narrowing of the oesophageal lumen at the suture site.

Operation for "Tumour Neck" (Chronic Yoke Abscess) in Cattle

ANAESTHESIA AND CONTROL

Local infiltration around the base of the tumour. Controlled in standing or lateral recumbency.

TECHNIQUE

An elliptical incision enclosing the necrotic areas of the skin over the swelling is made parallel to or slightly oblique the long axis of the neck. By blunt dissection, reach base of the swelling and enucleate the mass. The wound is closed by interrupted apposition ·sutures after assuring ıthat the bleeding points are arrested. The length and shape of the incision is adjusted for proper closure without pouch formation and the skin is trimmed, if necessary, before suturing. (See also page 114)

CHAPTER 72

Paracentesis Thoracis* in Bovine

INDICATIONS
(1) To relieve severe respiratory distress in moist pleurisy.
(2) Collection of fluid samples for diagnostic purpose.

ANAESTHESIA AND CONTROL
Local analgesia; standing position.

ANATOMY
The mediastinal septa in bovine is complete. The chest cavity thus is divided into two compartments and therefore paracentesis of one side does not affect the opposite side.

SITE
Left side: The sixth intercostal space and on a line with the point of the elbow close to the anterior border of the seventh rib.

Right side: The fifth intercostal space and on a line with the point of the elbow close to the anterior border of the sixth rib.

TECHNIQUE
A trocar and canula about 6 inch long and $\frac{1}{8}$ inch in diameter is used. The skin is punctured further behind the level of site chosen so that the points of puncture do not coincide. The trocar is withdrawn slowly to drain the fluid. The trocar is replaced before canula is withdrawn with it after paracentesis.

(While puncturing the thoracic wall, better to go close to anterior border of the rib, since intercostal vessels are situated near the posterior borders of ribs.).

---

*Tapping the Chest; Thoracocentesis, or Thoracentesis.

CHAPTER 73

Pericardiotomy in Bovine

INDICATIONS

(1) Accumulation of fluid in the pericardial sac. (2) To remove foreign bodies.

ANAESTHESIA AND CONTROL

Standing position with sedatives. Local infiltration anaesthesia along the line of incision and also into the soft tissue surrounding the portion of rib to be removed.

SITE

Along the fifth rib on the left side.

TECHNIQUE

Incise the skin over the fifth rib on the left side, starting from a little below the costochondral junction and extending upwards for about 6 inches. (See also page 339).

Reflect the skin edges and separate also the muscles overlying the rib. By careful dissection, separate the rib from underlying parietal pleura, avoiding injury to the intercostal vessels along the posterior border of the rib.

Pass a wire-saw between the pleura and the rib at the upper commissure of the incision and cut the rib at this point. Reflect the cut rib outward and remove it by breaking at the costochondral junction. The pleura and the pericardium underlying it are now visible. Incise the pleura at a point and extend the opening with scissors. Open the pericardial sac and drain fluid collection and foreign bodies, if any. Suture the pericardium, pleura and skin wound as separate layers.

CHAPTER 74

Paracentesis Abdominis (Laparocentesis) in Bovine

INDICATIONS
Ascites. For diagnostic and therapeutic purposes.

ANAESTHESIA AND CONTROL
Local analgesia; standing or recumbent position.

SURGICAL ANATOMY
The trocar and canula is to be directed through the skin, subcutis, aponeurotic part of the oblique abdominal muscle, rectus abdominis muscle, the deep facia and parietal peritoneum, to enter the peritoneal cavity.

SITE
Lateral to and behind the umbilicus.

PROCEDURE
The points of puncture on the skin and muscle should not coincide. A trocar and canula (one-eighth of an inch diameter and 6 inches long) is used.

To drain the peritoneal fluid, the trocar is withdrawn, leaving the canula *in situ*. After draining the fluid, the trocar is reintroduced and the two instruments are withdrawn together to avoid escape of fluid along the way.

CHAPTER 75

Puncture of Rumen
(Rumenocentesis)

INDICATIONS
: (1) Relief of acute tympany as an emergency measure.
: (2) Direct medication into the rumen.

ANAESTHESIA AND CONTROL
: Local infiltration analgesia; standing or recumbent position.

SITE
: Centre of the hollow of the flank on the left side.

TECHNIQUE

A trocar (and canula) of about $\frac{3}{8}$ inch diameter is used. The points of puncture on the skin, abdominal wall and the rumen are not allowed to coincide as the skin is punctured first and the point of the trocar is carried a little away from that point before puncturing the abdominal muscles and rumen. The trocar is removed to establish communication with the interior of rumen through the canula. The canula is removed only after replacing the trocar and withdrawing the trocar and canula together, keeping the flank pressed against the rumen by hand to prevent ruminal contents escaping into the peritoneal cavity.

Anatomy, Nerve Supply, Blood Supply: See under Rumenotomy.

CHAPTER 76

Paravertebral Nerve Block in Bovine

INDICATIONS

Regional analgesia of the flank. The thirteenth thoracic, and first, second and third lumbar spinal nerves are to be blocked.

ANATOMY

The nerve supply for the flank region is by the thirteenth (last thoracic) and first and second lumbar spinal nerves. In addition to this the third lumbar supplies a small cutaneous branch in front of the external angle of the ilium. The ventral aspect of abdomen receives branches also from the spinal nerves anterior to the thirteenth dorsal. Each spinal nerve has one dorsal and another ventral branch. The dorsal branch is mainly motor but supplies sensory fibres to the skin of the loins. The ventral branch is sensory and supplies the skin, muscles, peritoneum and viscera. The ventral branch travels below the inter-transverse ligament and hence the anaesthetic solution should be deposited below this ligament.

SITE

The last thoracic nerve (thirteenth) is blocked about 5 to 6 cm lateral to the mid-dorsal line at a point behind the level of the head of the last rib.

The sites for blocking the first three lumbar nerves are 5 to 6 cm lateral to mid dorsal-line and behind the transverse processes of the first three lumbar vertebrae, respectively.

ANAESTHESIA AND CONTROL

A skin weal is made by injecting a few drops of the local anaesthetic solution at each site. Controlled in standing position,

TECHNIQUE

A needle about 3 inches to 4 inches long is used to reach a depth of about 2 inches to 2½ inches at the sites chosen. The needle point hits slightly behind the head of last rib and the posterior borders of the first, second and third lumbar transverse processes for blocking thirteenth dorsal, and the first, second and third lumbar nerves, respectively. The skin and cutaneous muscle, the thick longissimus dorsi and the inter-transverse ligament are pierced before it reaches the point. The anaesthetic effect is manifested in about ten to fifteen minutes. The quantity of fluid injected is variable. A dose of 5 to 20 cc of a 2% solution of procaine may be used for each nerve.

CHAPTER 77

Rumenotomy

INDICATIONS
Exploratory. Foreign body reticulitis. Severe impaction.

SITE
Left flank, in the para-lumbar fossa, a vertical incision 6 to 8 inches long.

ANAESTHESIA AND CONTROL
Paravertebral or local infiltration analgesia. Control in standing position preferred.

ANATOMY
The muscle fibres of the obliqus abdominis externus run downward and backward and that of obliqus abdominis internus downward and forward. The fibres of transverse abdominis are directed vertically.

Nerve supply: Lumbar nerves. See under paravertebral analgesia.

Blood supply: The blood supply to the flank is contributed by the phrenico-abdominal and deep circumflex iliac vessels. The blood vascular channels of the rumen are located in the left and right longitudinal grooves and the anterior and posterior transverse grooves of it.

TECHNIQUE
A vertical incision about 6 to 8 inches long is made commencing about 2 inches below the level of the lumbar transverse process. The abdominal muscles and the parietal peritoneum are traversed by a direct incision corresponding to the skin incision. The wound is kept retracted and the rumen wall is fixed to the skin edges by a set of temporary through-and-through

mattress sutures before opening into the rumen. This is to prevent escape of rumen contents into peritoneal cavity. (Instead
of such fixation, the McLintock's method or Weingart's method
may be used). A short incision is made on the rumen and this
is extended enough to permit easy access by hand into the rumen
and reticulum. The rumen contents are removed without con-
taminating the peritoneal cavity by proper packing. The reti-culum
can also be examined by stretching the hand through the rumen.
The large rumeno-reticular passage, the oesophageal groove, and
the opening of oesophagus into the stomach are also palpable this
way.

The temporary fixation sutures of the rumen to the skin are
removed only after the incision on the rumen wall is closed by
inversion sutures. Connel's or Cushing's sutures are used to close
the rumen, commencing slightly above and extending a little
below the line of incision. A continuous Lembert's suture is also
placed over this. The parietal peritoneum is closed by continuous
suture. The incised muscles are brought into apposition by
continuous sutures. The skin incision is closed by vertical mattress sutures or ordinary interrupted apposition sutures.

Note: Instead of suturing the parietal peritoneum, muscles
and skin by separate layers of sutures described above, some
persons prefer a "figure-of-eight suture" to close these different
layers of tissues in the abdominal wall.

CHAPTER 78

Abomasotomy

INDICATIONS

(1) Obstruction due to foreign bodies. (2) Abomasal ulcers with haemorrhage.

ANAESTHESIA AND CONTROL

Field block and local infiltration. Dorsal recumbent position.

ANATOMY

The abomasum can be located on the right side of abdomen. The fundus of abomasum is near the Xiphoid cartilage and its pyloric part inclines dorsally and joins the duodenum at the level of the tenth rib.

Blood supply: Blood supply is derived from the coeliac artery and the veins join the portal vein.

SITE

No. 1: On the linea alba, about 2 inches behind Xiphoid cartilage of the sternum and extending up to the umbilicus.

No. 2: A 4 to 10 inches long paracostal incision is made about 2 inches behind the costal arch beginning at about 6 inches away from the mid-ventral line and extending caudo-dorsally. The lower commissure of the incision may be extended ventro-medially when found necessary to operate on the fundus.

TECHNIQUE

The abdominal cavity is entered by incising skin, abdominal muscles and parietal peritoneum. Introduce the hand into the abdomen towards the right side and pull out the greater curvature of the abomasum. Hold it through the incision by means of four temporary stay sutures passed through the wall of the abomasum. Any space left between the abomasum and the lips of the abdominal wound is packed off with moist sterile towels to prevent escape of abomasal contents into the peritoneal cavity. Incise the abomasum (3 to 6 inches) and perform the necessary operations by introducing the hand through the incision.

(For *abomasal ulcers* that are bleeding, the ulcerated surface on the mucus membrane with the bleeding vessel is enclosed in a series of stample type sutures placed along the base of the ulcer.)

The abomasal incision is closed by Cushing's suture. The temporary sutures are released and the laparotomy wound is closed as usual. (As already mentioned under rumenotomy.)

CHAPTER 79

Epidural Analgesia (Caudal Epidural Analgesia) in Bovine

INDICATIONS
Surgery of hind limbs and posterior regions of the body, chiefly obstetric surgery in cow, surgical manipulations of penis of bull, correction of vaginal prolapse, etc.

ANAESTHESIA AND CONTROL
Local infiltration before introducing the epidural needle; controlled in standing or recumbent position.

ANATOMY
The spinal cord in the bovine ends about the region of the last lumbar vertebrae. The epidural space is filled by loose fatty areolar tissue.

SITE
1. Sacro-coccygeal site (anterior caudal site), between sacrum and first coccygeal vertebrae.
2. Inter-coccygeal site (posterior caudal site), between first and second coccygeal vertebrae.

TECHNIQUE
The site is located with the tip of a finger when the tail is manipulated up and down with the other hand. The needle is introduced at an angle of 45° to a depth of about ½ to 1 inch to enter the vertebral canal. The solution is injected slowly.

Dosage: Small heifers: 40cc of 2% Procaine solution.
Large heifers: 50cc of 2½% solution.
For amputation of udder in cows: 40-50cc 3% solution.
To prevent straining: 8 to 10 cc of a 2% solution for a 1200

lb cow and 5 cc for a 500 lb cow if the cow should remain standing.

Note: To prevent straining in prolapse of vagina in the cow, 22% alcohol can be injected epidurally. The dose for a Jersey cow weighing 1200 lb is 7 cc. Never exceed this dose because paralysis of tail might result. (Approximate dose for local cattle: 600 lb=4 cc; 800 lb = 5 cc; 1000 lb=6 cc.)

Unlike lumbar epidural anaesthesia, caudal epidural anaesthesia is very commonly practiced.

CHAPTER 80

Castration of Bull

The various methods of castration in the bovine may be listed as follows:
1. Closed method (Burdizzo method)
2. Open method (1) "Open-uncovered" or "Open-Open" or "Open" method. (2) "Open-covered" or "covered" method.

INDICATIONS

To prevent breeding. For easy management and maintenance of working cattle. For quick and economic fattening of beef cattle.

ANAESTHESIA AND CONTROL

Spermatic nerve block or epidural analgesia. No analgesic is used under field conditions, for the Burdizzo method. Controlled in standing or recumbent position.

ANATOMY

The scrotum of the bull is long and pendulous with a well-defined neck. The testicles are elongated and oval in outline and are placed vertically in the scrotum along its long axis. The tail of the epididymus is located at the lower end and its head is on the superior aspect. The testicle, epididymis and the spermatic cord are enclosed by a layer of serous membrane called the tunica vaginalis. The spermatic cord consists of an anterior vascular bundle and a posterior bundle containing the vas deferens.

Blood supply: Spermatic vessels for the testes and the branches of the external pudic vessels for the scrotum.

Nerve supply: Spermatic nerves derived from the renal and mesenteric plexus supply the testes. Branches of the second and third lumbar spinal nerves supply the scrotum.

TECHNIQUE

(i) *Castration of bull with Burdizzo forceps*—The spermatic cord of each side is held outward against the scrotal skin and is crushed in such a way that the crush marks on either side do not coincide. Each side cord may be crushed twice, first at a higher level and then about an inch below, taking care to see that the testicle itself is not crushed. The sigmoid curve of the penis should not be included within the jaws of the forceps by mistake. The testicle is pushed upwards after removing the forceps to prevent adhesions at the points crushed.

(ii) *Castration of bull by the open (open-open) method*—The scrotal skin and tunica vaginalis over the testes are held tense by holding the testicle and are incised.

(The scrotum can be incised on its anterior, lateral or posterior aspects of each testicle. But in any case the incision is extended ventrally to provide drainage.)

The spermatic cord is exposed by traction on the exposed testicle. The vas deferens and tunica vaginalis are severed by scissors or emasculator as high as possible. The vascular bundle is ligatured as high up as possible and is severed a little distance below the ligature. (It can be severed by emasculator, by torsion or by hot iron, if ligation is not desired. If division is by torsion, it is held by clamps close to the abdominal wall and the portion below is twisted slowly and continuously by torsion forceps till it severs itself.) The incision on the skin may be left open. The excess skin may be trimmed if desired. If conditions for primary healing are satisfied, there is no objection to suturing the skin wound.

(iii) *Castration of bull by the open-covered method*—In this method ("open covered method" or "covered method") the testes with its covering of tunica vaginalis are removed after incision of only the scrotal skin. (See also pages 341, 345).

Vasectomy (See pages 341 and 348).

CHAPTER 81

Oopherectomy (Spaying) in Cow

INDICATIONS
(1) To prevent breeding and fattening for slaughter. (2) To prolong lactation period in milking cows which are not likely to be useful for further breeding.

ANAESTHESIA AND CONTROL
Epidural analgesia; standing or recumbent position.

SITE
Method 1—The vaginal method, possible in large sized heifers and cows: Vaginal fornix lateral to the cervix.

Method 2—Flank method: below and in front of the external angle of the ilium, preferably on the left side.

Method 3—Mid-line in front of pubis, in young heifers.

TECHNIQUE
1. *Vaginal method*: The right hand carrying a short bladed concealed knife is introduced into the vaginal canal. The vaginal fornix is stretched and the blade of knife is exposed in order to make a stab-opening lateral to the cervix so that the thickness of the vaginal wall with its anterior peritoneal lining is pierced at the same time. The opening thus made is stretched by fingers and enlarged enough to enable the hand to pierce without stripping the peritoneum in front. The ovaries are easily located and identified by following the uterine cornu on each side. The ovaries are then drawn into the vaginal canal and are severed by ecraseur and removed. The wound on the fornix is left unsutured.

2. *Flank method*: A vertical skin incision 4 to 6 inches long is made at the site described. The muscular wall, deep facia and parietal peritoneum are incised to permit the entry of the hand.

The ovaries are located and are severed and removed by ecraseur. The incision is closed as usual for laparotomy.

3. *Mid-line approach*: This is suitable in young heifers after pre-operative fasting and control in dorsal recumbent state with hind parts well-raised. The ovaries are removed by a laparotomy in front of pubis, along linea alba.

Vulval Suture TO PREVENT VAGINAL PROLAPSE IN COW

Method 1-A *purse-string suture* going around the vulva subcutaneously.

Method 2-One or more *mattress-sutures* passing through and connecting both lips of the vulva.

Mathod 3-"*Cross-lacing method*". This is found to be more efficient and causes less discomfort to the patient. A number of independent interrupted skin sutures are made with sterile um-bilical tape or similar suture material on one side (say, left side) of vulvar lip. A corresponding equal number of sutures are made on the opposite (right) side. Using these sutures as "loops", separate pieces of tapes are "laced through" them, so as to support the vulvar lips both diagonally (cross-wise) and transversely, and tied. The lacing tapes can be changed daily or whenever required, without damaging the loop sutures.

Note: In order to understand the cross-lacing method described above, the student may draw a diagram wherein the loops stitched on one side of the vulva may be represented as A, B, C, D and the loops at corresponding level on the opposite side marked as P, Q, R, S, respectively. If these loops are to be tied together by three independent tapes, the first tape should be passed through loops in the order of A, P, B, Q, before its two ends are brought back and tied at loop A. In a similar fashion, the second tape is passed through in the order of B, Q, C, R, B and is tied at B. Finally, the third tape is looped and tied in the order C, R, D, S, C.

CHAPTER 82

Hysterotomy
(Caesarian Section) in Cow

INDICATIONS

Delivering foetus when normal delivery is difficult or not desirable.

ANAESTHESIA AND CONTROL

Paravertebral or lumbar epidural; recumbent state.

SITE

There are many sites for this operation. (1) Between the mammary vein and the midline, either on the left or right side from the front of the udder forwards; (2) lateral to and parallel to milk vein; (3) oblique flank incision, .downward and forward from a little below external angle of ilium; (4) vertical incision in the paralumbar fossa (preferably of the *left* side to avoid the omentum and intestines).

Note: I prefer site No. 4.

TECHNIQUE

The skin and sub-cutis and the abdominal muscles and the parietal peritoneum are incised to expose the gravid uterine cornua. The incision on the uterus is made away from its attached border, big enough to deliver the foetus. The incision is so placed that only the minimum number of cotyledons are affected by it. The foetus is delivered. The umbilical cord is ligated and cut. The foetal fluids should be directed outwards by packing the uterus suitably. The uterine incision is closed by a double layer of Lembert sutures which do not include the foetal membranes. Suture the parietal peritoneum, muscles and skin separately.

ANATOMY

See under Rumenotomy regarding abdominal muscles.

Blood supply: The anterior, middle and posterior uterine vessels situated in the broad ligament of the uterus.

OPERATION FOR RECTO-VAGINAL FISTULA IN COW/MARE (FORSSEL'S OPERATION)

From 3 days before operation until about 10 days after it, reduce bulky feed, to reduce quantity of dung in rectum. Epidural anaesthesia. Immediately before operation, remove dung manually and clean rectum.

Put a transverse incision between rectum and vulva, and continue it forward upto about 5 cm anterior to the fistula, to visualise the fistulae on rectal and vaginal walls. Suture rectal wall by interrupted Lembert suture with non-absorbable material, leaving the ends of sutures long enough for removal on 10th day. Suture vaginal wall also with same type of sutures, but in *opposite directions*. Pack cavity between rectum and vagina with BIPP-gauze, and put retention sutures on skin. On third day remove gauze packings, thereafter daily clean the wound mopping with antiseptic lotion and treat it in a routine manner. By tenth day the inner sutures also can be removed and further healing is uneventful. For more details see Frank (1959).

CHAPTER 83

Amputation of Penis (Peotomy) in Bull

INDICATIONS

Irreparable injury. Paraphimosis. Permanent paralysis. Malignant disease.

ANAESTHESIA AND CONTROL

Epidural analgesia combined with local infiltration. Dorsal recumbency.

SITE

Proximal to the seat of lesion. The sheath is also removed with the penis.

ANATOMY

The cavernous tissue is very meagre towards the tip of the penis. The tunica albugenia is very thick and fibrous. The retractor penis muscles are inserted at the second flexure of the sigmoid curve. *Blood supply to the penis*: Branches of internal pudic artery supply the root of the penis. A branch of the external pudic artery constitutes the dorsal artery of the penis. Veins are external pudental, perineal, and internal pudic vessels.

TECHNIQUE

Two skin incisions are made parallel to the sheath on either side of it, starting from a point in front of the preputial orifice and meeting at the level of amputation. The portion of sheath so enclosed by incisions is undermined from the abdominal wall up to the posterior commissure of the resulting elliptical wound where portion of penis is exposed. A tourniquet is placed around the penis. The urethra which may be identified on the ventral aspect of the penis (by passing a catheter or sound, if necessary), is carefully dissected from the penis for a distance of about $\frac{1}{4}$ to $\frac{1}{2}$ inch at this exposed portion. A strong suture material is passed under the dissected portion of urethra and by it a tight ligature is placed around the penis *excluding* the urethra. The penis and the dissected portion of urethra are cut $\frac{1}{4}$ inch distal to the ligature to remove the distal portions and complete the amputation. The tourniquet is removed. The stump of penis is fixed to the posterior commissure of the skin wound by a suture to prevent its retraction. The skin wound is sutured leaving the stump containing urethra to protrude through the posterior commissure of the incision.

When it is desired to remove the penis completely, the operation is suitably modified to enclose the scrotum also in the initial skin incisions and the testicles and scrotum are also removed along with penis and sheath.

CHAPTER 84

Urethrotomy in Bull

INDICATIONS
Urethral obstruction.

ANAESTHESIA AND CONTROL
Epidural anaesthesia; controlled in standing or dorsal recumbent state.

SITE
1. *Post scrotal site*—for removal of obstruction at the sigmoid flexure. About 3 inches behind the scrotum along the median line.
2. *Ischeal site*—for obstructions close to ischeal arch. From two inches below the ischeal arch downwards along medial line.

TECHNIQUE
1. *Post scrotal method*—A midline incision 3 inches long is made about 3 inches behind the scrotum. The areolar tissue is dissected to reveal rectractor penis muscles on either side. These are separated and held retracted to expose the body of the penis. Palpate the urethra on the ventral aspect and incise it longitudinally along the exact midline. The blockage is relieved and the patency of the canal is established by a gum elastic catheter or a pliable metal probe. A thin plastic tube may be used as a catheter and left in situ for one or two days. The wound is left open to heal by second intension which ensues if the normal passage is clear.
2. *Ischeal urethrotomy*—A skin incision 2 inches long is made along the midline starting from about 2 inches below the ischeal arch downwards. This exposes the two retractor penis muscles. The remaining part of the operation is as already described. The incision can be started in level with the ischeal arch, but will cause unnecessary bleeding due to the cutting of the ischeo-cavernosus muscle.

Cystotomy in Bovine

INDICATIONS

Vesical calculi. Neoplastic growth.

ANAESTHESIA AND CONTROL

General anaesthesia; dorsal recumbent state.

SITE

The pre-pubic (ante-pubic or supra pubic) site is chosen along linea alba starting in front of the pubic symphysis to a length of about 3 to 4 inches forward. (In the male the skin incision is placed lateral to the sheath and subsequently operated along the linea alba.)

TECHNIQUE

After opening the abdomen, the bladder is brought over to the incision on the abdominal wall, turned over its neck and is isolated by packing suitably to prevent contamination of the peritoneal cavity. An incision about 2 to 3 inches long is made on the *dorsal surface* of the bladder towards its neck, to gain access into the bladder for necessary manipulations and removal of contents and neoplastic growth, if any. The incision on the bladder is closed by Cushing's inversion sutures. The opening on the linea alba is closed by interrupted apposition sutures reinforced by mattress sutures. The skin wound is closed by ordinary interrupted sutures or by vertical mattress sutures.

(It is sometimes difficult to bring out a collapsed urinary bladder in the bovine through the wound because of its deep retraction into the pelvic cavity.)

Blood vessels of the bladder: The arteries are derived chiefly from the internal pudic but branches also come from obturator artery. The veins terminate chiefly in the internal pudic veins.

CHAPTER 86

Ablation(Amputation) of Mammary Gland in Cow

INDICATIONS

Gangrene of the udder. Malignant diseases of the udder. Suppurative mastitis.

ANAESTHESIA AND CONTROL

Epidural anaesthesia with blocking third lumbar spinal nerve or local infiltration. Lateral recumbent posture.

TECHNIQUE

Either the right or left half or both halves of the udder may be removed. The animal is cast and secured in lateral recumbency with the affected side above. *Method (1)*: The two teats of the side affected are together enclosed in an elliptical antero-posterior incision. The base of the gland is reached by blunt dissection. The three major arteries and veins (mentioned below) are identified and sectioned between ligatures. Dissection is continued and the gland is removed completely with the two teats. The cavity is packed to control bleeding and retention sutures are placed. *Method (2)*: This method is chosen when it is desired to remove the glands leaving behind the teats. Here the amputation is effected through a T-shaped incision on the lateral aspect of the udder which is partially sutured leaving about 1 inch of the vertical incision for drainage.

ANATOMY

There is a superficial and deep facia covering the gland. The deep facia is made up of elastic tissue. Centrally two laminae detached from the abdominal tunic descend on either side of the median plane, forming a septum between the right and left glands, constituting the ligamentum suspensorium. The quarters of same side are not so well-separated by fibrous septum.

Blood supply: There are three major vessels supplying the udder: (1) the external pudic artery and vein coming through inguinal canal and entering through the base of the gland at its middle, (2) the perineal vein and an associated branch from the femoral artery entering through the posterior aspect, and (3) the subcutaneous abdominal or milk vein and branch of external pudic artery from the anterior aspect of the gland.

Nerve supply: The three sources of nerve supply to the udder are: (1) the anterior and posterior inguinal nerves coming through the inguinal canal, (2) the sympathetic nerves incorporated in the inguinal nerves but originating from the posterior mesenteric plexus, and (3) the cutaneous nerves originating from the ventral branches of the first, second and third lumbar and possibly the thirteenth thoracic nerves.

CHAPTER 87

Operation for Teat Fistula in Cow

ANAESTHESIA AND CONTROL
Local infiltration; standing position.

ANATOMY
The teat canal or lactiferous duct is lined by non-glandular mucous membrane, surrounded by unstriped muscular tissue, the bulk of the fibres being arranged in a circular manner to form the sphincter.

TECHNIQUE
Method (1): (*Moussu's method*)—The edges of the fistula are freshened and are then sutured by a set of mattress sutures passing through the skin and subcutis on one edge, and only the subcuticular tissue on the opposite edge.

The set of sutures may start from alternate edges. Another layer of ordinary interrupted opposition sutures may be put over this. The wound is sealed with Tr. Benzoin or Collodion. A teat syphon is introduced into the teat canal and is left in position with adhesive plaster for a few days so as to prevent escape of milk through the fistula until healing.

Method (2): (*Gold's method*)—A piece of tissue from each side of the fistula is cut out and the edges of the fistular opening are thus freshened. A series of mattress sutures are placed through the mucular coat and skin of either side, going close to the mucous membrane but not piercing it, thus causing a slight eversion of skin edge and inversion of mucous edge. The suture line is sealed and a teat syphon or tubing is kept. It is necessary to provide some artificial contrivance to drain milk for at least 72 hours post-operatively, to facilitate healing. (See page 504).

CHAPTER 88

Operation for Stricture of Teat in Cow
(Sphincterostomy)

INDICATIONS
Tight milking, natural or acquired.

ANAESTHESIA AND CONTROL
Local infiltration; standing.

TECHNIQUE
In tight milking due to narrow teat sphincter, the tip of the teat is cut across, holding it between the thumb and index finger, by a sharp blade. A grooved director like Stinson's teat director is useful to direct a thin blade or scalpel. Alternatively, McLean's teat knife or Hall's teat knife or Hudson's teat knife may be used for cutting the sphincter. The cutting is done twice, to form a crucial shape.

Note: A simple method to drain milk post-operatively after open-teat surgery, by passing a poly-ethylene tube 2 to 3 mm diameter with an outer air-cuff made out of an ordinary balloon, has been described by Pande and Kulkarni, 1985.

Ref: Pande. S.V., and Kulkarni, P.E. (1985). The use of polyethylene tube with rubber balloon in open-teat surgery in goat. Indian J. Vet. Surg. 6(2): 131-133.

CHAPTER 89

Digital Nerve Block of fore-limb in Bovine

INDICATIONS

Surgical interferences on the digits.

ANATOMY

In the bovine the digital nerves of fore-limb are derived from the continuation of radial, medial and ulnar nerves. Each of the two digits gets innervation through four digital nerves.

TECHNIQUE

Each of the chief digits is supplied by four digital nerves.

The best site for blocking these nerves is above the fetlock. Five to 10 cc of a 3 to 4% Procaine solution is injected at each of the five points described below. Anaesthesia develops in about ten minutes and lasts for about half to one hour.

Point 1. On the inner aspect of the limb about 2 inches above the fetlock joint and in the groove between the flexor tendon and suspensory ligament. This is to block the terminal branch of the median nerve which supplies the posterior portion of the lateral aspect of the inner digit. (Lateral volar digital nerve of the inner digit.)

Point 2. Similar to (1) on the outer aspect of the limb to block the lateral volar digital nerve of the outer digit which is constituted by the branches of median and ulnar nerves.

Point 3. Similar to (2) on the outer aspect of the limb, but in front of the suspensory ligament in order to block the anterior branch of the ulnar nerve which also supplies the lateral aspect of the outer digit. (Lateral dorsal digital nerve to the outer digit.)

Point 4. About 3 inches above the fetlock on the anterior aspect of the limb, on a line with the interdigital space, in order to block the radial nerve which forms the common dorsal digital nerve of both digits and also forms the lateral dorsal nerve of the inner digit.

Point 5. Similar to (4) on the posterior aspect of the limb but only about ½ inch above fetlock. This is to block the common medial volar digital nerve of both digits. (See also page 267)

CHAPTER 90

Pudic (Internal Pudental) nerve Block in Bull

INDICATIONS

To expose the penis.

SITE

The ischeo-rectal fossa of either side (the depression between the anal orifice and the ischeal tuberosity).

ANATOMY

In the region of the sacro-sciatic foramen, the nerve is situated between the sacro-sciatic ligament and the coccygeus muscle. It can be palpated per rectum as a cord close to the pulsating internal pudic artery.

TECHNIQUE

For blocking the nerve of the right side, the left hand is introduced into the rectum to locate the lesser sciatic notch by the index finger and keeping this finger as a guide, a long needle is introduced through skin at the ischeo-rectal fossa, medial to the sacro-sciatic ligament, till the needle tip reaches the lesser sciatic foramen. The anaesthetic solution is injected. To block the middle haemorrhoidal nerve which may carry some sympathetic fibres to the penis, some anaesthetic solution is also injected a little above and behind this point.

For blocking the internal pudental nerve of the left side, the right hand is introduced per rectum to locate the lesser sciatic notch and the injection is made with the left hand, following the same procedure.

The penis is let down within about half an hour and the effect is maintained for a few hours (up to twelve hours even).

CHAPTER 91

Patellar Desmotomy
(Section of Internal Straight
Ligament of Patella)
In Bovine

ANATOMY

The 3 straight ligaments of patella are: (1) Lateral (outer or external) straight ligament; (2) Median (middle or anterior) straight ligament; (3) Medial (internal or inner) straight ligament. The word *desmos* (Gr.) means ligament.

INDICATIONS

In chronic subluxation (upward fixation; dorsal fixation; recurrent fixation; or upward displacement) of patella, the patella gets fixed above the trochlea of femur and the medial straight ligament is tightly overstretched behind the medial trochlear ridge, which prevents the downward return of the patella. The object of the operation is to mechanically bring down the patella by cutting the tensed medial ligament.

CONTROL

The animal is cast and secured in lateral recumbency on the *same side* of the affected limb. A rope is tied to the affected limb at its pastern and is pulled backwards in the extended position. The other 3 limbs are tied and secured together.

ANAESTHESIA

Local infiltration anaesthesia or epidural anaesthesia.

SITE

A skin incision, 1 to 2 cm., is made close to and parallel to the posterior border of the medial straight ligament

at the site chosen out of the following 3 sites:
Site No. 1: Close to the insertion of the medial ligament to the anterior tuberosity of tibia. This is the *most suitable site* as it is easier to locate, causes lesser bleeding and there is no danger of injuring the joint capsule. *Site No. 2*: At the middle portion of the medial ligament. Since there is a thick padding of fat here between the ligament and the joint capsule which (although protects the joint capsule from any injury during surgery), is likely to protrude through the incision. There is also chance of causing injury to articular vessels in this area. Hence this is a less desirable site than the former. *Site No. 3*: Close to the origin of the medial ligament from the patella. This site is not at all recommended because there is added chance of causing injury to the joint capsule, adjacent vessels and musculature.

TECHNIQUE

Either the open technique or the closed technique may be followed: (1) *Open technique*: A sufficiently long vertical incision, 2 to 3 cm., is made at the site described above, cutting through the skin and subcutaneous facia, and through it the ligament is pulled out with a tenaculum and is cut. Instil about 1 ml. of Tr. Iodine into the wound before it is sutured. (2) *Closed technique (Blind technique)*: A small incision or stab wound is made at the site, through the skin and subcutaneous facia, and a scalpel (or, a probe-pointed tenotomy knife) is introduced flat-wise under the ligament from its posterior aspect until the tip of the scalpel/knife can be palpated anteriorly under the skin in the space between the medial and median patellar ligaments. Afterwards turn the sharp edge of the knife towards the ligament to cut it by a sawing movement. Then the knife is turned back to the flat-wise position and is withdrawn. Protruding fat-tissue, if any, is snipped off and a few drops of Tr. Iodine are instilled into the incision before it is sutured. No suture is necessary if the wound is small. *Note*: Three common mistakes to be avoided during the operation are: 1. Avoid injury to the prominent cutaneous vein; 2. Do not mistake the thick subcutaneous facia for the ligament; and 3. Avoid injury to the joint capsule.

Chapter 92

Amputation of Digit (Claw) in Bovine

Indications

Irreparable injury. Foul-in-the foot of the digit. Gangrenous dermatitis.

Anaesthesia and Control

Blocking plantar nerves; recumbent state.

Anatomy

The three bones of the digit are: (1) os-suffragins or first phalanx, (2) os-corona or second phalanx, and (3) os-pedis or third phalanx. The respective interphalangeal joints are: (1) the suffragino-coronal (first interphalangeal) joint, and (2) the corono-pedal (second interphalangeal) joint.

Site

1. Through the 'corono-pedal joint, leaving the coronary band intact.

2. Through the lower third of the os-suffraginis.

Technique

A tourniquet is applied above the knee to control bleeding.

Technique 1: For amputation through the second interphalangeal joint: The wall of the hoof is pared, leaving only a thin layer of horn. A horizontal incision over the thinned hoof, close to and below the coronary band, cutting through the horny tissue and sensitive laminae, is made; and the interphalangeal joint is reached. Disarticulate through the joint and complete the amputation of the digit.

Technique 2: Amputation through the lower third of the first phalanx, above the first interphalangeal joint: In this method, the skin is incised horizontally above the coronary band and another vertical incision on the lateral aspect of the pastern is made to join it, so as to raise two skin flaps and expose the lower portion of the first phalanx. The first phalanx is cut horizontally with a saw and the amputation is completed.

After amputating the digit by any one of the above 2 methods, the tourniquet is removed and further haemorrhage is controlled by ligaturing the bleeding vessels and by gauze packings. The skin flaps are sutured and a bandage is applied.

The sutures are partially removed, to remove the gauze packings the next day, and afterwards the wound is treated on general principles.

CHAPTER 93

Amputation of Limb in Bovine

INDICATIONS
Irreparable injury. Gangrene. Malignant disease.

ANAESTHESIA AND CONTROL
General anaesthesia; recumbent state.

ANATOMY
The cross-section of the fore and hind limbs at the levels mentioned may be referred.

SITE
(1) *Fore-limb*: Common site is junction of the lower and middle third of the radius (fore-arm).
(2) *Hind limb*: Common site is the middle third of the leg region (tibia).

TECHNIQUE
A tourniquet is applied below the elbow or the stifle, as the case may be. Semi-circular or V-shaped skin incisions are made, on the medial and lateral surfaces at the site chosen, to obtain two flaps of skin which will cover the stump after amputation. The muscles are cut and reflected from below and the bone is sawed off at the desired level. The tourniquet is released, bleeding vessels are ligatured.

The bone stump is then covered by suturing the muscles over it and finally the skin flaps are sutured.

Note: However, if artificial limb is to be fitted after amputation, it is advantageous to preserve maximum possible portion of the limb. (Nayak and Mohanty, 1994).

CHAPTER 94

Amputation of Tail

INDICATIONS
Irreparable injury. Malignant diseases.

ANAESTHESIA AND CONTROL
Epidural; standing or recumbent position.

SITE
Above the seat of injury. Enough length to cover the vulva in cows and anus in bulls is left, if possible.

ANATOMY
Cross-section of the tail reveals the *muscles*: (1) Sacrococcygeus dorsalis, (2) sacrococcygeus lateralis, (3) intertransversales caudae, (4) sacrococcygeus ventralis, and (5) compressor coccygeus; and the *vessels*: middle coccygeal and lateral coccygeal vessels.

TECHNIQUE
"V" shaped skin incisions are made on the dorsal and ventral surfaces of the tail to raise two triangular flaps of skin, the bases of which flaps should correspond to the intervertebral space through which the disarticulation is to be effected. Cut through the intervertebral space. Haemorrhage during the operation is controlled by a tourniquet which is released subsequently and the bleeding points are ligatured or torsioned. The skin flaps are sutured by a series of simple interrupted sutures or mattress sutures.

CHAPTER 95

Maxillary Nerve Block in Canine

INDICATIONS

To desensitise the teeth, gum and alveoli of the upper-jaw.

SITE

1. *Upper site*: The maxillary foramen to be reached by inoculation needle through the site 2 to 4 cm below the external canthus of the eye and between the posterior border of malar and coronoid process of mandible.

2. *Lower site*: The infra-orbital foramen reached through the gum, above the level of the third upper cheek tooth.

ANATOMY

The maxillary nerve which is a branch of the trigeminal nerve (fifth cr.) after its emergence through the foramen rotundum, passes forwards in the pterygo-palatine fossa and enters the maxillary foramen and the infra-orbital canal. It emerges through the infra-orbital foramen and continues thereafter as the infra-orbital nerve.

The maxillary nerve gives the sensory supply to the teeth. The branches supplying the molars are given off before the nerve enters the infra-orbital canal. The other branches supplying the pre-molars, canine and incisor teeth are given off during the course in the infra-orbital canal. Blocking the nerve through the infra-orbital foramen (Site No. 2) desensitises canine and incisors together with their alveoli and gums and also that half of the upper lip.

TECHNIQUE

1. *Upper site*: The skin at the site is punctured and when the tip of the needle is behind the edge of the malar it is directed

forwards and inwards in a horizontal level to reach the maxillary foramen. The needle travels a depth of 2.5 to 4 cm depending on the size of the dog before the tip of the needle reaches the maxillary foramen. Two to 4 cc of a 2 to 3% solution of novacaine is injected.

2. *Lower site*: The rim of the infra-orbital foramen is palpated through the gum at the root level of the third pre-molar tooth (this will be about the midpoint of a line joining the naso-maxillary notch and the inner canthus of the eye). The needle is introduced through the foramen to a depth of 1 cm and 2 to 3 cc of the anaesthetic solution is injected.

Anaesthesia develops in about five to ten minutes and lasts for about twenty to thirty minutes.

CHAPTER 96

Mandibular and Mental Nerve Blocks in Canine

INDICATIONS

Desensitising of the teeth, alveoli and gum of the lower jaw and the lower lip.

SITE

1. Mandibular nerve block: The mandibular foramen on the medial aspect of vertical ramus.
2. Mental nerve block: The mental foramen on the lateral aspect of the horizontal ramus.

ANATOMY

The mandibular branch of the trigeminal (fifth cr.) enters the mandibular foramen on the medial aspect of the vertical ramus of the mandible and emerges through the mental foramen on the lateral aspect of the mandible. During its course sensory branches are given off to the cheek teeth, canines and incisors.

TECHNIQUES

(1) *Mandibular nerve block*: The depression on the ventral border of the mandible (head horizontal position) in front of the angular process of the mandible, is located. The skin at about the middle of this depression is punctured by the needle with its tip directed upwards and along the medial aspect of the mandible for a distance of 1.5 to 2 cm, according to the size of the dog, and 2 to 3 cc of a 2% procaine solution is injected. (2) *Mental-nerve block*: Palpate the mental foramen through the gum, just below the level of the anterior root of the second pre-molar tooth of the lower jaw and on a line corresponding to the direction of the root of the canine tooth. The tip of the needle is introduced

into the foramen and 2 to 3 cc of a 2% procaine solution is injected thrusting the needle about 0.7 cm into the foraman.

Analgesia develops in about five to ten minutes and it persists for twenty to thirty minutes.

CHAPTER 97

Nerve Block for Eye Operations in Canine

INDICATIONS

Desensitising for surgical manipulation. The concerned branches of the facial nerve, the oculomotor nerve, and the naso-ciliary nerve fibres, are to be blocked.

Facial Nerve

SITE

Half inch below the temporo-maxillary articulation, along the posterior border of the vertical ramus.

TECHNIQUE

The lower jaw is moved by one hand keeping the other hand thumb over the articulation. The thumb is moved down to feel the cord-like trunk of the facial nerve as it crosses over the posterior border of the vertical ramus on to the face.

About 5 cc of a 2% to 4% local anaesthetic solution is infiltrated under the skin at the point perineurally.

Note: To facilitate examination of the eye (by preventing closure of eyelids), the auriculopalpebral nerve supplying the orbicularis oculi muscle may be blocked. This nerve is a branch of the facial nerve. The site is along the upper border of the posterior third of the zygomatic arch. About 1 cc of the anaesthetic solution is injected.

Oculo-motor and Naso-ciliary Nerve Fibres

TECHNIQUE

The needle is introduced deep into the orbit through the skin or conjunctiva at the temporal canthus and anaesthetic solution is deposited in the space between the Tenon's capsule and the bony orbit.

The tendon of the superior rectus muscle is held with tissue forceps applied over the conjunctiva (or skin) and the needle is introduced between the eyeball and orbit and the anaesthetic solution is infiltrated.

CHAPTER 98

Canthotomy

1. A temporary canthotomy may be done during surgical operations of the eye when the lids are to be kept wide open, by simply incising the skin at the lateral canthus which is sutured after the operation.

2. Canthotomy for correction of Ectropion consists of removing a V-shaped skin piece in addition, and suturing to correct the deformity.

CHAPTER 99

Extirpation of Harder's (Harderian) Gland in Canine

INDICATIONS

In cases where the gland protrudes due to enlargement and displacement from beneath the free border of the third eyelid making it unsightly.

ANAESTHESIA AND CONTROL

Local application of 4% cocaine or 2% anethaine gives satisfactory results.

ANATOMY

The Harder's gland is situated on the inner surface of the border of the third eyelid. The secretion of the healthy gland has a lubricating action on the cornea. The nictitating membrane (third eyelid) is a semi-cartilaginous structure situated at the inner canthus of the eye. The cartilage is roughly triangular, the exposed portion of which is covered by a fold of conjunctiva. The deep portion of the cartilage is embedded in the fat in the medial aspect of the eyeball.

Blood supply: Branches from ophthalmic and facial arteries.

Nerve supply: Branches of ophthalmic and maxillary divisions of the fifth cranial nerve (sensory supply).

TECHNIQUE

The enlarged gland is held by tissue forceps or by suture thread around its base and it is snipped off. Haemorrhage is not serious except in very rare cases when it will have to be arrested by crushing with a haemostat.

CHAPTER 100

Haematoma Operation of Ear (Surgical Treatment for Haematoma of Ear) in Canine

ANAESTHESIA AND CONTROL

Surface anaesthesia or local infiltration anaesthesia; or, general anaesthesia in the case of difficulty in restraining the subject.

ANATOMY

The blood collection (haematoma) will be between concha and skin layer either on the inner or outer aspect of the ear.

TECHNIQUE

Incise the skin and drain out haematomal contents. To prevent future effusion into the cavity, the space between skin and conchal cartilage is obliterated by sutures and/or bandage. Before incising, the ear opening is plugged with cotton wool. The incision should extend to the full length of the haematoma. The edges of the incision may be trimmed for better drainage. Remove contents and swab the cavity with Tincture iodine.

Method 1: Turn the ear flap over the head and apply a pressure bandage. Or,

Method 2: Apply a series of through-and-through mattress sutures through the concha and skin on its inner and outer aspect; and then put pressure bandage as described. Or,

Method 3: Instead of mattress sutures, put a series of button sutures to compress skin and conchal surfaces more effectively. Bandage then is not essential. Sometimes, mattress sutures tear through tissues; but button sutures generally dont.

CHAPTER 101

Ear-trimming or Ear-cropping in Canine

INDICATIONS

Owners' fancy. (The best age for trimming is two to two-and-a-half months.)

When there is irreparable injury or gangrene.

TECHNIQUE

The ear is trimmed to the desired shape. The skin is sutured over the cartilage by continuous sutures, after the cartilage is trimmed short of the skin edges. The usual standards for ear-trimming are given elsewhere in this book.

Blood supply: Anterior auricular branch of the superficial temporal artery and the posterior auricular branch of the external carotid.

Auricular veins drain chiefly into the superficial temporal and jugular veins.

Nerve supply: *Motor supply*—Chiefly auricular and auriculopalpebral branches of the facial nerve.

Sensory supply: Superficial temporal branch of the mandibular nerve and auricular branch of vagus.

CHAPTER 102

Zepp's Operation for Chronic Otorrhoea in Canine

INDICATIONS
To facilitate good drainage through the external ear canal.

ANAESTHESIA AND CONTROL
General anaesthesia; lateral recumbent state.

ANATOMY
The external ear canal is not a straight tube. It has a horizontal portion and a vertical portion formed by the tubular portion of concha. The object of this operation is to out open the vertical portion to facilitate drainage.

Blood and nerve supply to the external ear: Anterior auricular branch of the superficial temporal, posterior auricular branch of external carotid, and anterior branch of occipital artery. Veins go chiefly to superficial temporal and jugular veins. Sensory nerve supply derived from superficial temporal branch of mandibular nerve and auricular branch of vagus.

SITE
The tubular portion of the antero-external aspect of the concha and the skin below it.

TECHNIQUE
Two long curved clamps or forceps (like Rochester-Carmalt forceps) are applied to control haemorrhage. Each of these forceps holds the conchal portion within its jaws and are applied at an angle to each other, making out a V-shaped area of the concha, the apex of the "V" being towards the external auditory meatus. The part thus isolated is cut close to the jaws of the forceps, the two incisions not being allowed to meet. These two

incisions are later extended a little downwards independently and diverging from each other cutting through the skin only and at the terminal part a third incision is made to connect them. The triangular skin flap thus isolated is reflected upwards and over the conchal cartilage. The triangular cut piece of conchal cartilage is then pulled downwards and is fixed to the sides of the skin incision after trimming the excess length of the cartilage, so that the ear canal now drains directly downwards through this open channel.

Before removing the forceps, continuous sutures are loosely passed through the skin and cartilage including the jaws of the forceps and as the forceps is drawn out the sutures are tightened over the incision.

Note: It is also possible to do this operation without prior clamping of concha with the forceps.

CHAPTER 103

Ventriculo-cordectomy (De-barking) in Canine

INDICATIONS

Partial muting or silencing in very noisy dogs between four to six months of age.

ANAESTHESIA AND CONTROL

General anaesthesia; ventral recumbent position; head extended and mouth kept open with an oral speculum.

ANATOMY

The vocal cords are two in number. Each of them is a membrane or ligament connecting the process vocalis of the arytenoid cartilage and the junction of the wing and body of the thyroid cartilage. At its point of insertion to the body of the thyroid cartilage it is in contact with the cricothyroid ligament and is close to its fellow of the opposite side.

TECHNIQUE

The mouth is held fully open with the speculum. The tongue is drawn outwards holding the tip over a layer of gauze. The epiglottis is held by a long-handled tissue forceps and light from outside is directed into the oropharynx to illuminate the larynx. The vocal cords on each side are held by forceps and are snipped off by scissors. The operation is much simplified if a laryngoscope and long-handled biopsy forceps are available. The Gruenwald's nasal punch forceps is best suited.

REFERENCES

1. Ormrod, Noel A. (1966). *Surgery of the Dog and Cat*. Baillers, Tindall and Casell.

2. *Canine Surgery* by 38 authors.

Note: A similar operation called *De-bleating* is done in sheep after performing laryngotomy. For details see Frank (1959) pp. 159-60.

CHAPTER 104

Tonsillectomy in Canine

INDICATIONS

In chronic inflammatory conditions of the tonsils, which do not respond to other methods of treatment. The operation is not recommended in the acute stage.

ANAESTHESIA AND CONTROL

Intravenous anaesthesia with pre-anaesthetic sedation. The mouth is kept open with a mouth gag. If the general condition of the animal is not good for intravenous anaesthesia, local infiltration anaesthesia may be adopted. But if the animal is uncontrollable, inhalation anaesthesia, through a tracheotomy tube may be tried.

ANATOMY

The tonsils are situated in the pharynx, one on each side. Each tonsil is located in the space between the two folds of mucous membrane of the soft palate, called the anterior and posterior pillars or arches. The tonsil in the dog has a thick capsular covering and is situated deeply. It is not easily visible during examination of the throat.

Blood supply: Branches from external and internal maxillary and external carotid arteries, with satellite veins.

TECHNIQUE

For the success of the operation, the tonsillar tissue should be removed completely. On account of the thick capsular attachment, the wire-loop method adopted in human surgery is not very satisfactory in the dog.

The anterior pillar of the soft palate is held with a long tissue-forceps or artery forceps, to facilitate better view of the tonsil. The tonsil is held with an Allis tissue forceps and carefully dissected with scissors. The bleeding is controlled by swabbing with 1 in 1000 Adrenaline. If any larger bleeding vessel could be located, it is clamped and ligatured with fine catgut. Bleeding can be further controlled by keeping a gauze piece soaked in Adrenaline pressed over the area for sometime. The position of the animal should be adjusted to avoid aspiration of blood into the trachea.

CHAPTER 105

Extraction of Teeth (Exodontia) in Canine

Extraction of Temporary Incisors and Canines

INDICATIONS
Persistent milk teeth even after the permanent ones are cut. Damaged or diseased teeth.

ANAESTHESIA AND CONTROL
In cases where there is difficulty in controlling the patient, short-acting general anaesthetics like pentothal sodium may be required. Otherwise no anaesthesia is necessary.

TECHNIQUE
The tooth is held by its neck by means of suitable dental forceps, and it is pulled out by swift and slight rotary traction without undue violence.

Extraction of Permanent Incisors

INDICATIONS
Fractured tooth. Infected alveoli. Tumours (Myeloma; Epulis).

ANAESTHESIA AND CONTROL
Maxillary/mandibular nerve block combined with local infiltration or short duration general anaesthesia. The mouth is kept open by means of tape or by oral speculum.

ANATOMY
All the incisors have single roots; their labial surfaces are convex.

Blood supply: The incisor branch of the mandibular alveolar artery supplies the lower incisors and canines; Infra-orbital artery supplies branches to the upper incisors. Both these are subsidiary branches of internal maxillary. Drained by corresponding veins. *Nerve supply*: The sensory nerves to the teeth are derived fɪ ɔm the maxillary and mandibular divisions of the fifth cranial nerve. The branches supplying the upper incisors and canine are given off immediately before the exit of the maxillary nerve from the infra-orbital foramen. Similarly, the mandibular nerve immediately before its emergence from the mental foramen supplies the branch to lower incisors and canine teeth.

TECHNIQUE
    Forcible extraction by suitable dental forceps can be tried if the whole tooth can thus be removed without breaking. Otherwise the external alveolar plate is cut through the gum, to expose the root and the tooth is levered out by a "Tooth Elevator" (Tooth Gouge).

Extraction of Permanent Canine Tooth

TECHNIQUE
    1. The gum is cut along the outline of the alveolus of the tooth and the alveolar plate is cut along the same line using chisel and mallet to expose the root to its depth. The tooth is then levered out by means of a tooth gouge.
    2. Same as method (1), but the gum covering the alveolus is incised and reflected to a side before-hand which is later sutured in position after extraction of the tooth. This method of preserving the gum, however, has no major advantage.

Extraction of Cheek Tooth

INDICATIONS
    Alveolar periostitis. Caries. Pus in the antrum with or without dental fistula.

ANAESTHESIA AND CONTROL
    Short duration general anaesthesia; lateral recumbent position; mouth kept open with oral speculum.

ANATOMY

The number of roots for each cheek tooth are as follows:

Single rooted: Upper first; Lower first and seventh teeth;

Three rooted: Upper fourth, fifth and sixth (each of these teeth has two large roots on its buccal aspect and one small posterior root on the lingual aspect).

Two rooted: All other teeth. (The roots are anterior and posterior, of which the posterior one is longer.)

Blood supply: Alveolar branches of the internal maxillary artery.

Nerve supply: *Upper row*—Branches from the maxillary branch of fifth cranial given off along its course in the infra-orbital canal.

Lower row: Branches from the mandibular branch of fifth cranial before its exit through the mental foramen.

TECHNIQUE

For the extraction of a tooth having two roots, using dental forceps, traction with an inward and outward rocking motion (instead of a to-and-fro rotary motion in the case of single-rooted ones), is applied.

Removal of the external alveolar plate is usually necessary to remove a large cheek tooth especially the fourth upper cheek tooth. The gum over the external alveolar plate is incised and reflected. The external alveolar plate is removed by using chisel till the lateral aspect of roots are fully exposed. The cement substance between the roots is scooped out using the angle or corner of the chisel. The whole root is removed with the tooth. In odd cases the tooth breaks and then the fragments are removed separately.

CHAPTER 106

Oesophagotomy in Canine

INDICATIONS

Oesophageal obstruction. The common points of obstruction in the dog are: (1) at the entrance of oesophagus into the thorax, (2) above the heart, and (3) close to the diaphragm at the entrance of oesophagus into stomach.

ANAESTHESIA AND CONTROL

General anaesthesia; dorsal recumbent state in the case of cervical oesophagotomy and lateral recumbency for thoracic approach.

SITES

The site is chosen according to the level of obstruction.

(a) *Cervical (pre-sternal) site*: Mid-ventral line of neck in front of sternum.

(b) Thoracic approach, when the obstruction is in the thoracic portion of oesophagus.

(c) Obstructions close to the gastric end are relieved better through gastrotomy, than by oesophagotomy.

TECHNIQUE

(a) For cervical approach the procedure is on similar lines as in the bovine except that the approach is through mid-ventral line of neck. The sternocephalicus and sternothyrohyoideus muscles of either side are separated along midline to expose the trachea and oesophagus. (b) For thoracic approach see under thoracotomy.

CHAPTER 107

Thyroidectomy in Canine

INDICATIONS

Goiter. Hyper thyroidism. Malignancy of the gland.

ANAESTHESIA AND CONTROL

General anaesthesia; dorsal recumbency with the head well-extended.

ANATOMY

The thyroid in the dog chiefly consists of the two lobes connected by an isthmus which is variable in its development. Each of these lobes are situated lateral to the trachea extending between the first and seventh tracheal rings. Laterally the lobe is in close proximity to the recurrent laryngeal nerve, carotid artery and the vagus. The parathyroids are chiefly two in number, one placed at the anterior pole and the other ventro-medially at about the centre of the lobe, and are very small greyish pink bodies on each lobe.

Blood supply: Derived from the carotid artery. Usually there are two branches entering the lobe, one through the posterior extremity along the dorsal aspect of the gland and other through the anterior extremity.

Nerve supply: Derived from the sympathetic system.

SITE

Mid-ventral line of neck, beginning from the thyroid cartilage backwards to a distance of about 1 inch.

TECHNIQUE

After making the skin incision at the site described, and cutting through the sub-cutis, the sterno-hyoideus muscle of either side is separated along the midline and is held retracted to expose the trachea. The two lobes of the thyroid gland are then traced on the dorse-lateral aspect of trachea. Grasp the lobe to be removed by means of tissue forceps and isolate it from surrounding structures by blunt dissection, without causing injury to the recurrent laryngeal nerve. The anterior and posterior thyroid arteries entering the two poles of the gland are identified. The vessels are ligatured and thyroid lobe of that side is removed. The sternohyoideus muscles are replaced into position to eliminate the formation of pockets and the skin is sutured. If the lobes of both sides are removed, see that the parathyroids are retained.

CHAPTER 108

Paracentesis Thoracis in Canine

INDICATIONS

For tapping the pleuritic fluid in moist pleurisy accompanied by respiratory distress. For collection of the fluid samples for diagnostic purpose. As a route for administration of therapeutic agents.

ANAESTHESIA AND CONTROL

Local infiltration anaesthesia; standing position.

ANATOMY

The intercostal artery is situated along the posterior border of the rib (in the vascular groove). To prevent injury to this, the needle is directed close to the anterior border.

The thorax is divided into two compartments by the mediastinum. But the anterior mediastinal fold is very flimsy in the dog and hence pneumo-thorax of one side causes collapse of lungs on both sides.

SITE

The seventh intercostal space on the left side and the sixth intercostal space on the right side, above the level of the point of the elbow of the respective side in the standing position. The needle is introduced close to the anterior border of the rib concerned.

TECHNIQUE

A small trocar and canula or a hypodermic needle is used. In order to prevent pneumothorax, a rubber tube, the free end of which is kept dipped in water, is attached to the needle; or the needle is attached to a syringe.

CHAPTER 109

Thoracotomy in Canine

INDICATIONS

Surgery of the thoracic portion of the oesophagus. Exploration of the thoracic viscera. Thoracic approach for repair of diaphragmatic hernia. Surgery of the lungs and heart.

ANAESTHESIA AND CONTROL

General anaesthesia; lateral recumbent state with the fore and hind limbs extended.

SITE

Usually the sixth or seventh intercostal space. The side chosen and the actual site depends on the purpose for which thoracotomy is performed.

ANATOMY

The origin of the obliqus abdominis externus muscle is in close association with intercostal muscles, covering the lower half of the ribs from the fifth rib backwards. The latissimus dorsi muscle covers almost the upper half of the ribs. The posterior deep pectoral muscle covers the lower portions of the ribs, from the fifth rib forward.

TECHNIQUE

A cuffed oral endo-tracheal tube (Magill's) is introduced into the trachea up to the middle cervical level. (The tongue is drawn outwards by holding the tip of the tongue by a piece of gauze, the epiglottis is depressed by a long forceps and the tube is introduced into the larynx and trachea.) The free end of the tube is fixed by a tape to the upper jaw.

The cuff of the tube now in the trachea, is inflated with air by a syringe and the inflating side tube is clamped. Connect the tube to a respiration pump or other device for positive pressure ventilation of the lungs.

The skin over the intercostal space is incised parallel to the ribs. The serrated border of the muscle latissimus dorsi is first incised. A short incision is made through the middle of the intercostal muscles and parietal pleura, when the lung is in a deflated state. The incision is extended over finger introduced through it to protect the lungs. The rate and stroke volume of air inflated is adjusted according to the need. The ribs are retracted by self-retaining thoracic retractors and that side lung can be packed off with towels for mediastinal surgery.

The thoracotomy wound is closed by interrupted sutures passed around the adjacent ribs. The last suture is tied with the lung inflated to its full capacity so that negative pressure would be restored as the lung deflates.

Another method of establishing negative pressure is by closing the intercostal incision with a thin long rubber tube in the wound, the free end of which is kept below a water seal in a trough kept at a lower level, so that when the lung is inflated the air retained in the chest cavity is expelled through the tube whereas sucking air back is prevented by the water seal. The tube can then be removed.

The next layer of muscle is also brought into apposition by sutures and the skin incision is also closed.

Note: Thoracoplasy involves resection of a rib or ribs. Greater retraction of thoracotomy incision can be brought about by dividing the adjacent ribs. The rib in front may be divided close to the lower commissure and the rib behind it close to the upper commissure of the incision.

Paracentesis Abdominis in Canine

Similar to the bovine except that a proportionately small trocar and canula should be used. In most cases a hypodermic needle will suffice.

Laparotomy (Coeliotomy) in Canine

INDICATIONS

Laparotomy or opening of the abdomen may be undertaken for any of the following purposes:

1. Gastrotomy
2. Enterotomy and Enterectomy
3. Cystotomy
4. Hysterotomy (Caesarian section)
5. Hysterectomy
6. Ovariotomy (Spaying)
7. Splenectomy
8. Ventropexy
9. For diagnostic purpose (Exploratory laparotomy)

ANAESTHESIA AND CONTROL

General anaesthesia; Control in lateral or dorsal recumbency, depending on the site chosen.

ANATOMY

The abdominal cavity is limited anteriorly by the diaphragm and posteriorly by the pelvic inlet. The lateral wall is formed by the three abdominal muscles, viz., (i) *the obliqus abdominis externus* whose fibres are directed downwards and backwards. It originates from the fifth to the last rib and is inserted on to the pubic tubercle and external angle of ilium. The ventral aponeurotic portion joins the linea alba, (ii) *the obliqus abdominis internus* whose fibres are directed in the opposite direction get attached to the lumbodorsal facia, the inguinal ligament (Poupart's ligament) and the last two ribs. Ventrally the muscle is continued as an aponeurosis getting inserted on to the linea alba, (iii) *the transverse abdominis muscle* fibres run at right angles to the long axis originating from the lumbar transverse processes and from the medial surface of the last four or five ribs and their cartilages. The ventral aponeurotic portion blends with the deep part of the internal oblique and joins the linea alba. The aponeurotic portion of these last two muscles go to the formation of the deep sheath of rectus abdominis muscle.

The ventral abdominal wall is formed by the aponeurotic portions of the oblique and transverse muscles, the rectus abdominis muscle, and the linea alba. The linea alba is formed by the blending of these muscular aponeuroses in the midventral line. The rectus abdominis muscle lies parallel to the midline of the abdomen, getting inserted on the anterior part of the pubic symphysis.

Blood supply: The blood supply to the flank is contributed by the lumbar vessels. Lower portions of the abdominal wall is supplied by the cranial and caudal epigastric vessels and branches of external pudic artery.

Nerve supply: Branches from the thirteenth thoracic, first, second and third lumbar spinal nerves.

SITE

1. *Flank site*: Vertical or oblique incision on the hollow of the flank.

2. *Mid-line site*: Incision through the linea alba between the xiphoid cartilage of sternum and pubic symphysis.

3. *Para-median site*: Parallel to the linea alba along the belly of rectus abdominis muscle.

4. *Para-rectal site*: Parallel to the rectus abdominis muscles close to its lateral border.

5. *Para-costal site*: Parallel to the costo-chondral arch.

TECHNIQUE

1. *Flank site*: The skin is incised to the required length and avoiding division of lumbar spinal nerves the incision is extended through the external and internal oblique abdominal muscles and the transverse abdominal muscle. The parietal peritoneum is picked up by tissue forceps and is first snipped open by scissors and this opening is then extended by scissors

over finger or grooved director introduced into it to protect the viscera.

2.   *Mid-line site:* The skin over the white line is incised to the length required. The sides of the white line are held by tissue forceps and lifted so that a small opening is made by cutting with scalpel between the forceps, through the white line and the adherent parietal peritoneum. A finger is introduced into the opening and the incision is extended to the required length by scissors over the protecting finger.

3.   *Para-median site:* The incision here is made parallel to the linea alba, through the skin, outer and inner coverings and belly of the rectus abdominis muscle and the parietal peritoneum. During the dissection through abdominal muscles (in the paramedian site), it is better to separate the muscles along the direction of their fibres, rather than cutting/incising across.

4.   *Para-rectal site:* In this case the skin and oblique abdominal muscles and aponeurotic sheath and the parietal peritoneum are to be incised, the incisions being parallel to the rectus muscle.

5.   *Para-costal site:* The incision is through the skin, oblique and transverse abdominal muscles, and the parietal peritoneum, parallel to the costochondral arch.

For closing the incision in all these cases the parietal peritoneal layer is closed by continuous sutures and muscles separately, except in case of the mid-line incision at which site the peritoneum is adherent to the abdominal aponeurosis.

The skin wound is closed by interrupted sutures, preferably by vertical mattress sutures.

Note: The length of incision necessary for major abdominal surgery is variable. A little longer incision is better than a shorter incision.

CHAPTER 112

Gastrotomy in Canine

INDICATIONS

Removal of foreign bodies from the stomach or from the gastric end of the oesophagus.

ANAESTHESIA AND CONTROL

See under laparotomy.

ANATOMY

The left fundic portion of the stomach lies under the vertebral ends of eleventh and twelfth ribs. The pyloric portion is situated towards the right of the median plane and lies almost ventral to the ninth intercostal space, between the Xiphoid cartilage and costal arch of right side, in contact ventrally with the right central lobe of liver.

BLOOD SUPPLY

Branches of the coeliac artery. Veins drain into the portal vein

NERVE SUPPLY

Vago-sympathetic.

SITE

1. Mid-line incision between the Xiphoid cartilage and the umbilicus.

2. Para-costal incision on the *left* side in large and deep-chested animals.

TECHNIQUE

Perform laparotomy. The stomach is exterioised through the laparotomy wound and is packed off with surgical towels.

The foreign body in the stomach wall is isolated in a pouch (the pouch may be clamped below with bowel clamps). An incision depending on the size of the foreign body is made along the length of the pouch or across it avoiding division of gastric vessels to the extent possible. The foreign body is extracted and the mucous membrane that pouts through the incision is trimmed level with the edges of the incision. The incision is closed by a set of Connel's sutures followed by continuous Lembert's suture over it (or by Cushing's suture).

The surface of the stomach is cleaned with sterile saline solution and it is returned to position after removing the packing towels. The laparotomy wound is closed as usual.

CHAPTER 113

Enterotomy in Canine

INDICATIONS
Intestinal obstructions.   Foreign bodies.

ANAESTHESIA AND CONTROL
General anaesthesia; lateral or dorsal recumbent state.

ANATOMY
The intestine is suspended by mesentery which is a double fold of peritoneum encasing the bowel. The mesentery attached to it along one border only, conveys the blood vessels supplying the intestine which are segmentwar or circumferential in distribution. The intestinal wall has a serous layer on the outside and a mucous lining facing the lumen with an intervening muscular coat.

Blood supply: Branches from coeliac and anterior mesenteric arteries. Veins go to the portal vein.

Nerve supply: Vagus and sympathetic fibres from the coeliac plexus.

SITE
1. Mid-ventral site.
2. Flank site.

TECHNIQUE
Perform laparotomy at the site chosen. The laparotomy wound is retracted and the intestinal coils are examined to locate the foreign body by drawing the coils between thumb and fingers. The affected segment of intestine is exteriorised and isolated by packing with surgical towels and is clamped before and behind with bowel clamps. The free (antimesenteric) border is incised to the required length to exract the foreign body. The opening

is closed by Cushing's sutures, or by continuous Lambert's sutures. Size 3/0, medium chromic, catgut with atraumatic needles is suitable for intestinal suture. The towels are removed after cleaning the bowel surface with saline solution. The laparotomy wound is closed after returning the bowel into the abdomen.

CHAPTER 114

Enterectomy and Enteroanastomois in Canine

INDICATIONS

(1) Gangrene. (2) Intussusception with obstruction and adhesion.

TECHNIQUE

Perform laparotomy. The segment affected is clamped at two points, before and behind. The mesenteric vessels supplying the isolated segment are ligatured. The triangular piece of mesentery distal to the ligatures is torn towards the attached border of the segment and the bowel is divided close to the clamps and removed. The divided clamped ends are mopped clean and the stumps are closed by temporary continuous inversion sutures applied over the jaws of either clamp separately. The free ends of each thread are held and pulled as the forceps is withdrawn thereby closing each cut end of the intestine with this temporary suture.

The closed ends are brought together and are united by Lembert's or Cushing's sutures all around. The temporary sutures are then drawn out and removed to establish patency of the ends after re-union. Patency is confirmed by feeling with the tips of fingers. The mesenteric tear is repaired. No part of the bowel wall should be left without blood supply.

To complete the operation return the bowel into the abdomen and close the laparotomy around.

CHAPTER 115

Caecectomy in Canine
(Typhlectomy)

INDICATIONS

Heavy infestation with whip worms (Trichuris vulpis).

ANAESTHESIA AND CONTROL

General anaesthesia; dorsal recumbent state.

ANATOMY

The caecum is situated in level with the umbilical region mid-way between the right flank and the median plane, ventral to the duodenum. It is a short spiral or bent tube, its blind end lateral to the ileo-colic orifice. It is closely attached to the ileum by means of the meso-caecum.

Blood supply: Branches from the ileo-caeco-colic artery which is one of the branches of the cranial mesenteric artery.

SITE

Mid-ventral abdominal incision in level with the umbilicus.

TECHNIQUE

Perform laparotomy at the site. The caecum is exposed with the adjacent portion of ileum and colon. Then the branches of the ileo-caeco-colic artery supplying the caecum are ligatured as it enters the caecum on each side. The meso-caecum (ileo-caecal ligament) is severed and the caecum is lifted up to its base. The base of the caecum is clamped with two clamps placed a little apart from each other. It is cut and removed along with the distal forceps. The stump is inverted by Cushing's suture.

CHAPTER 116

Spleenectomy in Canine

INDICATIONS

Neoplastic abnormalities. Treatment of choice in rupture of spleen.

ANAESTHESIA AND CONTROL

General anaesthesia; right lateral or dorsal recumbent position, according to the site chosen.

ANATOMY

The spleen extends from the left lumbo-costal angle along the greater curvature of the stomach.

The splenic artery is the largest branch of the coeliac artery and the splenic vein lying behind in the hilus drains into the portal vein.

SITE

1. Midline incision between Xiphoid and umbilicus.
2. Left para-costal site.

TECHNIQUE

The spleen is brought out of the laparotomy incision and it is wrapped in moist saline gauze to prevent drying and shock.

(The volume of spleen can be reduced if so desired, by injection of adrenalin 1 to 2 cc into the splenic *artery*.)

The splenic artery is tied off first and is followed by ligaturing of the splenic vein.

The gastro-splenic omentum is then divided after ligaturing stage by stage the many vessels that pass through all along its length.

The abdominal wound is closed as usual.

CHAPTER 117

Perineal Herniorrhaphy (Reconstruction of the Pelvic Diaphragm) in Canine

INDICATIONS
Perineal hernia.

ANAESTHESIA AND CONTROL
General anaesthesia; ventral recumbency with the hind parts elevated and the body inclined downwards at an angle of about 45°, being kept in this position by means of pillows or other supports.

ANATOMY
The pelvic diaphragm is formed by the Levatores ani muscles and the coccygeus groups of muscles situated between the lateral wall of the pelvis and rectum. It is firmly supported by the perineal facia which is closely adherent to its posterior aspect. The perineal facia is continuous with the facia of the leg and gluteal region. It supports the pelvic diaphragm and continues as a lining to the lateral pelvic wall and blends itself with the sacrosciatic ligaments. The medial and lateral coccygeal muscles of each side originate from the shaft of ilium, the pubis and pelvic symphysis and pass upward and backward in a fan-like fashion to become attached to the first few coccygeal vertebrae and the sphincter ani externus. In *perineal hernia* a separation is created between the medial (posterior) border of medial coccygeus muscle and the sphincter muscle and "hernial ring is formed. The blood and nerve supplies to the anus are derived from the internal pudic vessels and the pudic nerve of the respective sides. These vessels have anastomotic branches between them.

The other important muscles are: *medial coccygeal m.*, (also called *middle coccygeal m.*, or *levator ani m.*, or *retractor ani m.*); and *lateral coccygeal m.* (*lateral coccygeus m.*). (See also Addm. p. 660).

SITE

Lateral to the anus.

TECHNIQUE

The anus is closed by a pure-string suture for the duration of the operation, to prevent contamination of the site.

A slightly curved skin incision is made over the hernial swelling between the base of the tail and ischeal tuberosity. The skin edges are retracted medially and laterally so as to allow maximum exposure of the field of operation. The hernial sac constituted by the perineal facia is incised with the skin incision.

A band-like structure seen between the pelvic wall and the rectum, containing the branches of interanal pudic vessels and pudic nerve supplying the anus, may be either pushed aside or cut between ligatures to facilitate manipulation and reduction of hernial contents.

The protruding retro-peritoneal fat may be removed. The hernial passage (hernial ring) is seen in the space outlined by the rectum medially, the ano-coccygeal muscles laterally and the obturator internus muscle ventrally, after pushing back the hernial contents. *Suturing the hernial ring*: The posterior border of the median coccygeus muscle is sutured to the sphincter ani internus muscle to the extent the former muscle lends itself for reapproachment. Thereafter the medial surface of the sacrosciatic ligament and the obturator internus muscle on the pelvic floor are made use of to anchor the sutures and to unite them to the border of the sphincter muscle and thereby to close the hernial ring completely. *Suturing the perineal facia*: The perineal facia is mobilised by careful dissection from the pelvic side of the gluteal muscles and is sutured on to the outer portion of the anal sphincter so as to form a covering and support over the sutures already placed. If the facia is in excess, the free edge may be trimmed before suturing. *Suturing the skin*: Finally the skin wound is sutured after trimming the edges suitably.

On completion of the operation the purse string suture of the anus is removed.

CHAPTER 118

Ablation of Para-anal Sacs in Canine

INDICATIONS
Infection with abscess formation.

ANAESTHESIA AND CONTROL
Local infiltration; or epidural anaesthesia; or general anaesthesia; ventral recumbency with hind parts raised.

ANATOMY
The anal sacs are two in number situated one on either side of the anal opening. Each anal sac is situated between the external sphincter muscle and the rectal wall.

SITE
Linear incision 1 inch long, lateral to the anal orifice.

TECHNIQUE
The anal sac is filled before hand with a paste of *plaster of paris,* paraffin wax, Indian ink or distilled water to make the outline of the anal sac defined. A skin incision is placed lateral to the anal orifice close to the anal sac. The anal sac is manipulated outwards through the incision by separating the fibres of the sphinter muscle and it is dissected out carefully without rupturing, and is extirpated.

The skin wound is sutured with interrupted apposition sutures.

Note: Instead of injecting *plaster of paris*, a probe passed into the anal sac may be sufficient to identify its outline during dissection.

CHAPTER 119

Epidural Anaesthesia in Canine

INDICATIONS

Regional anaesthesia of the pelvis and hind parts of the body for surgical purposes.

CONTROL

Lateral recumbent state, in a state of pronounced flexion of the vertebral column.

ANATOMY

The spinal cord in the dog ends at the junction of the sixth and seventh lumbar vertebrae. Therefore, beyond this level solutions can be injected epidurally without risk of entering the subarachnoid space.

SITE

Through the intervertebral space between the last lumbar vertebra and sacrum, or the sixth and seventh lumbar vertebrae. The lumbo-sacral site is preferred, being wider.

TECHNIQUE

An imaginary line connecting the iliac crests will pass over the supra-spinous process of the last (or seventh) lumbar vertebra. The tip of the needle with styllette is introduced through the midline immediately behind this line in a direction slightly forward. As the interarcual ligament is punctured a sensation of yielding in resistance is felt when the needle is at a depth of about 2 to $2\frac{1}{2}$ cm from the skin surface. The styllette is withdrawn and the anaesthetic solution is injected.

CHAPTER 120

Puncture of Bladder in Canine

INDICATIONS

In emergent cases of urine retention as a temporary measure of relief.

ANAESTHESIA AND CONTROL

Local or surface anaesthesia; standing or lateral recumbent position.

ANATOMY

The empty bladder is a pelvic organ but when distended the fundus is abdominal in position. Part of it is lined outside by the parietal layer of peritoneum.

SITE

In front of the pubic symphysis. (Supra-pubic or pre-pubic or ante-pubic site.)

TECHNIQUE

A fine trocar and canula or an epidural needle with stylletts is used to puncture the distended bladder. The canula is pressed against the abdominal wall and the trocar is removed to permit the escape of urine. After removing urine, the trocar is re-introduced, and the two together are withdrawn.

CHAPTER 121

Vasectomy in Dog

INDICATIONS
Prevention of procreation.

ANAESTHESIA AND CONTROL
Local infiltration; dorsal recumbent position with the hind limbs stretched fully backward with the stifle pressed outwards.

ANATOMY
See under castration described on page 556.

SITE
Groin region, close to the external inguinal ring where the spermatic cord is palpated by manipulating from the testes.

TECHNIQUE
A ½ to 1 inch long incision is made cutting through the skin and sub-cutis to expose the spermatic sheath (Tunica vaginalis) and contents. The spermatic sheath is incised. The vas deferens is seen along the posterior aspect of the spermatic cord as a distinct tube, whitish or pink in colour. It is isolated along its length to permit ligation at two points and division between. The spermatic sheath and the skin are sutured.

Castration (Orchiectomy) in Dog

Open Method

INDICATIONS

1. Prevention of breeding nuisance.
2. Neoplastic growths or crushing injuries affecting the testicle.
3. In enlarged prostate.
4. Perineal hernia.
5. To make the animal more docile (and domesticated).

ANAESTHESIA AND CONTROL

Local infiltration; spermatic block or epidural anaesthesia; dorsal recumbent state.

ANATOMY

The epididymis is attached to the dorso-lateral aspect of the testis, the head of the epididymis pointing anteriorly. The testes, epididymis and spermatic cord are enclosed by the serous sac, the tunica vaginalis. The spermatic cord consists of the anterior vascular bundle and a posterior bundle consisting chiefly of the vas deferens.

Blood supply: Spermatic vessels supply the testes and branches of the external pudic vessels supply the scrotum.

Nerve supply: Spermatic nerves derived from the renal and mesenteric plexus supply the testes and branches of the second and third lumbar spinal nerves supply the scrotum.

SITES

1. Pre-scrotal site: Mid-line in front of the scrotum.
2. Longitudinal incision on the ventral aspect of the scrotum,

lateral and parallel to the median raphe on either side.

3. Longitudinal incision parallel to the median raphe on one side to remove that testicle and a second incision (through the first one) on the mediastinum testes to remove the other testicle.

TECHNIQUES

1. (Pre-scrotal site)—One testis is pushed forward to bring it under the skin over the ventral aspect of sheath. An incision is placed over it in the mid-line and the testis is squeezed out by mild presssure between thumb and finger. The cord is severed after ligation and the testis is removed. The other testis is removed similarly through the same opening. The skin wound is closed preferably by subcuticular sutures.

2. Each testis is tensed against the skin of the scrotum between the thumb and index finger and an incision is made anteroposteriorly parallel to the median raphe, cutting through the skin, dartos and tunica vaginalis. The testicle slips out through the wound. The spermatic cord is then separated into the anterior vascular bundle, and the posterior bundle containing the vas deferens. The posterior bundle (vas deferens) is divided by scissors. The vascular bundle is ligatured and then divided to remove the testes. The skin wound is left open. (The vascular bundle can be severed by torsion in young animals without ligaturing. The cord is fixed above by artery forceps and another forceps is applied half-an-inch below after milking the cord downwards for slow torsion till it is severed.)

3. After removal of one testis as in technique 2, the other testicle is extracted through the same opening by making an incision through the median septum of the scrotum.

Covered Method

The difference in procedure here as compared to the open method is that the testes are removed along with the tunica vaginalis. The spermatic cord is severed after ligaturing it over the tunica vaginalis. See also page 341

CHAPTER 123

Urethrotomy in Dog

INDICATIONS
Urethral obstruction.

ANAESTHESIA AND CONTROL
Epidural or local infiltration; dorsal recumbent position.

ANATOMY
The urethra at the ischeal arch is covered by the well-developed corpus cavernosum urethrae which is covered by the bulbocavernosus muscle. The urethra is encircled throughout by the corpus cavernosum urethrae (corpus spongiosum). In the region of the os-penis urethra is placed in a groove on the ventral aspect of the os-penis.

SITE
At the seat of obstruction. (The commonest seat of obstruction is behind the os-penis.)

TECHNIQUE
A sound or catheter is passed through the urethral opening to the level of obstruction to facilitate location of correct site. The glans penis is fully exposed and held in position and an incision is made along the mid-ventral line of the penis to enter the urethra on its ventral surface at the level of obstruction. The calculi are picked up and removed. A catheter is passed into the bladder through the normal opening to ensure patency of passage. The glans penis is then restored to its normal position in the sheath. The catheter is retained for a few days. There might be some leakage of urine through the incision for some days, but it ultimately closes up.

CHAPTER 124

Amputation of Penis in Dog

INDICATIONS
1. Neoplastic growths.
2. Fracture of os-penis.
3. Gangrene or crushing injuries.
4. Paralysis.

ANAESTHESIA AND CONTROL
Epdiural anaesthesia or general anaesthesia. Dorsal recumbent state with hind limbs secured wide apart.

ANATOMY
The glans penis of the dog contains the os-penis which is nearly four inches long. Os-penis is regarded as an ossified portion of corpus cavernosum penis.

Blood supply to the penis: The dorsal arteries of either side of the penis are branches of the external pudic artery. They lie lateral to the veins of the same name. The obturator artery forms the arteria profunda penis (deep artery of the penis) which ramifies in the corpus cavernosum penis. The internal pudic artery terminates at the base of the penis, and is called the artery of the bulb of the penis, and breaks up into number of branches.

Nerve supply: Branches of the pudental nerves lying lateral to the dorsal vessel and sympathetic fibres form the pelvic plexus.

SITE
Proximal to the seat of lesion. In paralysis, nearest to the root of the penis.

TECHNIQUES
A probe is passed into the urethra to identify it during dissection. An elliptical incision is made enclosing the sheath begin-

ning from the preputial orifice to a point just posterior to the level of amputation. The penis and sheath are lifted by dissection. Bleeding points from the divided branches of the external pudental vessels are ligatured. The urethra as defined by the probe is felt on the ventral aspect of the body of the penis. The penis at the site is incised longitudinally on either side of urethra for a distance of ½ inch to isolate the urethra for a length of about ½ inch. A ligature is passed through and tied around the penis at the place, excluding the isolated urethra. At a point distal to the ligature the body of the penis is divided and the urethra is also cut around the probe at that point, and the probe is withdrawn leaving the short stump of the urethra free. The cut end of the penis is fixed to the commissure of the skin incision by one or two sutures, so that the urethra will protrude out.

Note: If the amputation is to be done at the root of the penis the scrotum and testes also will have to be removed by extending the incision backwards to meet at the level of the ischeal arch.

CHAPTER 125

Nephrectomy (Removal of Kidney) in Canine

INDICATIONS

Injury or diseases of the kidney. Tumour affecting the kidney.

ANAESTHESIA AND CONTROL

General anaesthesia; controlled in lateral or dorsal recumbency, depending on the site chosen.

ANATOMY

The kidneys are located ventral to the thick sublumbar muscles. They are somewhat movable. The right kidney is slightly anterior in position than the left. The parietal peritoneum covers the ventral aspect of the kidneys. The kidneys are bean-shaped and the *hilus* is situated medially. The renal vessels and ureters enter the kidney through the hilus.

Blood supply: The renal arteries and veins.

SITES

1. An incision about 3 inches long, about 1 inch behind and parallel to the last rib.

2. A mid-line laparotomy incision extending from about one inch behind the Xiphoid cartilage and extending up to the pubic symphysis.

TECHNIQUE

After laparotomy through any one of the sites mentioned above, the intestines are packed off to make the kidney visible.

The peritoneum and fat covering the kidney are separated by blunt dissection. A small tear in its capsule is made in the anterior or posterior pole of the kidney and the capsule is then completely torn and separated from the kidney. At the hilus.

the vessels and ureter are separated from surrounding fat and peritoneum for a distance of about 2 inches and the ureter is clamped and severed first. Then the vessels are ligatured together or separately by the 3-forceps technique, and the kidney is removed. The abdominal wound is closed as usual.

TECHNIQE FOR PROSTATECTOMY IN DOG

Pass a catheter through the urethra. Incise skin from umbilicus to pubis in a slightly curved manner to reflect sheath sideways and incise linea alba and enter abdomen. Pack off intestines; pull bladder forwards with prostate. Cut vessels of prostate between ligatures (usually 2 on each side). Turn to dorsal aspect of bladder; cut between ligatures the 2 *vasa deferentia* close to their entrance to prostate. With catheter in situ, carefully cut urethra anterior to prostate, close to its junction with neck of bladder. (Do not cut the catheter which is only to guide). Clamp bladder neck with Allis tissue forceps. Cut and remove prostate after similarly cutting urethra posterior to it. Remove Allis forceps and re-introduce the catheter into the bladder. Apposition sutures are put to re-unite the urethra to neck of bladder. Leave the catheter *in situ* until 48 hours post-operatively. Suture abdominal and skin wounds as usual.

REFERENCE

Markowitz *et al.* (1959); Miller, M.E. (1952).

CHAPTER 126

Oopherectomy (Spaying) in Bitch

INDICATIONS
1. To prevent breeding and to prevent heat in bitches (Oopherectomy).
2. Neoplastic or cystic changes (ovariotomy or removal of diseased ovaries).

ANAESTHESIA
General anaesthesia or epidural anaesthesia.

ANATOMY
The ovaries are situated behind the kidneys, below the second and third lumbar vertebrae on the left side, and a little in front on the right side. The ovaries are enclosed in a peritoneal pouch called ovarian bursa. The bursa has a slit-like opening ventrally. The ovary may be as big as a pea or a bean.

Blood supply: Anterior ovarian artery which is a branch of the utero-ovarian artery from the posterior aorta.

Nerve supply: Renal and aortic plexus of the sympathetic system.

SITES
1. From a point a little behind the umbilicus backwards along the midline over a length of 3 to 5 inches.
2. In small-sized animals before the onset of first heat a 1 to 1½ inches incision on either flank, parallel to the last rib, below the lumbar transverse processes, at the level of the posterior lobe of the kidneys. The incision may be ½ inch behind the last rib on the right flank and about 1 inch behind on the left flank. If a single flank incision is to be made for removal of both ovaries a larger incision of about 3 inches is made on the right flank as described.

TECHNIQUE

Perform laparotomy through the site chosen. The ovary with its bursa is held with fingers. A ligature is applied anterior to the ovary and another one behind it, around the respective vascular connections. The ovarian bursa is opened and the ovary is removed leaving the bursa. The other ovary also is removed in a similar manner and the laparotomy wound is closed as usual. See also Panhysterectomy (p. 566).

CHAPTER 127

Hysterotomy (Caesarian Section) in Bitch

INDICATIONS

Surgical removal of a full term foetus/foetuses other than by the normal vaginal route. Caesarian section should normally be a planned operation and not an emergency operation.

ANAESTHESIA AND CONTROL

General anaesthesia, or epidural anaesthesia combined with local infiltration; dorsal recumbent position.

SITE

From a point 1 inch behind the umbilicus backwards along the midline for a distance of about 4 inches.

TECHNIQUE

Perform laparotomy. After laparotomy the gravid uterine cornua are exteriorised and packed off from the abdominal cavity by sterile towels. An incision is made on the *dorsal* aspect of the uterus close to the bifurcation of horns, avoiding the placental belt, if possible. The foetus nearest to the incision is removed. The umbilical cord is severed by torsion or by scissors and the pup is rolled in a dry towel by assistants, to stimulate respiration. The next adjacent foetus is brought to the same opening and is delivered similarly. The pups from the other cornu are also removed through same incision and finally the incision is closed by continuous double Lembert's sutures. The uterine cornua are mopped clean with saline and are replaced into position and the abdominal wound is closed as usual. (See also page 355).

ANATOMY

See under Panhysterectomy.

CHAPTER 128

Panhysterectomy (Ovaro hysterectomy) in Bitch

INDICATIONS
1. Chronic endometritis or pyometra.
2. Neoplastic or other incurable lesions affecting the uterus.

ANAESTHESIA AND CONTROL
General anaesthesia; if the patient is debilitated or toxaemic, epidural anaesthesia combined with local infiltration; dorsal recumbency.

ANATOMY
The canine uterus consists chiefly of two tubular horns (cornua) diverging from a vestigeal body towards each kidney. The body and horns are suspended by peritoneal reflections from the sub-lumbar region, known as broad ligaments. The broad ligaments are attached to the dorsal borders of the cornua and the lateral borders of the body of uterus. From the lateral surface of each broad ligament arises the cord-like round ligament of the uterus which goes down the inguinal canal to end in the region of the vulva by blending with the skin.

Blood supply to the ovaries and uterus: The utero-ovarian artery arising (similar to the internal spermatic artery in the male) as a direct branch from the abdominal aorta, supplies the ovary and also gives off a branch to anastomose with the posterior uterine artery. The (posterior) uterine artery in the bitch is a branch of the umbilical artery which is a branch of internal pudic artery, and it ramifies in the body of the uterus and vagina and anastomoses with the utero-ovarian artery in front.

SITE
Same as for hysterotomy but length of incision may be extended depending on need.

TECHNIQUE

Perform laparotomy. The anterior ovarian ligament is cut. Ligature the anterior utero-ovarian vessels. The ovarian bursa is cut across its middle to expose the ovary. The ovary is disconnected from its anterior attachment. After both ovaries are freed in this manner, the posterior uterine arteries are ligatured and cut in level with the cervix. The broad ligament of the uterus is torn to liberate the uterine cornua. Apply two clamps anterior to the cervix and cut in between them to finally disconnect and remove the uterus with the ovaries. (This amputation can be done posterior to the cervix, instead of anteriorly, if so desired.) The stump can be either closed by inversion sutures when the clamp is removed ('Parker-Kerr" sutures), or may be just ligatured. The stump may then be covered with a fold of omentum stitched to it (Omentalisation). The laparotomy wound is sutured as usual. (See also Addendum on page 658)

CHAPTER 129

Ablation of Mammary Gland (Amputation of Mammary Gland) in Bitch

INDICATIONS

Mammary abscesses or tumours.

ANAESTHESIA AND CONTROL

Local infiltration; dorsal recumbent state.

ANATOMY

The mammary glands of the canine are eight to ten in number (four or five pairs). They are arranged along the ventral aspect of thoracic, abdominal, and pelvic regions.

Blood supply: Mammary artery (external pudic artery) after its emergence through the inguinal canal. The anterior glands also receive branches from external thoracic artery.

TECHNIQUE

The gland to be removed is enclosed within an elliptical incision parallel to the long axis of the body. After cutting through the skin and subcutis, the gland is separated by blunt dissection. It will be better to ligature the main vessels before cutting. In the case of ablation of the posterior glands the mammary artery can be ligatured at the inguinal ring. After removing the gland and controlling haemorrhage, the edges of the wound are united by interrupted apposition sutures, or preferably by vertical mattress sutures. A tight bandage with padding is advisable to prevent post-operative haematoma.

CHAPTER 130

Episiotomy in Bitch

INDICATIONS

1. To enlarge the external genital orifice for extirpation of neo-plastic growths like vaginal polypi.

2. To enlarge the vulval opening to aid copulation with selected stud dogs.

3. To facilitate catheterisation in bitches kept for certain experimental purposes.

ANAESTHESIA AND CONTROL

Epidural anaesthesia; Ventral recumbency with hind parts raised.

ANATOMY

During the operation the upper vaginal wall is incised after cutting through the skin and sub-cutaneous connective tissue at the upper commissure of vulva.

Blood supply: Branches of the internal pudic arteries and veins, vaginal and perineal arteries.

Nerve supply: Branches of the pudic nerve supply the perineal region. The vaginal wall is supplied by the sympathetic nerves from the pelvic plexus.

SITE

From the dorsal commissure of vulva upwards, according to the requirement.

TECHNIQUE

Clamps are applied at the dorsal commissure of the vulva one on each side parallel to the mid-line. These clamps include the skin, subcutaneous tissue and the vaginal wall. Incise between the clamps to expose the vaginal canal for necessary manipulation. After completing the manipulations, the lips of the wound are brought into close apposition and the two edges of mucous membrane are sutured separately and the skin edges separately.

If closure like this is not desired immediately (and the vulval opening is to remain like that permanently), the skin and mucous membrane of same edge are sutured together.

CHAPTER 131

Intravenous Injection in Canine

INDICATION

For introduction of drugs directly into circulation.

SITE

The common sites chosen are: (1) The *cephalic vein* on the anterior aspect of the forearm.

(2) The *external saphenous* (external metatarsal or recurrent tarsal) vein above the hock on the external aspect of the leg region.

TECHNIQUE

The vein is raised by pressure around the proximal part of the forearm for cephalic vein and by pressure around the back of the thigh for the tarsal vein. The skin is punctured with intravenous needle, directing the needle tip against the vessel wall. A mild thrust into the vessel causes blood to escape through the needle into the syringe and the solution is injected after releasing pressure on the vein.

Puncturing the vessel wall transmits a characteristic popping sensation to the finger tips, like that of puncturing a thin-walled, mildly inflated, balloon.

After completing the injection, the needle is withdrawn and the site of puncture is held under pressure for a couple of minutes to prevent local extravasation.

Note: The therapeutic introduction of a fluid, like saline solution, into a vein by allowing it to flow by gravitational force, is called *infusion.*

CHAPTER 132

Amputation of Limb in Canine

INDICATIONS
Crush injuries, septic fractures; Gangrene etc.

ANAESTHESIA AND CONTROL
If general anaesthesia is not advisable due to the toxaemic condition of the patient, local infiltration of the skin combined with blocking of the brachial plexus in the case of fore-limb and epidural anaesthesia in the case of hind-limb, may be done.

SITE
Through the shoulder or stifle, as the case may be, so that the stump will not drag on the ground during progression.

TECHNIQUE
(a) *Fore-limb*: By disarticulation of shoulder joint. A semi-circular incision is made on the outer as well as inner aspect of the limb, about 2 to 3 inches below the shoulder joint. The skin flaps are reflected upwards. The muscles mentioned below are sectioned, at their tendinous portions as far as possible, to expose the shoulder joint. The important muscles divided are the following: (1) Deltoid muscle where it is inserted on to the deltoid tuberosity of humerus; (2) Infra-spinatus where it is attached to the lateral tuberosity of humerus; (3) Teres minor where it is inserted on to a tubercle on the upper part of the deltoid ridge; (4) Supra-spinatus inserted on the lateral and medial tuberosities of the humerus; (5) Coracobrachialis, Latissimus dorsi, and Teres major, where they are inserted on to the proximal third of the medial surface of humerus; (6) Sub-scapularis where it is inserted on to the medial tuberosity of

humerus; (7) The biceps brachii where it is originating from the tubar scapula (this is cut at the point of origin); (8) Long head of triceps brachii where it is inserted on to the summit of olecranon; and (9) Tensor faciae antibrachii where it is inserted on to the olecranon.

Immediately after reflecting the skin and before dividing of these muscles, the cephalic vein is seen superficially; and the brachial artery, vein and median and radial nerves are noticed while separating the pectoral and latissimus dorsi muscles. These vessels are ligatured and severed. The nerves are severed and their ends crushed.

The portion of the limb below the joint is amputated by opening the joint capsule and disarticulation of the shoulder joint. The synovial surface of the glenoid cavity of scapula is scraped. The cut ends of muscles are brought to cover the scapular end and the skin is sutured by means of mattress sutures.

(b) *Hind-limb*: By disarticulation through stifle. Elliptical incisions are made on the lateral and medial aspects of the limb about two inches below the stifle so as to lift two semi-circular skin flaps. The skin flaps are reflected. The dorsal metatarsal artery and external saphenous vein which are seen subcutaneously are ligatured. The gastrocnemius muscle parts at their insertions on the tuber calcis are cut and are separated and lifted from their underlying muscles; The gracilis, biceps femoris and semitendinosus muscles are disconnected from their attachments on the anterior tibial crest; The sartorious and semitendinosus muscles are liberated from their insertions on the medial surface of tibia; The femoropatellar ligaments are separated at their attachments on the femur; The attachment of sartorious, vastus medialis, biceps femoris, vastus lateralis and rectus femoris muscles on the patella are separated and the joint capsule is incised at its dorsal border; The origin of the long digital extensor muscle on the extensor fossa of the femur and of plantaris muscle close to it are sectioned; The popliteus muscle is then separated from the joint capsule and lateral condyle of femur; and the insertion of semi-membranosus on the medial condyle of tibia is separated.

The portion of the limb below the stifle is thus separated and removed. During the course of dissection the poplitial artery on the posterior aspect of the distal extremity of femur and the large branch from the femoral artery on the lateral aspect of the thigh are ligatured and cut.

The synovial surface of the articulating extremity of femur is scraped and it is covered with the already isolated gastrocnemius muscle, by suturing the muscle tendon to the facia in front of femur. The skin is sutured, with mattress relaxation sutures combined with simple apposition sutures (or, by vertical mattress sutures).

CHAPTER 133

Amputation of Digit in Canine ("Filletting")

Removal of the terminal phalangial bone in the dog and then suturing the skin incision, has been called "filleting". (The word 'fillet' literally means a boneless piece of meat or fish).

INDICATIONS
Phalangeal fractures. Sprain of inter-phalangeal joints. Infection of toe nails, crushing injuries of the toe, etc.

ANAESTHESIA AND CONTROL
Local infiltration, recumbent position.

SITE
The joint above the seat of the lesion.

TECHNIQUE
Method No. 1: By disarticulation of the 2nd interphalangeal joint (Removal of the claw or removal of terminal phlanx):

A so-called "tennis-racket incision" is made by placing a vertical incision along the dorsal aspect of the digit which is continued downwards by two divergent incisions along the base of the terminal phalanx.

The incisions are extended downwards to meet at the level of the foot pad below the claw. The claw is flexed and it is disarticulated and removed.

The foot pad is pressed upwards and is sutured to the corresponding skinedges. The vertical skin incision is also sutured to complete the operation. This method of removing the terminal phalanx is also called 'Filleting'.

Method No. 2: The procedure when 1st or 2nd phalangeal bones are also to be removed is similar. The vertical incision is started immediately above the joint to be disarticulated.

Amputation of Dew Claw (First Digit) in the Canine

INDICATIONS

In breeds like the Alsatian, dew claws are not permissible especially in hind limbs and hence the need for this operation. Supernumerary dew claws or diseased ones are also removed.

ANAESTHESIA AND CONTROL

Local infiltration. Lateral recumbency.

TECHNIQUE

In puppies the claws are snipped off between the third and fifth day. No anaesthesia is necessary at this stage. In adults the claw is removed through an elliptical skin incision at its base. The wound is sutured.

CHAPTER 134

Amputation of Tail (Docking) in Canine

For puppies docking is done according to breed fancy and specifications, eg.,

Terriers—— 2/3 length is retained.

Spaniels—— 1/3 length only is retained.

Poodles—— 1/2 length is retained. (See also page 578).

Age: Before the fifteenth day after birth. (No anaesthetic is required at this age.) Disarticulation is effected through the intervertebral cartilage at the site chosen, by cutting through with a scalpel. The skin is pushed forwards towards the base before cutting, so that enough loose skin will be available to form a cover for the stump afterwards. One or two stitches may be necessary to keep skin edges in apposition.

For adult animals the technique is similar to amputation of tail in the bovine, already described (p. 513).

CHAPTER 135

Standards for Ear-trimming and Docking in Canine

Breed	Ears	Tail
I: Sporting breeds		
Golden Retriever	No	No
Labrador Retriever	No	No
English Cocker Spaniel	No	Leave 1/3
II: Hounds		
Afgan Hound	No	No
Beagle	No	No
Dachshund	No	No
English Fox Hound	No	No
III: Working breeds		
Belgium Sheepdog	No	No
Boxer	Yes	Leave 2 coccygeal vertebrae
Collie	No	No
Bull Mastiff	No	No
Doberman Pinscher	Yes	At second joint
German Shepherd (Alsatian)	No	No
Great Dane	Yes	No
Mastiff	No	No
English Sheepdog	No	Remove completely, or leave not more than 2 inches in adult
St. Bernard	No	No
IV: Terriers		
Airedale Terrier	No	Remove 1/3
Bull Terrier	Optional	No
Irish Terrier	No	Leave 3/4
Scottish Terrier	No	Never
V: Toy breeds		
Chi hua hua	No	No
English Toy Spaniel	No	Cut to 1½ inches.
Pekingese	No	No

Breed	Ears	Tail
Pomeranian	No	No
Toy Poodle	No	Remove half
VI: Non-sporting breeds		
Boston Terrier	Yes	No
Bull Dog	No	No
Chow Chow	No	No
Dalmatian	No	No
Poodle	No	Tailless or ½ inch allowed

Ear-trimming and docking are not done in Hounds like Basset hound, Bassingee, Grey hound, Pointer and Whippet; and in Spintz (a non-sporting breed); and also in Indian breeds. Fox Terriers and Bull Terriers are sometimes ear-trimmed.

Note: (1) Three Indian breeds recognised by the Kennel Club of India are: Bhotia (Himalayan Sheep Dog), Rampur Hound (Origin is Rampur in U.P.), and Rajapalayam (Origin Tamil Nadu). Other Indian breeds of dogs are: Chippipare, Kombai, Sindh-hound, Tripuri, Patti, Poligar, Banjara, Mudhol-hound (Origin is Mudhol in Karnataka), etc.

(2) Of all domestic breeds of dogs, St. Bernaud is perhaps the biggest sized. It has its origin in Switzerland. Also called Barri-hound.

(3) The Spitz breed of dog is incorrectly referred to as Pomeranian. Though there is some similarity in external features, Spintz is a much larger-sized dog compared to Pomeranian.

CHAPTER 136

Some Methods for Immobilisation of Fractures

1. Gum Bandages: Useful for fractures in birds.

2. Splints made up of wooden pieces or light metal plates supported by bandages.

3. Plaster of paris bandages ("plaster casts").

4. Plaster of paris splints and gutters.

5. Thomas splints (modified Thomas splints).

6. Mason metasplint: For fractures in the metacarpal or metatarsal region.

7. Suturing the bone fragments with stainless steel wires.

8. Vitellium bone plates and screws.

9. By using bone pins: There are two methods of bone pinning.

(a) External pinning (Examples: Kirschner splint, Stadar splint). (b) Intramedullary pinning.

(a) *External pinning*: (Cortical pinning; External fixation)—Two pins are driven through the sides of each bone fragment, at an angle of about 40° to each other, using a chuck. The pins are driven through skin and other soft tissues covering the bone and then into the bone. The pinpoints should get firmly embedded in the cortex. The pins fixed to each fragment are connected by assembling pins. External pinning is done from that aspect of bone where it is superficial. For example: Postero-lateral aspect of femur; Antero-lateral aspect of humerus; Medial aspect of tibia; Medial aspect of radius etc.

(b) *Intramedullary pinning*: (Internal fixation)—In this method the pin is driven through the medullary cavity of the bone. There are two methods for doing this: viz, the open method (open reduction) and the closed method (closed reduction).

In the *open method* a pin pointed at both ends is used. The seat of fracture is opened surgically and the pin is first driven through the proximal fragment until the pinpoint comes out through the other end of bone and skin for short distance. The point of the pin at the fracture site is rhen directed and driven through the distal fragment until it gets firmly embedded in the epiphysis. The wound is sutured, the excess length of the pin left outside is cut and removed. After healing of fracture, the pin may be retained or removed.

In the *closed method* the fracture site is not opened. The pin is driven from the upper (proximal) end of the bone by following certain landmarks.

Examples

1. For fracture of the shaft of *Femur*, the pin is driven through the trochanteric fossa which is located by feeling the trochanter major and directing the pin along its medial aspect.

2. For fracture of the shaft of *Humerus*, the pin is introduced through a point ¼ inch below the ridge on the *lateral* tuberosity.

3. For *Tibia* the pin is driven ¼ inch below the *medial* meniscus and between the anterior and medial tuberosities. (See also chapter on Fractures, p. 166.)

Bone plates and screws are specially useful in certain oblique fractures where intramedullary pin or external immobilisation will not hold the bone fragments properly in position.

Note: While applying a plaster cast when there is an open wound on the skin, a window may be left to facilitate drainage.

Plaster casts are usually removed after *six weeks*. However, removal and reapplication may be necessary to attend to complications like excessive swelling, pus formation, etc., whenever such complications develop.

CHAPTER 137

Euthanasia by Shooting, Horse

INDICATIONS

Incurable diseases, old age etc., when it is uneconomical to maintain the animal. For experimental purpose.

SITE

Point of intersection of two imaginary lines drawn on the forehead, connecting the base of each ear with the middle of supra-orbital process of the opposite side. This point will usually be the lowest limit of the fore-lock.

TECHNIQUE

The animal is shot through this point. (The bullet will pierce through the cerebrum, the medulla and the proximal portion of spinal cord and immediate death results.)

CHAPTER 138

Euthanasia by Pithing, Horse

INDICATIONS
As for shooting.

SITES
1. the occipito-atlantal space.
2. The atlo-axoid space.

TECHNIQUE
The head is flexed. For pithing through the occipito-atlantal space, a pithing knife or a long-bladed scalpel is introduced at the point where an imaginary line connecting the anterior borders of the wings of atlas meets the crest of the neck.

The knife is passed through the skin and ligamentum nuchae and the interarcual ligament between vertebrae, to gain entrance into the vertebral canal and sever the spinal cord.

For pithing through the atlo-axoid space the site is at the point where an imaginary line connecting the posterior border of the wings of atlas meets the crest of the neck. The procedure is similar.

Mandibular Nerve Block in Equine

INDICATIONS

Desensitisation for surgical manipulation of lower lip and incisors.

ANATOMY

The mandibular division of the fifth cranial nerve gives off the alveolar branch which enters the mandible through the mandibular foramen on the medial aspect of the vertical ramus, and emerges through the mental foramen situated on the external aspect of the body of the mandible. During its course within the bone the nerve supplies branches to the teeth of the lower jaw analogous to the infra-orbital nerve of the upper jaw.

TECHNIQUE

1. Mental nerve block—Locate the mental foramen on the lateral aspect of the mandible above the middle of the interdental space. The foramen can be palpated under the skin by pushing the tendon of depressor labii inferioris muscle. About 2 to 3 cc of the analgesic solution is injected into the foramen, using a hypodermic needle.

2 Mandibular nerve block—The *level* of mandibular foramen which is on the *medial* aspect of the mandible is assessed from lateral aspect of mandible as the point of intersection of an imaginary line passing vertically downwards from the lateral canthus of the eye (head horizontal position) and a line drawn backwards along the tables of the teeth of the lower jaw. The needle is passed along the *medial* aspect of the mandible to reach the foramen at this point after penetrating the skin about 3 cm below the temporo-mandibular articulation and behind the posterior border of the vertical ramus and directing it forward. About 4 to 6 cc of solution is injected.

CHAPTER 140

Supra-orbital Nerve Block in Equine

INDICATIONS

Operation on the upper eyelid.

ANATOMY

Supra-orbital nerve (frontal nerve) is one of the terminal branches of the ophthalmic division of the fifth cranial (trigeminal) nerve. It is accompanied by the artery of the same name. It is sensory to the upper eyelid.

SITE

The root of the supra-orbital process.

TECHNIQUE

The supra-orbital foramen is easily palpable as a depression at the root of the supra-orbital process. The needle is introduced under the skin and 5 cc of the analgesic solution is injected at the site.

CHAPTER 141

Infra-orbital Neurectomy in Equine

INDICATIONS

Continuous and spasmodic twitching of unidentified etiology of the upper lip and nostril. For temporary relief, blocking of the nerve can be done instead of neurectomy.

ANAESTHESIA AND CONTROL

Nerve blocking; standing position.

ANATOMY

The infra-orbital nerve is the terminal branch of the maxillary division of the trigeminal nerve (trifacial or fifth cranial). The nerve crosses the pterygo-palatine fossa, and enters the infra-orbital canal (superior dental canal) and emerges through the infra-orbital foramen where it is broad and partly covered by the levator naso-labialis muscle and is accompanied by the infra-orbital artery. It is the sensory nerve supplying the upper lip, muzzle and nostrils of that side, but also receives a few motor fibres from the terminal branches of the superior buccal nerve.

SITE

The level of bisection of a line connecting the facial tuberosity and the nasomaxillary notch.

TECHNIQUE

The nerve trunk as it emerges from the infra-orbital foramen is palpated and a longitudinal incision is made on the skin. The naso-labial muscle is pushed aside. This exposes the nerve and it is picked up and divided. The proximal end of the nerve is crushed by artery forceps before its division and a bit of the nerve distal to it is cut off. Trauma to the lateral nasal artery accompanying the nerve is avoided. The skin wound is closed as usual. (See also page 267.)

LIGATION OF STENSON'S DUCT

The ligation of stenson's duct in the equine is similar to what has been already described for bovine (p. 460).

CHAPTER 142

Trephining of Facial Sinuses in Equine

INDICATIONS

(1) Empyema; (2) Removal of tumours, cysts; (3) In depressed fractures; (4) For removal of isolated fragments of bone; (5) For punching out the fourth or fifth upper molars, the maxillary sinus is trephined.

ANAESTHESIA AND CONTROL

Local infiltration; standing position.

ANATOMY

(a) *Frontal sinus*: The frontal sinus in the horse consists of two portions, the frontal part bounded chiefly by the frontal bone; and the turbinate part located in the posterior part of the turbinate bone with the nasal and lachrimal bones forming the outer boundaries. It is separated from the frontal sinus of the opposite side by the median septum. Other boundaries of the sinus are as follows when head is in the vertical position. Superior limit: A line connecting the zygomatic arches of either side. In the upper portion, the cavity is very narrow. Inferior limit: The frontal part extends up to a line joining the inner canthii of the eyes; and the tubinate part is limited by a line connecting the mid-point of the facial crest of either side. Lateral limit: Line connecting the medial canthus of the eye and the naso-maxillary notch of the same side.

Note: Unlike in cattle the turbinate part of the frontal sinus in equine is separated from the nasal cavity by the thin plate of dorsal turbinate bone and therefore it has no direct communication with the nasal cavity; The frontal and maxillary sinuses of equine comn inicate with each other.

(b) *Maxillary sinus*: The maxillary sinus in the horse is

divided into two compartments, the superior maxillary sinus and the inferior maxillary sinus, by a thin bony septum. The septum is usually situated at about 2 inches above the lower limit of facial crest but its exact position may vary in individuals. The septum is either partially or wholly absent in the mule.

The bony infra-orbital canal passes through the superior maxillary sinus.

The superior maxillary sinus communicates with the nasal cavity through a very narrow slit located at the posterior limit of the middle nasal meatus.

The inferior maxillary sinus communicates with. the middle meatus of the nasal cavity.

For removal of third, fourth and fifth cheek teeth, a trephine approach can be made through the maxillary sinus. The root of the third cheek tooth projects partially into the inferior maxillary sinus. The roots of the fourth molar also project into the maxillary sinus.

Roots of the fifth cheek tooth are placed in the superior maxillary sinus. The sixth is rooted in the superior maxillary sinus but is situated below and behind the orbit and hence cannot be approached through a trephine opening from the sinus.

SITES

Sites for trephining frontal sinus—(1) *Upper site*: The inferior angle of intersection of two imaginary lines; one line joining the middle parts of the roots of supra-orbital processes of either side and the other drawn along the mesial suture. (2) *Middle site*: The superior angle of intersection of the two lines, one line joining the inner canthi of the eyes and the other line drawn along the mesial suture. (3) *Lowest site*: One inch medial to a point marked 2½ inches below the inner canthus of eye on a line joining the inner canthus of the eye and the naso-maxillary notch.

Site for trephining superior maxillary sinus—Half to 1 inch inwards from a point at the centre of the facial crest.

Site for trephining inferior maxillary sinus—About ½ to 1 inch inwards from the lower end of facial crest.

TECHNIQUE

An estimate of the circumference of the trephine head is made on the skin with the trephine head itself. A cruciate incision slightly bigger than the diameter is made, and the resulting four triangular flaps of skin are cut around and removed to create a circular area.

The surface of the bone (frontal bone in the case of frontal sinus and maxilla in the case of maxillary sinus) in the exposed area is scraped with scalpel. The levator labii supertoris proprius muscle will have to be pushed outwards if it comes in the way while trephining maxillary sinus.

The trephine head is fixed on the bone and is rotated to-and-fro, applying pressure till the thickness of the bone yields. The isolated piece of bone comes off with the trephine head, or it is picked out to open into the sinus.

REPULSION OF TOOTH (TOOTH EXTRACTION) IN EQUINE

The operation tooth extraction (repulsion of tooth) is similar to extraction of teeth in the bovine already described (p.472).

CHAPTER 143

Amputation of Tongue in Equine

INDICATIONS
Irreparable injury. Gangrene.

ANAESTHESIA AND CONTROL
General anaesthesia.

ANATOMY
There is an outer covering of mucous membrane. The tongue s composed largely of intrinsic muscular fibres dorsally and extrinsic muscles ventrally. There is a median dorso ventral septum dividing the tongue tissue symmetrically.

Blood supply: Lingual and sub-lingual branches of the external maxillary artery. The veins drain into the internal and external maxillary veins. The pharyngeal lymph nodes govern the lymph circulation of the tongue.

Sensory nerve supply: Lingual branch of trigeminal (fifth cranial) and Glosso-pharyngeal (ninth cranial) nerves.

Motor nerve supply: By the hypoglossal (twelfth cranial).

SITE
Proximal to the seat of lesion.

TECHNIQUE
A series of haemostatic mattress sutures passing through the thickness of the tongue are applied about ½ inch proximal to the desired level of amputation. The distal part of tongue is divided in front of suture line and is removed.

CHAPTER 144

Surgical Drainage from Guttural Pouch in Equine

INDICATIONS
Empyema of guttural pouch.

ANAESTHESIA AND CONTROL
Depends on the site chosen. For hyovertebrotomy, general anaesthesia is required. Local analgesia may be adequate for opening the pouch at the Viborg's triangle. The horse is cast and secured on the opposite side with head extended.

ANATOMY
The guttural pouches are diverticula of the eustachian tubes and present in the equine species. *Relationship of guttural pouch*:

Dorsally: Base of cranium and atlas;

Ventrally: Pharynx and oesophagus;

Medially: Medially the two guttural pouches are in contact with each other with a little separation above due to the ventral straight muscles of the head. (Rectus capitis ventralis);

Laterally: Laterally it is overlapped by many important structures, viz., Pterygoid, Levator palati, Tensor palati, Stylohyoideus, Occipito-hyoideus, Occipito-mandibularis, and Digastricus muscles; the parotid and mandibular (sub-maxillary) salivary glands; the Glosso-pharyngeal, Hypoglossal and Anterior laryngeal nerves; and the great cornu of the hyoid bone;

Dorso-medially: The Vagus, Spinal accessory and Sympathetic nerves; the anterior cervical ganglion; the internal carotid artery, and the ventral cerebral vein.

SITE
1. Over the antero-inferior border of the wing of atlas called the *Dieterich's Method of Hyo-vertebrotomy*.

2. In the *Viborg's triangle*, which is outlined by the posterior border of the vertical ramus in front, tendon of sternomaxillaris above and the sub-maxillary vein below.

TECHNIQUE

Site No. 1: Make a 3 to 5 inches long skin incision along the antero-inferior border of the wing of atlas. Reflect the parotid gland forward by freeing it from areolar attachments. In a distended state the pale wall of the guttural pouch would become visible immediately. Normally it is under cover of the digastricus, stylo-maxillaris and occipito hyoideus muscles. A fold of the guttural pouch is held by tissue forceps and an opening is made into it. A probe or a sound is then introduced into the pouch towards the Viborg's triangle so that a counter opening can be made at that level to facilitate drainage and introduction of a seton, if required.

Site No. 2: Through the Viborg's triangle by a simple incision and blunt dissection.

CHAPTER 145

Roaring Operation (Ventriculectomy; Stripping of Ventricles; Hobdaying) in Horse

INDICATION
"Roaring" or "whistling".

ANAESTHESIA AND CONTROL
Ordinarily local infiltration combined with 20% cocaine spray on the laryngeal mucous membrane; standing position.

General anaesthesia may be required in certain cases and then the animal is secured in dorsal recumbency.

ANATOMY
The cricoid cartilage of the larynx is connected to the body of the thyroid cartilage by the crico-thyroid ligament. The vocal fold (vocal cord) connects the vocal process of each arytenoid cartilage to the body of the thyroid cartilage.

There are two lateral ventricles, one on each side. Each lateral ventricle is a saccular space leading to the laryngeal saccule situated between the arytenoid cartilage and the wing of the thyroid cartilage. Thus the lateral ventricle is bounded laterally by the wing of the thyroid cartilage and medially by the arytenoid cartilage and the vocal fold. In the standing position the lateral ventricle opens downwards and forwards.

SITE
A midline incision on ventral aspect of neck, along the crico-thyroid ligament.

TECHNIQUE
A midline cutaneous incision is made over the site described.

The sterno-hyoideus muscles of either side are separated to expose the crico-thyroid ligament. The ligament is incised from the cricoid cartilage to the body of the thyroid cartilage. Using a laryngeal dilator the edges of the incision are retracted exposing the interior of larynx for any further surgical intervention.

With the larynx laid open, the mucous membranes of the lateral ventricles of either side are stripped by using the burr. The head of the burr is introduced into the lateral ventricle and is rotated so that the lining mucous membrane gets attached to its rough surface. The burr covered by mucous membrane is now drawn out and the mucous membrane is severed by scalpel or scissors and removed with the burr. The dilator is then removed. The wound is not sutured.

CHAPTER 146

Muting Operation in Equine

INDICATION

To avoid horses and mules on front line duties in the army making noises by crying aloud.

TECHNIQUE

Perform laryngotomy as described under roaring operation. The vocal cords are held by tissue forceps and a part of each vocal cord containing the vocal cartilage is snipped and removed.

Note: The operation *tracheotomy* in the equine is similar to tracheotomy in the bovine. But permanent tracheotomy tubes like Field's Tracheotomy Tube or Pape's Tracheotomy Tube are used in the equine, instead of simple rubber tubing. Elliptical pieces from adjacent annular cartilages are removed to introduce the tube. The tube is periodically cleaned of discharges, daily or on alternate days.

CHAPTER 147

Oesophagotomy in Horse

INDICATION
Oesophageal obstruction.

ANAESTHESIA AND CONTROL
Local or general anaesthesia; controlled either in the standing or right lateral recumbent state.

ANATOMY
The oesophagus is a musculo-membranous tube about 5 ft long and is continuous with the pharynx and lies above the larynx and trachea at its commencement and then slides down the left side at the level of the third or fourth cervical vertebra. It is almost ventral to the trachea immediately behind the sixth cervical vertebra. At the level of the third thoracic vertebra it is dorsal to the trachea, and crossing the aortic arch it is shifted to the right of median plane. It continues its further course along the dorsal surface of the trachea and later to left of trachea.

Blood supply: The oesophagus is supplied by branches from the carotid artery in the cervical course; broncho-oesophageal branches in the thoracic region; and branches from the gastric arteries towards the terminal part.

Nerve supply: Vago-sympathetic fibres and glossopharyngeal branches.

SITE
1. At the level of obstruction.
2. At the base of the neck if the obstruction is at the entrance to the thorax.

TECHNIQUE
A 3 to 4 inches long longitudinal incision is made through the

skin, cutaneous muscle and facia along the superior (or, inferior) border of the jugular furro. The jugular vein is pushed aside by separating it from adjacent muscle. The areolar tissue is torn through by blunt dissection towards the trachea. The oeso- phagus is recognised by its distinct light pink colour and the feeling of the lumen when held between fingers. An incision is made through the oesophageal wall after raising it through the wound. Remove the obstruction. To complete the operation the mucous membrane is sutured by apposition sutures and the outer muscular and fibrous coats of oesophagus by a set of closely placed interrupted sutures. Finally the skin wound is closed.

CHAPTER 148

Paracentesis Thoracis in Horse

The indications, procedure etc., are similar to what has been described in the bovine except for the following differences.

SITE IN THE HORSE

Left side: Through the eighth intercostal space, just above the spur vein and close to the anterior border of the ninth rib.

Right side: Through the seventh inter-costal space, just above the spur-vein and close to the anterior border of eighth rib.

ANATOMY

The anterior mediastinum in the horse is open unlike in cattle and dogs.

CHAPTER 149

Caecocentesis (Caecal Puncture) in Horse

INDICATIONS

Acute tympany of the caecum and colon.

ANAESTHESIA AND CONTROL

Local infiltration; standing position.

ANATOMY

The caecum in the horse occupies the ventral floor of the abdomen chiefly to the right of the median plane with its base towards the right flank. Its apex lies about a hands-breadth behind the Xiphoid cartilage and the base extends up to the tuber coxae or external angle of ilium.

SITE

The hollow of the flank on the right side.

TECHNIQUE

A point equidistant from the posterior border of the last rib, lumbar transverse processes and the external angle of the ilium is chosen. A trocar and canula of about 1/16 inch diameter and about 6 to 10 inches long is used to puncture through the skin and muscles, the peritoneal lining, and wall of caecum. The trocar is withdrawn to permit escape of gas. The trocar is replaced before removing canula. Trocar and canula are withdrawn together in the same way as they were introduced.

CHAPTER 150

Cystotomy in Equine

See cystotomy in the bovine and also note the anatomical descriptions noted below.

ANATOMY

The urinary bladder of the horse has a fundus (or vertex), body and neck. It is situated in the floor of the pelvic cavity behind pelvic inlet, but may change its position, shape and size according to the amount of its contents. The dorsal surface in the male is related to the rectum, the genital fold, the terminal parts of the ductus deferentes, the vesiculae seminalis and the prostate. The posterior portion of the bladder is not covered by peritoneum. The retroperitoneal part of the bladder is attached to the surrounding parts by loose connective tissue in which there is a quantity of fat.

TECHNIQUE

A method of cystotomy in the horse is described in the operative surgery book by Berge and Wasthues, translated into English by Siller and Fraser.

In this method an incision is placed lateral to the anus to dissect through the intervening perineal and perirectal tissues and get at the urinary bladder. The bladder is then incised close to its neck after manipulating the calculus to that point. The bladder in this region has no peritoneal covering and hence no danger of peritonitis. After removing the calculus, no suture is put on the bladder or the external wound. Post-operative care includes free drainage for the leaking urine. Wound on the bladder closes in about two weeks and subsequently the external wound also heals in about ten days. For details refer Berge, Ewald, and Wasthues, Melchior (1966).

CHAPTER 151

Castration of Horse

INDICATIONS

To make the horse docile and easily manageable in the presence of mares. Malignant diseases or irreparable injury to the testes. Cases of inguinal hernia or scrotal hernia.

ANAESTHESIA AND CONTROL

Nacrosis and spermatic blocking and local infiltration; or general anaesthesia; perferably lying position.

ANATOMY

The scrotum from without inwards is made up of skin, dartos, the scrotal facia and parietal layer of tunica vaginalis. The epididymis is adherent to the dorsal border of the testicle with its enlarged anterior end termed the head, and its posterior end called tail. The narrow part between its head and tail constitutes the body of the epididymis.

The spermatic cord has the covering of the spermatic sheath formed by the tunica vaginalis and cremaster externus muscles. Spermatic cord consists of an anterior vascular bundle and a posterior bundle containing the vas deferens.

Blood supply: Blood supply to the scrotum is derived from the external pudic vessels. Testicle is supplied by the spermatic artery. Veins form a plexus and drain into the spermatic vein. The right spermatic vein joins the posterior vena cava while the left one joins the left renal vein.

Nerve supply: Ventral branches of second and third lumbar nerves supply the scrotum. Nerve supply to the testes are derived from the renal and posterior mesenteric plexus.

TECHNIQUE

There are different methods for castration:

(1)   Closed method; and (2) Open method:
(a)   Uncovered or open method; and
(b)   Covered method.

1. *Closed method*: Each spermatic cord is held firmly under skin of the neck of the scrotum and is crushed only once with a Burdizzo forceps. Not recommended.

2. *Open method*: (a) *Uncovered*—The testicle of the side nearer to the ground in the cast position of the animal is removed first. It is held between thumb and fingers and is tensed against the skin of the scrotum. Using the castration knife, a longitudinal incision is made antero-posteriorly to expose the testicle. The anterior and posterior bundles of the spermatic cord are separated. The vas deferens and the tunica vaginalis are severed as high up as possible. The anterior vascular bundle is ligatured at the highest point accessible and is divided distal to the ligature to remove the testicle. (Instead of ligaturing and cutting, this vascular bundle could be severed by using ecraseur or emasculator or by torsion. In the torsion method, the cord is fixed by clamps and torsion forceps is applied a little away for slow twisting and severing. The spermatic cord can also be severed by using a dull red-hot line-firing iron, by drawing the iron repeatedly over the desired point of division, so as to prevent bleeding.) The other testicle is also removed in a similar manner.

(b) *Covered*—This method is adopted for castration as a remedial measure for scrotal hernia.

The incision is limited to skin and subcutis, the testicle being exposed with its covering of tunica vaginalis intact. The spermatic cord is severed after ligaturing outside its covering. See also page 341; 342

CHAPTER 152

Amputation of Penis in Horse

INDICATIONS

Malignant diseases. Irreparable injury. Permanent paralysis.

ANAESTHESIA AND CONTROL

General anaesthesia; dorsal recumbency.

SITE

In paralysis, amputation of the excess portion hanging outside the sheath. In malignant diseases amputation as close to the root as possible; in other cases proximal to the seat of lesion.

TECHNIQUE

The glans penis is hooked out of the sheath by the tip of the index finger introduced into the *Navicular fossa* (urethral sinus) at the tip of the penis. A metal sound is introduced into the urethra and a tourniquet is applied around the penis posterior to the level of amputation. On the ventral aspect of the penis a transverse incision is placed involving about half its circumference. The sides of this transverse incision are extended backwards to converge at a point 3 inches behind. Remove the superficial tissues from the triangular area so demarcated, so that the urethra is visible. The urethra is then incised in front corresponding to the transverse incision; and then longitudinally within the triangle.

The sides of the urethral wall thus opened are sutured on to the two corresponding edges of the triangular incision originally made, to allow free drainage for urine. The tourniquet and sound are now withdrawn and a tight ligature is placed in level with the transverse incision. The penis is now cut at a point distal to the ligature and is removed.

Note: In malignant disease, the sheath, scrotum and testis may also be removed with the penis.

Blood supply to the penis: See under amputation of penis in the bovine.

CHAPTER 153

Urethrotomy in Horse

INDICATIONS

Urethral obstruction and for removal of calculi.

ANAESTHESIA AND CONTROL

Epidural anaesthesia or general anaesthesia; dorsal recumbent state.

SITE

The median line of perineal region at or below the level of the ischeal arch.

TECHNIQUE

A median cutaneous incision is made in the perineal region at (or, starting immediately above) the ischeal arch, 3 to 4 inches long. Go between the retractor penis muscles and cut through the accelerator urinae muscle, corpus spongiosum and the urethral wall Confine to the exact median line to avoid branches of the internal pudic artery. The wound may be left open, or, alternatively, the urethra may be sutured to correspond to the skin edges, to keep the opening patent.

CHAPTER 154

Oopherectomy (Spaying: Ovariotomy) in Mare

INDICATIONS
1. Bad temperament and behaviour.
2. To prevent nuisance of heat.
3. Diseases of the ovary. (Removal of diseased ovary is called ovariotomy.)

For other details of the operation refer spaying in the bovine.

Note: The ovaries are located near the antero-internal aspect of the middle of the iliac shaft on each side. The uterine cornua diverge at right angles from the uterine body and are short and stout. The cervix in the mare is a limpid finger like process and the vaginal fornix is more capacious.

Caslick's Operation of Suturing Vulva in Mare/Cow

This is an operation to prevent *wind-sucking* or *pneumovagina*. The lips of the vulva are united by sutures at its upper part, leaving about 3 to 4 cm at the lower commissure unsutured, for passage of urine and for breeding purposes. Local anaesthetic solution is injected along the muco-cutaneous line and the mucous membrane elevated by the injections is snipped off with scissors to provide raw surfaces. The lips are sutured with interrupted apposition sutures. Sutures should *not* be tightened as they may tear through. They can be removed in 7 to 10 days.

CHAPTER 155

Operation for Blemished Knee in Equine (Cherry's Operation)

SITE

Anterior surface of the knee where the scar (blemish) is situated.

TECHNIQUE

The scar or cicatrix is removed by including it in an elliptical skin incision vertically on the anterior aspect of the knee. This wound is closed by interrupted apposition sutures after relaxing the skin by placing additional vertical skin incisions on either side of it. After healing, the three wounds will only appear as three narrow streaks of scar covered by hair.

CHAPTER 156

Median Neurectomy in Equine

INDICATIONS

As a palliative last resort measure to prolong the utility of working animals in incurable, aseptic, chronic inflammatory lesions without serious structural alteration. e.g. Navicular disease before advanced structural alterations set in.

ANAESTHESIA AND CONTROL

General anaesthesia and cast position, or regional anaesthesia combined with narcosis.

SITE

The point below the medial radial tuberosity, in the groove between the posterior border of radius and the flexor metacarpi internus.

TECHNIQUE

A two-inch long incision is made at the site parallel to the bony edge. This exposes the posterior superficial pectoral muscle which is incised next. (If the operation is performed lower down, only the aponeurotic portion of the muscle is met with.) The wound is retracted and the nerve is usually found with the artery and vein. Separate the nerve which is flat, is yellowish white in colour, and is striated longitudinally. The nerve is then pulled out and is held by artery forceps at the proximal end. A piece of nerve distal to the forceps and the distal commissure of the wound is cut and removed. The skin wound is closed by interrupted apposition sutures. (See also page 267)

CHAPTER 157

Median Nerve Block in Equine

INDICATIONS

Surgical interference in the distal portion of the limb: To test for certain lamenesses.

The site for *median nerve block* is the same as for median neurectomy. The anaesthetic solution (7 to 10 cc) is injected over the nerve (perineural injection).

For complete anaesthetisation below the carpus, blocking of ulnar and musculo-cutaneous nerves also are necessary. Site for *ulnar block* is same as for ulnar neurectomy. The *musculo-cutaneous nerve is blocked* on the medial aspect of the middle of the fore-arm immediately in front of cephalic vein.

CHAPTER 158

Ulnar Neurectomy in Equine

INDICATIONS

As for median neurectomy. Usually done in combination with median neurectomy, e.g. in splints.

ANAESTHESIA AND CONTROL

See under median neurectomy.

SITE

About 4 inches above the upper border of pisiform bone (Accessory carpal bone), along a line joining the point of the elbow with the pisiform.

TECHNIQUE

A longitudinal incision about 2 inches long is made at the site. The nerve is superficial. Common mistake is to go deep.

(See also page 267)

Ulnar Nerve Block in Equine

The site for *blocking ulnar nerve* is the same as described for ulnar neurectomy. See also median nerve block.

Volar and Plantar Neurectomies in Equine

INDICATIONS

Ring bone. Chronic osteo-periostitis of the os-pedis.

ANAESTHESIA AND CONTROL

See under median-neurectomy.

ANATOMY

Fore-limb: The *volar* or *metacarpal** nerves are the terminal branches of the median nerve. The external plantar nerve merges with the terminal branches of the ulnar nerve. The medial plantar nerve is accompanied by the large metacarpal artery and internal (medial) metacarpal vein. Similarly the external nerve is accompanied by the external metacarpal vein and the small lateral volar metacarpal artery. The internal plantar nerve gives off a branch at about the middle of the metacarpal region which joins the external plantar nerve at the level of the button of the splint. Below the fetlock each plantar nerve divides to form the three digital nerves (anterior, middle and posterior) in close association with the digital vessels.

Hind-limb: The *plantar or metatarsal* nerves in the hind-limb are terminal branches of the posterior tibial (or, tibial) nerve. Each plantar nerve is accompanied by the metatarsal *vein* of that side and by a slendar artery from the vascular arch at the back of the tarsus. (Note that the large metatarsal artery does not follow a course similar to the large metacarpal artery.) Below the fetlock region the distribution of digital nerves is similar to the fore-limb.

SITE

(i) *Fore-limb*—(a) *outer aspect*: Half inch below the button of the splint, in the depression between suspensory ligament and flexor tendons.

(b) *Inner aspect*: In level with the button of the splint, in the depression between suspensory ligament and flexor tendons.

(ii) *Hind-limb*—(a) *outer aspect*: One inch below the button of the splint bone, in the depression between the suspensory ligament and flexor tendons.

(b) *Inner aspect*: Same as in the fore-limb.

TECHNIQUE

Make a longitudinal cutaneous incision about an inch long The nerve is picked up by tenaculum and is separated from the accompanying artery and vein (placed in the order *van* from the front). Proceed as usual for neurectomy. (See also page 267).

Volar and Plantar Nerve nerve Blocks in Equine

The sites for volar nerve block (in fore-limb) and plantar nerve block (in hind-limb) are the same as for respective neurectomies.

Local anaesthetic solution (e.g. Procaine solution 2% two to four ml) my be injected around each nerve (perineurally) at sites described.

*NOTE:— Although some veterinary text books use the term "plantar" while referring to flexor aspect of either the metacarpal region (in fore-limb) or metatarsal region (in hind limb), the correct equivalent terminology for the region in fore-limb is "volar" and not "plantar", vide Sisson (1958).

CHAPTER 161

Digital Neurectomies ("Low Volar" and "Low Plantar" Neurectomies) in Equine

ANAESTHESIA
Local infiltration, subcutaneously.

ANATOMY
See page 613 under volar/plantar neurectomy.

SITE
There are *two* sites (medial and lateral) for each limb. The sites are similar whether in the fore-or hind limbs or whether on the medial or lateral aspect of each limb:—

The depression on the lateral/medial aspect immediately below fetlock, which can be palpated between the posterosupero-lateral aspect of os-suffraginis (first phalanx) and the deep flexor tendon of the digit.

TECHNIQUE
On incising the skin at site described, the digital nerve which is situated on the edge of the flexor tendon, and which is more superficial than the accompanying artery and nerve, is identified. Then proceed as for other neurectomies. (See also page 267).

Anterior Tibial (Deep Peroneal) Neurectomy in Equine

INDICATIONS

Spavin. In most cases of spavin both anterior tibial and posterior tibial neurectomies are indicated.

ANAESTHESIA AND CONTROL

As for median neurectomy.

SITE

Two inches below and behind the lateral tuberosity of tibia, in the groove between extensor pedis (long digital extensor) and peroneus (lateral digital extensor) muscles.

TECHNIQUE

Make an incision of about $1\frac{1}{2}$ to 2 inches through the skin and subcutis. Beneath the aponeurotic sheath is the peroneal cutaneous and on separation of the extensor pedis and peroneus muscles the anterior tibial nerve will be found as a distinct white, thin, cord-like structure lying close to the bluish fleshy part of flexor metatarsi. The anterior tibial nerve is cut.

(See also page 267)

CHAPTER 163

Posterior Tibial (Internal Poplitial or Tibial) Neurectomy in Equine

INDICATIONS
Spavin, chronic sprained tendons.

ANAESTHESIA AND CONTROL
General or epidural anaesthesia.

ANATOMY
The posterior tibial nerve (internal poplitial or the *tibial nerve*), is a direct continuation of the sciatic nerve. At a varying level in the distal third of the leg, the posterior tibial nerve divides into the lateral and medial plantar nerves. In the proximal third of the leg, the nerve is under cover of the medial head of gastro-cnemius and lies along the medial aspect of superficial flexor; lower down, it is covered by the common deep facia (aponeurosis) and is situated in the space between the deep flexor and the medial border of tendo-achilis. It is accompanied by the recurrent *tibial* vein and artery. By doing posterior tibial neurectomy, the object of plantar neurectomy also is achieved.

SITE
On the medial aspect of the leg, about a hands breadth above the point of the hock and ½ inch in front of tendo-achilis. (In the flexed position of the hock the nerve can be palpated under skin.)

TECHNIQUE
A cutaneous incision of 1 to 1½ inches is made along the course of the nerve. Extend the incision through the strong aponeurosis covering the nerve and expose it. Proceed as described for other neurectomies. Occasionally the nerve is seen branching into plantar nerves at this site. In that case both the branches are to be divided. (See also page 267)

CHAPTER 164

Plantar Tenotomy
(Sections of Perforans and
Perforatus Tendons) in Equine

INDICATIONS

Knuckling. If the fetlock only is involved, perforatus (superficial flexor) tenotomy will suffice.

ANATOMY

The flexor tendons are situated posterior to the suspensory ligament on the posterior aspect of the metacarpus/metatarsus. See under plantar neurectomy for details. The perforans tendon (deep digital flexor) is situated in front of the perforatus tendon (superficial digital flexor).

Plantar Tenotomy in Fore-limb

ANAESTHESIA AND CONTROL

Local infiltration; cast on the side of the affected limb. The upper fore-limb is taken backwards by a rope above the knee and is secured with the upper hind-limb above the hock.

SITE

The *inner* aspect of the limb, a little below the middle of metacarpus and along the anterior border of the tendon.

The inner aspect of the fore-limb is chosen because the large metacarpal artery which is close to the site can be seen and avoided. On the external aspect of the limb the corresponding vessel is the lateral volar metacarpal artery which is comparatively small.

TECHNIQUE

A cutaneous incision about 1½ inches long is made to identify the plantar nerve, large metacarpal artery and vein of the side. Keeping the fetlock and phalangeal joints flexed in order to relax the tendon, a blunt-pointed curved tenotome is introduced flatwise along the anterior border of the perforans (deep flexor) tendon until its point can be felt on the opposite side under the skin. The cutting edge is now turned against the tendon and with a sawing movement and the limb stretched, the tendon is divided. If the division is complete it leaves a gap and the snapping sound of cutting the tendon fibres can also be appreciated. If the knuckling is still not corrected, the *peroratus* (*superficial flexor*) *tendon* is also cut by the tenotome from behind forwards. The skin wound is sutured and the leg is immobilised in extension.

Plantar Tenotomy in Hind-limb

ANAESTHESIA AND CONTROL

Local anaesthesia; cast position. Hind-limb fixed together above the hock.

SITE

On the outer aspect of the limb about the middle of the metatarsus and along the lateral border of the tendon.

The outer aspect is chosen for easier access.

TECHNIQUE

Similar to the fore-limb.

CHAPTER 165

Cunean Tenotomy and Periosteotomy in Equine

INDICATIONS
Typical bone spavin lameness.

ANAESTHESIA AND CONTROL
Local anaesthesia; cast on the affected side.

ANATOMY
The cunean tendon is one of the two tendons of insertion of the flexor metatarsi (Tibialis anterior) muscle. It is situated on the medial aspect of the hock and it crosses the hock diagonally (from the supero-antero-internal aspect of the hock) to get inserted on to the cuneiform parvum (second tarsal) bone.

SITE
Medial aspect of the hock, in front of and in level with the chestnut. where the cunean tendon can be palpated.

TECHNIQUE
A 1 to 2 inches long vertical skin incision is made across the cunean tendon after palpating it. The cunean tendon is divided by sawing movement of the knife against the tarsal bones. The skin wound is sutured.

CHAPTER 166

Ligation of Digital Artery in Equine

INDICATIONS
Per-acute laminitis.

ANAESTHESIA AND CONTROL
Local or regional anaesthesia; standing or cast position.

SITE
The depression between the suspensory ligament and flexor tendons at the level of the button of the splint. The artery is between the vein and nerve.

TECHNIQUE
An inch long skin incision is made to locate the vessel which is picked up and ligatured.
Note: For a description of the Operation for the Removal of Lateral Cartilage of the Foot in Equine, see page-231.

CHAPTER 167

Peroneal Tenotomy (Boccar's Operation) in Equine

INDICATIONS
Stringhalt.

ANAESTHESIA AND CONTROL
Local anaesthesia; standing position.

ANATOMY
The peroneal tendon is the tendon of peroneus (lateral digital extensor) muscle. This tendon joins the tendon of the long digital extensor (extensor pedis) along proximal and antero-external aspect of the metatarsal region.

SITE
Supero-antero-external aspect of the upper third of the meta-tarsus before the lateral digital extensor tendon merges with the long digital extensor tendon.

TECHNIQUE
The lateral digital extensor tendon is palpated and a skin incision 1 inch long is made parallel to its posterior border. The tendon is divided with a tenotomy knife passed underneath in the usual manner. The skin wound is sutured to complete the operation.

CHAPTER 168

Docking (Amputation of Tail) in Equine

INDICATIONS

Fancy purpose, e.g., in carriage horses. Irreparable injury. Malignant disease. Paralysis.

ANAESTHESIA AND CONTROL

Local or epidural anaesthesia; standing position.

SITE

Above the seat of injury. In malignant disease and in paralysis of the tail amputation at the root of the tail. For fancy purposes enough length of tail is retained to cover the anus in the male and vulva in the female.

TECHNIQUE

The hair above the site of operation are turned up and bandaged. The hairs at the site of operation are clipped short and shaved clean. The distal part of tail is bandaged to avoid contamination. For other details see amputation of tail in the bovine.

CHAPTER 169

Epidural Anaesthesia in Equine

INDICATIONS

For desensitising the pelvis and hind part of body for surgical intervention.

ANAESTHESIA AND CONTROL

Local infiltration at the site; standing or cast position.

ANATOMY

The spinal cord in the horse extends only up to the level of the lumbosacral area (Conus Medullaris and Cauda Equina). The epidural injection is given posterior to this and therefore the solution does not get into the cerebrospinal fluid.

SITE

No. (1): Anterior site—Sacro-cococcygeal space. Move the tail up and down while palpating for the space between last sacral vertebra and the first coccygeal vertebra.

No. (2): Posterior site—First inter-coccygeal space (which is about 1 inch anterior to the first tail hairs at the level of the caudal folds immediately behind the first coccygeal spine). This can also be palpated as for site No. 1.

TECHNIQUE

A skin puncture is made at site with a hypodermic needle before introducing the epidural needle. About 1 cc of analgesic solution may be injected subcutaneously. Withdraw the hypodermic needle and the epidural needle with stillette in position is introduced in a direction at right angles to the fall of the tail. The required volume (as mentioned below) of a 1 to 2.5% solution of procaine solution is injected. The quantity injected varies according to the area to be anaesthetised.

In *anterior anaesthesia* the field of anaesthesia is more extensive whereas in *posterior anaesthesia* it is limited to the tail and hind-limbs only. The area anaesthetised will depend on the volume of solution injected in the epidural space so that if a arger volume is injected it travels more anteriorly and a larger area is therefore desensitised. (The terms anterior and posterior anaesthesia should be differentiated from anterior site and posterior site.) Quantity of solution required:—

For posterior anaesthesia: 15 to 20 cc of a 2% procaine solution.

For anterior anaesthesia: 30 to 80 cc of a 2% solution or 50 to 120 cc of a 1% solution of procaine.

For amputation of tail in foals 3 to 5 cc of a 2% solution is adequate.

Note: (1) While introducing the needle, bleeding may be encountered if the dorsal coccygeal vein is punctured. This can be ignored. (2) On either side within the vertebral canal and along the floor of it are the two basivertebral veins and their interconnecting branches located over the vertebral bodies. If the needle is introduced at an acute angle to touch on the floor of the vertebral canal, there is likelihood of puncturing one of these interconnecting branches, and blood may be seen escaping through the needle. In that case withdraw the needle slightly to get it out of the vein and then only inject the anaesthetic solution.

CHAPTER 170

Caponisation of Fowl (Chicken)

INDICATIONS

For fattening broiler cockerels and for improving the quality of meat. To prevent indiscriminate breeding. To avoid fighting among cockerels.

Best age for caponisation—Between third and fourth months, i.e. about six to eight weeks prior to slaughter for meat purpose.

ANAESTHESIA AND CONTROL

Local infiltration anaesthesia; lateral recumbency; the wings are spread and held backwards, two fingers are put around the base of neck, and the legs are held stretched backwards.

SITE

The last intercostal space. Incise close to the anterior border of the last rib.

Pre-operative preparation—The bird is preferably starved for about thirty hours prior to operation. The feathers in the region are plucked.

TECHNIQUE

The space between the last two ribs is palpated with the fingers. An inch long cutaneus incision is made parallel to the ribs. This intercostal space is covered by a thin strip of the muscle Tensor facia lata. It is retracted backward away from the site and a stab incision through the intercostal muscle (close to the anterior border to avoid the inter-costal vessels) of the last rib is made. A rib-retractor is used to dilate the opening. The parietal peritoneum is now torn with the caponising hook to see the maggot-like testes placed anterior to the kidney. (In older birds the testes are large, soft, yellowish bodies richly supplied with blood vessels.) Using the caponising forceps the testis is held and then removed as the forceps are withdrawn. (Damage to the posterior vena cava should be avoided.) The retractor is removed and the opening on the intercostal space gets automatically covered by the muscle strip when it is released. The wound on the skin need not be sutured (unless it is very big). The same procedure is repeated on the opposite side for removing the other testis. See also page 414

OVARIECTOMY (Ovariotomy; Oophorectomy)

Ovariectomy has little commercial application in meat production, but may be required for certain experiments. An ovariectomised female bird is called a "poulard".

The site and operative technique for ovariotomy are same as for caponisation. Note that the ovary in young birds may resemble the testis, but in older birds it might look like a bunch of grapes due to presence of developing ova. Only the left ovary may be available for removal, since the right one normally would have atrophied and disappeared in early embryonic life After removal of the left ovary, the right ovary may hypertrophy and produce androgens resulting in plumage changes of the bird; but subsequent production of oestrogens causes reversal of plumage changes. Occassionally, the ovary may also take up ovulatory function.

CHAPTER 171

Ingluviotomy (Incising the Crop) in Fowl (Chicken)

INDICATIONS

Impaction of the crop or ingluvius.

ANAESTHESIA AND CONTROL

The bird may either be lifted and held suspended by the pelvic limbs at a suitable height and the head and neck are stretched; or can better be placed in the lateral recumbent position; local infiltration anaesthesia.

ANATOMY

The crop (ingluvius) is a diverticulum of the oesophagus before it enters the thorax, at the base of the neck.

SITE

Base of the neck, over the distended crop.

TECHNIQUE

A longitudinal incision 1 to 2 inches long is made through the skin and wall of the crop. Contents are emptied. The incisions on the skin and crop are sutured separately by interrupted apposition sutures.

CHAPTER 172

Amputation or Dubbing of Comb and Wattles in Fowl (Chicken)

INDICATIONS

Amputation of either the comb or wattles or both becomes necessary when these structures are extra-large and interfere with movement of the head or feeding.

ANAESTHESIA AND CONTROL

Local or surface anaesthesia.

TECHNIQUE

To control bleeding, a series of mattress sutures passing through the thickness of the structure to be amputated is placed proximal to the level of amputation. Amputation is effected by cutting with scissors or scalpel distal to the line of sutures. Bleeding is little or absent, if the sutures are placed properly.

Note: In practice it is seen that no serious haemorrhage results even if the amputation is done without suturing.

APPENDIX 1

(Form of Soundness Certificate for Horse)

No............

CERTIFICATE

CERTIFIED that I have this day examined at the request of

....

(Name and address of the person on whose request the animal was examined)

................, a ...., ...

                    (colour)   *(breed)*

..................................., aged...............................

(horse/stallion/gelding/mare)

height...........................

The said..is

                      (horse/stallion/gelding/mare)

having ....

(mention here disease conditions or abnormalities, if any)

The said animal is in my opinion.................................

                         (sound/unsound)

Identification marks of the animal

(*Natural marks*)..

(*Artificial marks*)...

Signature............

Name of Veterinary Surgeon...........B.V.Sc.,

Official designation.............................

Place............   Address..

Date..............   ....

APPENDIX 2

(Specimen of Soundess Certificate for Horse)

No. 18/77

CERTIFICATE

Certified that I have this day examined a bay, Australian, gelding, aged eight years, height 19 hands.

The said gelding is having a small splint on the left fore-limb, outer aspect, away from knee.

The gelding is, in my opinion, sound.

Identification marks:—Star. Left hind pastern white.

Branded AQ

Sd/-

Anthicad,   Dr. C.N. Victor, B.V. Sc.
Dated: April 27, 1977.   Veterinary Surgeon,
                                       Anthicad.

APPENDIX 3

(Specimen of a Wound Certificate)

No. 7/77.

CERTIFICATE

This is to certify that I have this day examined at the request of *the Sub-Inspector of Police, Periamangalam, vide his letter No. 126/77 dated 18-4-77, a brown, Scindhi, cow, aged about five years,* sent to me in charge of *Police Constable No. 187, Sri. M. Chinnappan,* belonging *as stated in the letter* to *Sri. N. K. Vasudevan.*

 _ The said *cow* is found to have the following injuries: --

1. *Abrasions on abdomen, left side,*
2. *Wound, three inches long and half-an-inch deep on left thigh.*

I am of opinion that the *abrasions* could be caused by *the animal falling or rubbing against a rough surface and that the wound could be caused by a sharp object.*

In my opinion, the injuries mentioned are *not in the normal course serious enough to cause death of the cow.*

Identification marks of the animal :—

Horns, two numbers, both symmetrical, directed outward and upward, four inches long;

A star on the forehead.

Branded 234.

Sd/-

Periakulam,   Dr. P. E. Ahmed, B.V.Sc.
Dated: April 20, 1977.   Veterinary Surgeon
                                 Periakulam.

Some Terms Derived from Latin, Greek and French

ad hoc (L) for this special purpose.

ad interim (L) for the meantime.

ad manum (L) at hand, ready.

ad modum (L) after the manner (of).

ad nauseum (L) to the pitch of producing disgust.

ad referendum (L) to be further considered.

ad valorem (L) according to value.

ad vivum (L) to the life; life-like.

arbitrium (L) power of decision.

bona fides (L) good faith.

dei gratia (L) the grace of God.

de facto (L) in actual fact; really; actual.

de jure (Fr) by right, rightful.

de luxe (L) sumptuous.

de mal en pis (Fr) from bad to worse.

de novo (Fr) anew.

de mode (Fr) out of fashion.

D.V. (deo volente) (L) God willing.

en face (Fr) in front; in the face.

en masse (Fr) in a body.

ergon (Gr) work; business.

exceptio confirmat regulum (L) the exception proves the rule.

ex consequenti (L) by way of consequence.

ex gratia (L) as an act of grace.

ex officio (L) by virtue of his office.

ex parte (L) on one side; as a partisan.

extra modum (L) beyond measure; extravagant.

hoc anno (L) in this year.

hoc loca (L) in this place.

in absentia (L) in absence.

in malem partem (L) in unfavourable manner.

in situ (L) in the original situation.

inter alia (L) among other things

in toto (L) entirely.

in transitu (L) on passage.

in vitro (L) in glass.

in vivo (L) in the living organism

mutatis mutantis (L) with necessary changes.

APPENDIX 5

Some Abbreviations Used in Scientific Literature

anon. anonymous.

c., ca.—circa. (L) "about" used before approximate dates.

cf.—confer. (L) compare.

chap. chapter(s).

col., cols. column(s).

ed.
eds. }—editor(s), edition(s), edited by.

et al.—et alii (L) and others.

et seq—et sequens (L)
seqq— sequentia (L) } and the following.

f.
ff. } added to mean "and also the following page(s) or line(s)".

fig.
figs. } figure(s)

ibid.—ibidem. (L) the same place. This is used in place of a "ditto" when referring to some author and his work immediately above but not beyond that. If the page number in the work is different, *ibid* is followed by the page number. Dont use with name of author. Examples: *ibid.*, p-18.

illus. illustration(s), illustrated, illustrator.

loc. cit.—loco citato (L) the place cited. Refers to a specific passage cited much earlier than those referred immediately preceding. This abbreviation is used only to avoid repetition of title and page, and cannot replace name of author. Example: Wright, *loc. cit.*

n. d. no date on the book.

no.
nos. } number(s).

n.p. no place of publication.

op. cit.—opere citato. (L) in the work cited. Reference to a book previously cited but not immediately preceding. Used only in place of title only; authors name and page number to be suffixed. Example: Wright, *op. cit.*, p. 123.

p.
pp. } page(s).

par.
pars. } paragraph(s).

et passim. (L) here and there throughout the work. Means that whatever is referred to appears in various places in the book and not continuously. Example: Wright, pp. 14, 18, 21, *et passim.*

pl.
pls. } plate(s)

rev. ed. revised edition.

sic (L) thus. Used when there is some mistake in the material quoted by you which is there in the original. This abbreviation is noted within brackets after the quotation.

trans.—translation, translator, translated by.

vol.
vols. }—volume(s). The Roman numeral is used with this to indicate the volume number and the Arabic numeral when used to show total number of volumes. Example: Clinical Surgery, Vol. IV, 5 vols.

Cito totus salvus (L): Quick, complete, and safe.

APPENDIX 6

Cries of Animals

Cow—*bellow; moo*
Horse—*neighs*

Elephant—*trumpets*
Goose—*gaggle; cackle*

Donkey—*brays*
Dog—*barks*
Cat—*mews*; *purrs*
Sheep—*bleat*; *baa*
Pig—*squeal*; *grunt*

Duck—*quacks*
Hen—*cackle*; *cluck*
Chick—*peep*
Cock—*crows*
Monkey—*gibber*.

APPENDIX 7

Some Terms Pertaining to Animals

Stallion: Horse not castrated, male.
Gelding: A castrated horse, male.
Colt: Young horse, male.
Filly: Young horse, female.
Foal: Young one of a horse.
Bull: Male bovine, not castrated.
Bullock (Steer): Male bovine, castrated.
Ram (Tup): Male sheep, not castrated.
Ewe: Female sheep.
Wether (Wedder): Male sheep, castrated.
Lamb: Young sheep.
Buck: Male goat, not castrated.
Doe: Female goat.
Boar: Male pig, non-castrated.
Sow: Female pig.
Hog (Stag; Barrow): Male pig, castrated.
Gilt: Female young pig.
Farrowing: Parturition of the sow.
Whelping: Parturition of bitch.

Groups of Animals

Cattle—Herd
Sheep—Flock
Pig—Herd; Drove; Stock
Goat—Flock; Band

Fish—Shoal; School
Geese—Gaggle

Animal Houses

Cattle—Stall; Cow-shed; Bull-shed
Horse—Stable
Dog—Kennel
Sheep—Pen; Fold
Pig—Sty
Chicken—Coop
Rabbit—Hutch
Fish—Aquarium

APPENDIX 8

Number of Vertebrae in Different Species

Species	C	T	L	S	Cy	Total
Horse	7	18	6	5	15–21	51–57
Cattle	7	13	6	5	18–20	49–51
Dog	7	13	7	3	20–23	50–53
Goat	7	13	6–7	4	16–18	46–49
Pig	7	14–15	6–7	4	20–23	51–56
Elephant	7	19–20	4–5	4–5	26–30	60–67
Human	7	12	5	5	4	33

Note: The number of vertebrae in the goat is variable, except for the cervical vertebrae.

Number of Pairs of Ribs

Species	Sternal	A-sternal	Total
Horse	8	10	18
Cattle	8	5	13
Dog	9	3 + 1	13
Goat	8	5–6	13–14
Pig	7	7–8	14–15
Elephant	4	15–16	19–20
Human	7	5	12

Note: The last pair of ribs in dog and goat, being not connected to sternum directly or by cartilage, are called 'floating ribs'.

The head of the first rib articulates between last cervical and first thoracic vertebrae.

Conversion Table

Farenheit $= \frac{9}{5}$ C + 32.

Celsius (Centigrade) $=$ (F $-$ 32) $\times \frac{5}{9}$

Celsius	—	Farenheit (Approx.)
35	—	95
36	—	96.8
37	—	98.6
38	—	100.4
39	—	102.2
40	—	104
41	—	105.8
42	—	107.6
43	—	109.4

SOME MODEL QUESTIONS FOR OBJECTIVE TESTS

Many colleges and Universities have adopted the system of objective assessment. An objective-type question paper is expected to contain not only questions testing memory, but also those testing other specific outcomes of learning. The general view seems to be that a well-set question paper should ideally contain distribution of marks as follows:

Knowledge	15%
Understanding	20%
Application	38%
Analysis	9%
Synthesis	6%
Judgement	12%

Total   100%

The setting up of a properly balanced and effective objective-type question paper requires great deal of expertise and a lot of thoughtful planning.

Innumerable varieties of objective-type question are available. Some examples are: (1) True or False, (2) Enumeration, (3) Completion, and (4) Multiple-Choice.

A few objective-type questions are given here. Answers are given to most of them, at the end of the paper, except for the enumerative and short-essay types.

1. Cataract is a degenerative condition of the lens, and not an inflammatory phenomenon:
   (a) True (b) False
2. Enumerate the causes of facial paralysis in the horse.
3. Exostosis of phalangeal bone is called_____ .

4. In an upward and forward (antero-dorsal) dislocation of the hip in cattle, there is_____of the affected limb.
   (a) Lengthening (b) Shortening
5. Which of the following tissue changes are *absent* in surgical shock?
   (a) Increase in total leucocyte count
   (b) Increase in potassium content of *tissue* cells
   (c) Acidosis
   (d) Increase in ammonia content of blood
6. The five cardinal signs of inflammation are: Rubor, Calor, ...
7. Rearrange the letters to make the correct word: RIEBDE-MNDET (pertains to wound treatment).
8. The head of a horse during progression is_____when his lame fore-foot is put to the ground.
   (a) Lowered (b) Raised
9. Wound healing may be impaired by:
   (a) Severe anaemia
   (b) Bacterial infection
   (c) Zinc deficiency
   (d) Lack of immobilization
   (e) All of the above
10. Identify the word or statement *not* related or *least* related to key words "Abscess formation":
    (a) Pyogenic membrane
    (b) Pyaemia
    (c) Fluctuation
    (d) Maturation or ripening
    (e) Oedema
11. The presence of the following even without lameness is unsoundness:
    (a) Spavin
    (b) Splints in a young animal
    (c) Ring bone
12. Irregular hard work is the most common cause of navicular disease:
    (a) True (b) False
13. Shoeing of horse should be done at every_____ week intervals.
    (a) One (b) Two (c) Three (d) Four

14. Wound healing may be impaired by:
    (a) Foreign bodies in the wound
    (b) Inadequate blood supply
    (c) Frequent movements
    (d) Malignant growths
    (e) All of the above
15. Shock may be classified into four types: Cardiogenic,
    _____, _____ and _____.
16. It takes_____for the complete growth of new horn
    replacement of horse foot from the coronet.
    (a) One year (b) three months
    (c) three weeks (d) nine months.
17. The essential phenomena in shock are:
    (a) Increase in the vascular bed
    (b) Decrease in effective volume of blood in circulation
    (c) Imbalance between vascular bed and effective volume
        of blood in circulation
    (d) None of the above
18. Choking in cattle usually occurs at_____of oesophagus.
    (a) Upper third   (b) middle third
    (c) lower third   (d) gastro-oesophageal junction.
19. An ulcer is _____.
20. Which of the following is *not* a feature of hypovolemic
    shock?
    (a) Bradycardia   (b) Mental dullness
    (c) Tachycardia   (d) Peripheral vasoconstriction.
21. Identify the incorrect statement (or, the least related) to the
    key word:
    Atrophy: (a) Loss of innervation
             (b) Total loss of blood supply
             (c) Disuse
             (d) Diminished blood supply.
22. X-rays have their greatest harmful effects upon:
    (a) gonadal tissue   (b) skin
    (c) liver   (d) lung
    (e) bone.
23. In bovine rumenotomy what tissues are incised?
24. An open wound can be managed best during:
    (a) first week of injury
    (b) first six hours of injury

(c) first 12 hours of injury

(d) first day of injury.

25. Mark the sentence *least* related to the statement given:
Second intention healing differs from first intention healing in that:

(a) Takes more than two weeks to heal

(b) Healing by replacement of tissue

(c) Healing by granulation

(d) Takes less time to heal.

26. Failure of the cow to adduct the limb following the act
of parturition is due to injury to the following nerve:

(a) Femoral   (b) Obturator

(c) Anterior gluteal   (d) Radial.

27. Which of the following are most concerned in healing of
wounds?

(a) Vitamin-A   (b) Vitamin-C

(c) Vitamin-E   (d) Vitamin-B complex.

28. What is the age of a heifer when the two central incisors
are shed and replaced by permanents?

(a) Two years   (b) Four years

(c) Six months.

29. The most common type of coxo-femoral dislocation in
cattle is:

(a) Upward and forward (Antero-dorsal)

(b) Obturator dislocation

(c) Antero-medial

(d) Postero-dorsal

(e) Antero-ventral.

30. The space chosen for epidural anaesthesia in dog is:

(a) Sacro-coccygeal   (b) Lumbo-sacral

(c) Inter-coccygeal.

31. Calculi comprising *phosphates* of Ca/Mg/NH_4 are seen in
_____ urine.

32. Calculi made up of *oxalates* and *carbonates* of Ca/Mg/
NH_4 are seen in_____urine.

33. In a radiograph of horse foot in laminitis, one should
observe_____.

34. What is the best treatment of a valuable young cow with
a long-standing case of hygroma of the knee?

(a) Firing

(b) Extirpation

(c) Aspiration of contents

(d) Lancing (incision) and drainage

(e) Antiphlogistics.

35. Debridement of wound means:

(a) Excising the dead muscles

(b) Laying open all the layers of wound, excising of dead tissue, and thorough cleaning and dressing of the wound.

(c) Excising the dead skin.

36. Muscles paralysed in case of radial nerve injury are......

37. Enumerating-type questions similar to above may be asked with reference to Facial/Crural/Poplitial nerve injuries.

38. Match the statement/words *least* related to the key-words:

Acidic urine: (a) Ammonium carbonate

(b) Magnesium oxalate

(c) Calcium phosphate

(d) Magnesium carbonate.

39. To eliminate the problem of inguinal hernia in a herd of swine, it is better to   because it is inherited.

40. The posterior chamber of the eye is between_____.

41. The so called _____ is the most important diagnostic symptom of rupture of cruciate ligaments of stifle.

42. The "anterior drawer sign" manifested by forward gliding of tibia in the dog is diagnostic of rupture of_____cruciate ligament of stifle.

43. "Posterior drawer sign" is indicative of rupture of_____cruciate ligament.

44. The_____muscle forms the superior border of jugular furro in bovine.

45. The ventral border of the jugular furro in anterior one-third of the neck of horse is formed by _____muscle.

46. The fundamental cause of ranula is:

(a) Stenosis of duct   (b) Congenital anomalies

(c) Calculi   (d) Inflammation

(e) Traumatic injury.

47. Match the following:

A. Fibrosarcoma   P. Eye

B. Melanoma   Q. Grey horse

C. Epulis   R. Pharynx, bovine
D. Dermoid cyst   S. Alveolar periosteum
E. Adenoma   T. Glands
F. Perineal hernia   U. Dog.

48. In gastritis and pericarditis there are several symptoms which are similar; one differentiating symptom is_____.

49. Emergency splinting of fractured bone avoids_____.

50. Unilateral paralysis of lips is due to paralysis of_____ nerve.

51. Posterior dislocation of hip is characterised by:
    (a) Flexion, adduction and external rotation of hip joint
    (b) Flexion, adduction and internal rotation of hip joint
    (c) Flexion, abduction and internal rotation of hip joint
    (d) Only external rotation of hip joint.

52. In a calf with only one testicle in the scrotum, where will the other testicle most commonly be located?

53. In intervertebral disc disease of dog_____paralysis of hind limb is seen when the lesion involves middle and posterior lumbar discs.

54. Dog with spastic paralysis of hind limb is suspected of showing lesions in_____ part of spinal cord.

55. Locked jaw is seen in:
    (a) Rabies   (b) Tetanus
    (c) Dislocation of
        maxillary joint   (d) Trigeminal paralysis.

56. Fracture healing stages are (4 No.): . . . . . .

57. In cases of dislocation of shoulder in cattle, the head of humerus usually dislocates, in relation to glenoid cavity:
    (a) Upward and forward   (b) Anterior
    (c) Lateral   (d) Posterior
    (e) Superior.

58. In chronic subluxation of patella in cattle, the severity of lameness_____with exercise.

59. Divergent squint is seen due to paralysis of_____ muscle of the eye.

60. Intestinal gangrene may be caused by:
    (a) Incarcerated hernia   (b) Strangulated hernia
    (c) Volvulus   (d) Intusussception
    (e) All of the above.

61. Which of the following is *not* likely to happen in posterior dislocation of hip?
    (a) Sciatic nerve injury
    (b) Femoral nerve injury
    (c) Fracture of the rim of acetabulum
    (d) Avascular necrosis of femoral head.
62. In a dog showing abdominal breathing, short gasping breaths, and tucked up abdomen, the most logical thing to suspect would be:
    (a) Diaphragmatic hernia
    (b) Interstitial pneumonia
    (c) Lobar pneumonia
    (d) Pneumothorax.
63. The site for epidural anaesthesia in cattle is_____.
64. The chief cause of maxillary sinusitis in horse is_____.
65. Debridement of a wound is performed for what reason?
    (a) Cosmetic
    (b) Straighten suture line
    (c) Prevent infection
66. To make a confirmatory diagnosis of navicular disease, _____ nerve block is used.
    (a) median   (b) posterior digital
    (c) volar   (d) Ulnar
    (e) plantar.
67. The underlying cause for a pathological fracture may be:
    (a) Metabolic disorders
    (b) Infection
    (c) Malignancy
    (d) Any of the above.
68. The origin of cancer eye in cattle usually is from:
    (a) Lower lid and membrana nictitans
    (b) the orbit
    (c) the eye ball.
69. While administering epidural anaesthesia, the anaesthetic solution is injected into:
    (a) Sub-arachnoid space
    (b) Extradural space
    (c) Spinal cord
    (d) Subdural space.

70. Endotoxic shock is usually produced by:
    (a) E. coli   (b) Pseudomonas
    (c) Staphylococcus   (d) Streptococcus.

71. The X-ray view used to show anterior or posterior subluxation of tibia at the stifle joint is:
    (a) Antero-posterior
    (b) Lateral
    (c) Lateral with angle of cone tilted at 45 degrees
    (d) Medial
    (e) Postero-anterior.

72. In spaying a bitch through the mid-ventral site, the_____ ovary is comparatively easier to get at than the other ovary.

73. Catgut is prepared from the submucous layer of the intestine of:
    (a) Rabbit   (b) Cat
    (c) Sheep   (d) Horse
    (e) None of the above.

74. The binding material in wound healing is laid down by:
    (a) Blood vessels surrounding the wound
    (b) Fibroblasts
    (c) Eı dothelial cells
    (d) Epithelial cells.

75. The commonest organism of infection in an accidental wound is:
    (a) E. coli   (b) Staphylococcus
    (c) Pseudomonas   (d) Streptococcus
    (e) Pneumococcus.

76. In a surgical wound with imperfect aseptic precautions, infection usually appears during_____week post-operatively.

77. Citrated whole blood has an advantage over physiological saline in treating shock because:
    (a) It adds leucocytes to ward off infection
    (b) It maintains circulating fluid volume over a longer period of time
    (c) It supplies RBCs and increases the oxygen carrying capacity.
    (d) It provides added protein which replaces depleted supplies.

78. An "antibioma" is:
    (a) A tumour due to prolonged use of antibiotics
    (b) An antibiotic
    (c) An abscess treated with antibiotics and having excessive fibrous tissue around it
    (d) None of the above.

79. Maximum period for which a tourniquet may be applied safely for obtaining bloodless field in a limb is:
    (a) Thirty minutes
    (b) One hour and thirty minutes
    (c) One hour
    (d) Two hours
    (e) Any length of time till the operation continues
    (f) Twenty-four hours post-operatively.

80. In the normal bovine, jugular pulse is due to_____

81. The term "enzymatic debridement" is used for cleaning a wound with:
    (a) Hyaluronidase
    (b) Hydrogen peroxide
    (c) Streptokinase
    (d) None of the above.

82. Stenson's duct drains:
    (a) Sebaceous gland   (b) Parotid gland
    (c) Lacrymal gland   (d) Submandibular gland.

83. Ranula is:
    (a) A transparent, cystic swelling in the floor of the mouth
    (b) A renal tumour
    (c) A renal calculus
    (d) None of the above.

84. Which of the following renal stone does *not* cast shadow in plain X-ray:
    (a) Phosphate   (b) Uric acid
    (c) Oxalate   (d) None.

85. In a normal animal_____of total cardiac output of blood goes to brain.

86. Spot out the *incorrect* from the following:
    Atropine as a preanaesthetic agent:
    (a) reduces vagal effect on heart
    (b) induces sleep

(c) raises body temperature

(d) reduces bronchial secretions.

Answers

1. (a).
2. See page 205.
3. Ring bone.
4. (b).
5. (b).
6. Tumor, Dolar, and Vascular and exudative changes.
7. Debridement.
8. (b).
9. (e).
10. (c).
11. All three—(a), (b), and (c).
12. (a).
13. (c).
14. (e).
15. Vasogenic, Haematogenic, Neurogenic.
16. (d).
17. (c).
18. (a).
19. An inflammatory lesion of the skin or mucous membrane with loss of surface epithelium.
20. (a).
21. (b).
22. (a).
23. Skin, subcutaneous facia, external oblique abdominal muscle, internal oblique abdominal muscle, transverse abdominal muscle, parietal peritoneum, and ruminal wall.
24. (b).
25. (d).
26. (b).
27. (b).
28. (a).
29. (a).
30. (b).
31. Alkaline.
32. Acidic.
33. Relationship of third phalanx to hoof-wall.
34. (b).
35. (b).
36. Triceps brachii, and the extensors of the carpus and digits.
37. Vide pages 210 to 211 of text.
38. (c).
39. Change the breeding stock.
40. Iris and lens.
41. "Drawer sign"
42. Anterior.
43. Posterior.
44. Bracheo-cephalicus.
45. Sterno-cephalicus.
46. (b).
47. A-R; B-Q; C-S; D-P; E-T; F-U.
48. A distended jugular vein

with an evident pulse with
Swelling of sternum and
brisket.
49. Further trauma to tissues.
50. Facial.
51. (b).
52. Subcutaneously alongside
the penis.
53. Flaccid.
54. Anterior lumbar.
55. (b).
56. Formation of haematoma,
formation of soft callus,
formation of primary bone
callus, and formation of
secondary bone callus and
functional reconstruction.
57. (a).
58. Diminishes.
59. Internal (or medial) rectus.
60. (e).
61. (b).
62. (a).
63. Sacro-coccygeal/inter-
coccygeal.

64. Tooth infection.
65. (c).
66. (b).
67. (d).
68. (a).
69. (b).
70. (a).
71. (b).
72. left.
73. (c).
74. (b).
75. (b).
76. Second.
77. (b).
78. (c).
79. (b).
80. Rotation of the heart to
the right upon each
contraction.
81. (c).
82. (b).
83. (a).
84. (b).
85. *One-sixth*.
86. (b).

ADDENDUM TO PAGE 419

Pinioning in Birds

Pinioning is an operation on the wing of bird to prevent it from flying. It should be done only on one of the wings (and not on both wings), so as to make the bird incapable of maintaining the balance while attempting to fly.

METHODS

1. Temporary pinioning is done by plucking away or cutting off sufficient number of primary feathers of the wing (i.e., the so called flight feathers on the caudal border of the wing). In about 2 to 3 months the operation may have to be repeated, as the feathers regenerate.

2. Permanent pinioning can be done by tenotomy/neurectomy, but a better and more efficient and safe method is amputation of the distal portion of the wing as described below.

AMPUTATION

After plucking the feathers at the tip of the wing, the first digit or alula is located. Lateral to the articulation of the first digit, the carpometacarpus can be palpated. (The carpometacarpus which appears as two long bones fused together at their extremities enclosing a large interosseousspace between them, actually comprises the second, third, and fourth metacarpal bones).

The distal two-third of the carpometacarpus is to be amputated, without causing any damage to the adjacent first digit.

In small birds, amputation can be done by snipping off with a scissors and bleeding can be stopped by clamping with a haemostat. It is preferable to do the operation at a young age when the bird is less than a week-old. While doing in large adult birds, a tourniquet/ligature is desirable to control bleeding. The tourniquet/ligature can be passed through the interosseous space using sutureneedle, to make it more secure. Suturing the stump with a skin flap can be done, but is unnecessary even in large birds. The application of a suitable flyrepellant antiseptic to the wound is sufficient.

ADDENDUM TO PAGE 50

Treatment for snake-bite: The rational treatment is administration of polyvalent anti-venom which is effective against cobra, krait and viper venoms. It is available from Haffkine Institute, Bombay, in vials of 10 ml. and can be preserved at room temperature upto five years. The antivenom is administered slowly, mixed with saline, as a drip. Since anaphylactic reactions are common, it is advisable to keep simultaneously another intravenous needle and apparatus ready *in situ* for adrenaline administration. When anaphylactic reactions are noticed, the administration of antivenom is temporarily stopped and adrenaline is given. After the reaction is controlled, antivenom administration is re-started. A number of vials of antivenom will be required to treat a case as the administration must continue until symptoms of snake-bite are subsided.

ADDENDUM TO PAGE 197

Femoro-tibial luxation in the dog: Complete luxation is uncommon, but subluxations due to rupture of any of the following 4 ligaments may occur:
1. In Anterior (lateral) cruciate ligament rupture, what is called '*anterior drawer sign*' is noticed when the tibia is gently moved forward and backward keeping the femur fixed with the stifle in a semi-flexed state. The tibia can thus be manipulated only forwards and not backwards.
2. This is in contrast to the '*posterior drawer sign*' made

possible in similar manipulations in a case of posterior (medial) cruciate ligament.

3. In lateral collateral ligament rupture, medial and abductive movements of tibia are possible.
4. The rupture of medial collateral ligament of the femorotibial joint, permits only lateral and abductive movements of tibia.

Treatment: Surgical replacement of the ruptured ligament using facia, vide Leonard (1960).

ADDENDUM TO PAGE 425

Atropine: Available as 'Atropine sulphate injection' in 1 c.c (1 ml.) ampoules containing 0.065 gramme (65 mg.) of the drug. (i.e., 1/100 grain per millilitre). It may be given either subcutaneously or intramuscularly, in the following doses: Cat: $\frac{1}{2}$ ml.; Pig/Dog : $\frac{1}{2}$ to 2 ml. If quicker action is needed, intravenous or intraperitoneal injections may be done in half the above dose recommended for subcutaneous/intramuscular use.

ADDENDUM TO PAGE 638

Conversion Table for Weights:

	Imperial system (Apothecary)		Metric system
1 ounce (8 drachms)	(480 grains)	. . .	30 grammes.
1 drachm (60 grains)		. . .	4 grammes.
1 grain		. . .	65 mg.
			(0.065 grammes).

Conversion Table for Measures:

Imperial system	*Metric system*
1 minim	. . . 0.06 c.c. (0.06 ml.)
17 minims	. . . 1 c.c. (1 ml.)
1 fluid drachm	. . . 3.5 ml.
1 fluid ounce	. . . 28.5 ml.
1 pint (20 fluid ounces)	. . . 568 ml.
1 pint and 15 fluid ounces	. . . 1 Litre (1000 ml.)

Equivalents of Domestic Measures:

Domestic measure	*Imperial system*	*Metric system*
1 teaspoon	. . . 1 fluid drachm	. . . 3.5 ml.
1 dessertspoon	. . . 2 fluid drachm	. . . 7 ml.
1 tablespoon	. . . 4 fluid drachms	
	($\frac{1}{2}$ ounce) . . .	14 ml.

ADDENDUM TO PAGE 74

The following note may be added under the last para of page-74:

Note: In Heat-stroke the skin turns dry; whereas in Heat-exhaustion the skin goes moist. Both are medical emergencies. Heat-stroke demands urgent lowering of temperature as the first step, whereas Heat-exhaustion requires immediate fluid and salt replacement.

ADDENDUM TO PAGE 40

Contusions and *bruises* are treated initially with cold and astringent applications, to minimise extravasation. On the first day ice packs may be applied for about fifteeen minutes each time and repeated after an interval of another fifteen minutes. From the second day onwards, warm fomentations and topical application of ointments containing heparin (e.g. THROMBOPHOB), Iodex, etc., may help reabsorption of the extravasations.

ADDENDUM TO PAGE 42

(*After the first para*) Certain chemical dressings may in individual cases cause excessive granulation tissue formation. Frequent shifting from one chemical dressing to another is to be done with caution. Some owners sprinkle talcum powder on the wounds of their pets. This is not advisable because the Magnesium silicate contained in it stimulates formation of excessive granulations. Excessive granulation tissue formation in wounds (exuberant granulation or *'proud flesh'*), is also referred to as *'granuloma'*, although it is not a tumour in the real sense of the term.

ADDENDUM TO PAGE 47

(*Under treatment of maggot wounds*) A single subcutaneous injection of Ivermectin (Brand name: IVOMAC), which is a drug used against both endo-and ecto-parasites, is reportedly effective in eliminating maggots. Available as 10 mg. per ml. solution *Dose* : Dogs: lml. ; Cattle, goat, sheep: lml. per kg body weight; subcutaneously.

ADDENDUM TO PAGE 99

(*Under the subheading 'Acne'*) Acne is commonly known as *pimples* in human medicine, affecting mostly face, rarely the skin of shoulders, back and chest. It may be in the form of white-heads, black-heads, red bumps, cysts, or pustules (pus-pimples). The primary cause is occlusion of sebacious glandducts. Complications are due to infections, which usually result from expressing the contents under unhygienic conditions. The contents are called "comedones".

ADDENLUM TO PAGE 123

(*Under paragraph third*) Typically, sprain of a joint is a partial rupture of the joint capsule or any of its ligaments, without luxation of bones. Usually caused by over-extension/over-flexion of the joint. However, the term sprain is also used to denote partial rupture of tendons, as for example, sprain of flexor tendons. The term *strain*, though used in place of sprain, strictly confines to partial rupture of muscle fibres, due to overextension or overflexion.

ADDENDUM TO PAGE 397

(*Under treatment for Conjunctivitis*) Eye preparations (drops and ointments) containing corticosteroids may cause sudden and marked rise in intraocular pressure in a few individuals, whereas in others it may only cause a mild rise and that too only if treatment is prolonged for two weeks or more. In any case, topical corticoste-roids for the eye should not be used for more than one or two weeks for fear of complications like thinning of cornea and perforation of cornea, glaucoma, cataract, fungal infections, etc.

ADDENDUM TO PAGE 143

(*After the third para*) Some of the diagnostic imaging procedures, other than simple radiography dealt with in this chapter, are listed below:

1. *Computerised Axial Tomographic System (Popularly called 'CAT scanner' or 'CT scanner'):* The CT-scanner equipment has an array of circularly arranged detectors for measuring the penetrating X-rays absorbed by the exposed part of the patient, in multiple directions. These transmission readings are then converted to electrical signals which are processed and constructed by a computer. Using a narrow beam of x-ray source, the computer delivers the picture of the exposed body part in the form of several slices. Thus, true anatomical cross-sectional images of any desired area of the body can be obtained.

The x-ray radiation received by the patient in CT-scanning is *lesser* than in conventional radiography. In conventional radiography, only bones are clearly seen; In CT-scan three-dimentional pictures of bones as well as soft tissues and fluids are obtained which enables diagnosis of tumours of the brain, blood clots in the brain, hydrocephalus, extent of brain injury, etc.

2. *Positron Emission Transaxial Tomography (PETT):* In basic principles 'PETT-scan' is related to 'CAT-scan'. But while CAT-scan illuminates only bone and some of the soft tissues, PETT-scan presents more detailed information about them including their metabolic functioning and extent of damage, if any.

The assessment of tissue changes is made possible by using a particular type of radioisotope introduced into the tissues. The radioisotope emits positive charged electrons (Positrons) which attach themselves to glucose and other substances connected with tissue metabolism and thus become witnesses to tissue activity.

PETT-scanning has been used in human medicine specially for diagnosis of brain diseases like Alzheimer's disease, Schisophrenia, and Epilepsy.

PETT-scan is at present very costly and is beyond the reach of common man.

3. *Magnetic Resonance Imaging (MRI):* In MRI, the part to the imaged is exposed to very high magnetic field, which is about 10,000 times over that of the earth's. (Magnetic field is expressed as *'Tesla'* units or *'Gauss'* units or *'Oersteds'* units, named after the respective scientists. One *Tesla* is equivalent to 10,000 *Gauss* units or 10,000 *Oersteds*. The magnetic power of the earth is about one-third *Gauss*. MRI machines available vary in their capacities in the range of 0.02 to 2 *Tesla*.)

MRI is based on the principle called 'Nuclear Magnetic Resonance' (NMR). The cells of the body contain hydrogen atoms. And when body tissues are exposed to very high magnetic fields (over 10,000 times more than that of the earth), there will be sudden movements of the protons of the hydrogen atoms and they align themselves corresponding to the direction of the magnetic field. In the MRI-scanner, this temporary magnetisation of protons brought about by electromagnetic radiation of appropriate frequency, is reversed when the radio-frequency pulse is stopped; and then the protons will go back to align themselves in the original direction, though with a different velocity. This difference in velocity is analysed by powerful computers in the scanner equipment and based on that an image is produced.

There are differences between the proton NMR parameters of different tissues and also between same tissue of varying densities, and between normal and malignant tissues. This facilitates necessary tissue contrast in the image obtained.

There are three types of MRI equipments depending on the type of magnets used, viz., (1) Fixed magnet, (2) Electrical magnet, and (3) Low temperature superconductivity magnet. Of these three, the last mentioned type is the most efficient and costliest. Electromagnetic conductivity is increased as the temperature is lowered, and liquid helium or liquid nitrogen is used to lower temperature to as low as –269 degrees Celsius. Since the Helium evaporates very fast, it has to be replenished every three months or so.

The cost of an MRI-scanner is about 2 to 3 times more than that of a CT-scanner; but it has the following advantages:

(1) MRI produces sharper and clearer images with better tissue contrast;
(2) Pictures can be obtained in almost any plane without moving the patient;
(3) The technique is non-invasive, since no contrast media are required;
(4) There is no fear of radiation hazards because X-rays are not used; and
(5) No harmful effects have been reported so far for exposure to high magnetic field and it is safe for even pregnant women and children.

MRI is specially indicated in the investigation of diseases of the brain, spinal cord, musculo-skeletal system and blood vessels. However, patients with cardiac pacemakers, aneurism-clips, or such other metalic devices cannot be subjected to MRI for obvious reasons. Patients, technicians or others going near the equipment should not also wear or carry any materials susceptible to magnetic attraction.

4. *Ultrasonography:* This is a diagnostic procedure using sound waves. The ultrasonographic machines produce waves having velocity over 20,000 Hertz. Sound waves, like light waves, are governed by the laws of refraction and reflexion. The amount of reflexion while passing through a structure depends on: the thickness and type of structure, the frequency of the waves and, the angle of striking the structure. The mismatch between different structures in a given part of body provides their differentiation in imaging. Maximum information is provided when the beam hits the imaging structure at 90 degrees.

The advantages of ultrasonography as compared to radiography are: (1) better delineation of soft tissues; (2) absolutely safe, according to present knowledge, even in early stages of pregnancy; and (3) not very expensive.

Ultrasonography is generally used: (1) for detecting abnormalities of heart, uterus, pancreas, bladder, liver, stomach, kidneys, etc.; and (2) for detection of developmental stages and abnormalities of foetus. However, it cannot be used to study the lungs because the waves cannot penetrate the air present in the lungs. Bones, except their cartilaginous stages in the foetus, cannot also be studied by ultrasonography.

5. *Echocardiography* is ultrasonography as applied to the heart. It enables heart sounds to be 'seen', rather than heard, that too much more distinctly than heard with the stethoscope. The echo of the ultrasound waves passes into the heart and are converted into electricity by the machine and recorded on special photographic paper or ultraviolet paper. These recordings are called echocardiographs. An echocardiograph indicates three different factors, viz., the size and amplitude of the waves (A); the brightness (B); and the movement (M). To make a thorough study, these three factors are to be properly assessed.

ADDENDUM TO PAGE 567

Note : When ovariohysterectomy is performed in the bitch to avoid estrus and pregnancy, some Veterinarians have reported incomplete success due to the bitch still exhibiting estral bleeding, to the great annoyance of the owner. As such, the following additional points are worth remembering while performing the operation:

1. Preoperative starving for about twelve hours should be insisted. If the subject is weak or debilitated, you may resort to parenteral nutritive measures, but dont compromise on this prior starving.

2. Use general anaesthesia, and supplement it, if necessary, with muscle relaxants to reassure complete relaxation of abdominal muscles.

3. During surgery if you experience difficulty in pulling the ovary towards the abdominal incision, dont exert too much traction, as it may result in rupture of the ovarian artery and uncontrollable bleeding. Instead, first rupture the ovarian ligament with your fingers, or with a long curved scissors. (The scissors should be

properly guided with fingers to avoid accidental injury to adjacent vessels).

4. After the ovarian ligament is so severed, clamp the ovarian artery and vein together, with a long, curved hemostatic forceps, as much anterior to the ovary as possible. Ligature the vessels close to and anterior to the forceps. Clamp another haemostatic forceps behind the first one and cut between the two forceps for releasing the ovary for the remaining part of the operation.

5. The ovarian bursa is an antomical peculiarity in the canine species, and we can remove the ovary with or without its bursa. The leaving behind part of the bursa (vide technique mentioned above in the text), is an additional safeguard against slipping of the ligature on the ovarian vessels when the haemostat is removed. But the disadvantage in this method is the chance of leaving back part of the ovarian tissue unless the surgeon is quite skilful and careful. Whereas, in the other method of removal with the bursa, though devoid of the additional safeguard to the ligature, there is no chance of leaving back any part of the ovary. You can choose any of these two methods, considering the merits and demerits of each, and the suitability in every individual case.

6. If you could not succeed in removing the ovary completely, in spite of all the care taken, and the patient returns to you with the complaint of estral bleeding (which could happen even after months or years depending on the regeneration and multiplication of the left off ovarian tissue), there is the possibility of trying hormonal therapy to prevent/suppress the estrus.

REFERENCES

Adams, O.R. (1962). *Lameness in horses*. Lea & Febiger, Philadelphia.

Allen, James H. (1963). *Mayo's diseases of the eye*. William Wilkins Company, Baltimore.

Barger, Edger H., Card, Leslie B., and Pomery, B.S. (1958). *Diseases and parasites of poultry*. 5th ed. Scientific Book Agency, 22-Raja Woodmunt, Calcutta-1. pp. 56–70.

Barton-Wright, E.C. (1978). *Arthritis—a vitamin deficiency disease*. Roberts Publications (HHE), London.

Berge, Ewald and Westhues, Melchior. (Translated by Siller, Walter G., and Fraser, J.A.) (1966). *Veterinary operative surgery*. Medical Book Company, 7-Aaboulevard, Copenhagen.

Bojrab, M. Joseph (Ed.) (1975). *Current techniques in small animal surgery*. Lea & Febiger, Philadelphia.

Bradley, O.C. (1948). *Topographic anatomy of the dog*. 5th ed. Oliver & Boyd., London.

Burrows, W.H. (1936). The surgical removal of the gizzard from the domestic fowl. *Poultry Sci.*, 15: 290–293.

Carlson, William D. (1961). *Veterinary radiology*. Lea & Febiger., Philadelphia.

Cole, Warren H., and Elman, Robert (1952). *Text book of surgery*. Appleton Century Crafts. Inc., New York.

Delaplane, J.P., and Stuart, H.O. (1933). Caecal abligation of turkey by the use of clamps in preventing enterohepatitis (Black head) infection. *Jour. Am. Vet. Med. Assn.*, 238–246.

Dixon, J.M., and Wilkinson, W.S. (1957). Surgical techniques for the exteriorisation of the uterus of the chicken. *Am. J. Vet. Res.*, 18 : 665–667.

Douglas, S.W., and Williamson, H.D. (1963). *Principles of veterinary radiology*. Baillere, Tindall & Cox., London.

Durant, A.J. (1926). Caecal Abligation in Fowls. *Vet. Med.*, 21: 392–395.

Frank, E.R. (1959). *Veterinary surgery.* 6th ed. Burgess Publishing Company, Minneapolis 15, Minnesota.

Goligher, J.C., Duthie, H.L, and Nixon, H.H. (1975). *Surgery of the anus, rectum and colon.* 3rd ed. Baillere, Tindall, London.

Greig, J. Russel., and Boddie, George F. (Eds.) (1948). *Hoare's veterinary materia medica and therapeutics.* 6th ed. Baillere, Tindall & Cox, London.

Hall, L.W. (1966). *Wright's veterinary anaesthesia and analgesia.* 6th ed. Baillere, Tindall & Cassel, London.

Handfield-Jones, R.H., and Porrit, Sir Arthur (1957). *The essentials of modern surgery.* E & S Livingstone Ltd., London.

Harvey, J.D., Parrish, D.B. and Sandford, P.E. (1955). Improvements in the technique of deutectomy of newly hatched chicks, and the effect of the operation on their subsequent development. *Poul. Sci.,* 34: 3–8.

Hickman, John., and Walker, Robert G. (1973). *An atlas of veterinary surgery.* Oliver & Boyd, Edinburgh.

Hurov, L., Knauer, K., *Playter,* R., and Sexton, R. (1978). *Handbook of veterinary surgical instruments and glossary of surgical terms.* 1st. ed. W.B. Saunders Company, Philadelphia.

Knecht, Charles D., Welser, John R., Allen, Algernon R., Williams, David J., and Harris, N. Neil. (1975). *Fundamental techniques in veterinary surgery.* W.B. Saunders Company, Philadelphia.

Larrabee, M.G., and Posternak, J.M. (1952). Selective action of anaesthetics on synapsis and axons in mammalian sympathetic ganglia. *J. Neurophysiology,* 15: 91.

Leonard, Ellis P. (1960). *Orthopaedic surgery of the dog and cat.* W.B. Saunders Company, Philadelphia.

Mac Lean, Lloyd, D. (1972). Shock: causes and management of circulatory collapse. in *Text book of surgery* edited by Sabiston (q.v.).

Magrane, William G. (1977). *Canine ophthalmology.* 3rd. ed. Lea & Febiger, Philadelphia.

Malkani, P.G. (1933). Kumri. *Ind. Vet. J.,* 9: 184–192.

Manheimer, Martha L. (1973). *Style manual.* Marcel Dekker, Inc. New York.

Markowitz, J., Archibald, J., and Downie, H.G. (1959). *Experimental surgery.* 4th ed. William & Wilkins Company, Baltimore.

Mayer, Karl., Lacroix, J.L., and Hoskins, H. Preston. (Eds.) (1959). *Canine surgery by 38 North American authors.* 4th ed. American Veterinary Publications, Inc., California.

Miller, Malcolm E. (1952). *Guide to the dissection of the dog.* 3rd ed. Edward Brothers, Inc. Ann. Arbor, Michigan.

O'Connor, J.J. (Ed.) (1950). *Dollar's veterinary surgery.* 4th ed. Baillere, Tindall and Cox., London.

Oehme, Frederick, W., Prier, James E. (Eds.) (1974). *Text book of large animal surgery.* The William & Wilkins Company, Baltimore.

Prosser, Ladd C., Bishop, David W., Brown, Frank A., John, Theodorel., Wulff, Verner J. (1952). *Comparative animal physiology.* W.B. Saunders Company, Philadelphia & London. pp. 538–540.

Roberts, Stephen J. (1956). *Veterinary obstetrics & genital diseases.* Published by the author. New York State Veterinary College at Cornell University, Ithaca, New York.

Rothchild, I. (1947). The artificial anus in the bird, *Poul. Sci.,* 26: 157–162.

Sabiston, David C. Jr. (Ed.) (1972). *Text book of surgery. The biological basis of modern surgical practice.* 11th Asian ed. W.B. Saunders Company, Philadelphia.

Sahu, S., and Mithra, A.K. (1963). Bracheal plexus block in adult cattle. *Ind. Vet. J.,* 40(9): 578–581.

Schalm, Oscar W. (1961). *Veterinary haematology.* Lea & Febiger, Philadelphia.

Shuttleworth, A.C., and Smythe, R.H. (1960). *Clinical veterinary surgery.* Vol. II. Crosby Lockwood & Sons Ltd., London.

Sisson, S. (1958). *Scisson's anatomy of domestic animals.* Revised by J.D. Grossmann. 4th ed. W.B. Saunders Company, Philadelphia.

Sloan, H.J. (1936). The operative removal of the yolks from newly-hatched chicks. *Poul. Sci.,* 15: 23–27.

Smith, R.N. (1960). *Radiography for veterinary surgeons.* 1st ed. John Wright & Son Ltd., Bristol.

Smythe, R.H. (1956). *Veterinary ophthalmology.* Baillere, Tindall and Cox, London.

Smythe, R.H. (1959). *Clinical veterinary surgery.* Crosby Lockwood & Son Ltd., London.

Soma, Lawrence R. (Ed.) (1971). *Text book of veterinary anaesthesia.* The Williams & Wilkins Company, Baltimore.

Tasker, J.B., et al. (1958). Abomasal ulcers in cattle. *J. Amer. Vet. Med. Assn.* 133 (7).

Taylor, John A. (1959). *Regional and applied anatomy of domestic animals.* Parts I and II. Oliver and Boyd, London.

Wright, John G. (1957). *Veterinary anaesthesia.* William & Wilkins Co., Baltimore.

Wybar, Kenneth (1966). *Ophthalmology.* Baillere, Tindall and Cassel, London.

Additional references advised:

1. Nayak, S., Patnaik, R.N., and Mishra, A. (2000) *Surgical treatment of hard milker cows by single Sphincterostomy incision.* Ind. vet. J. 77(10): 893-894.

2. Pande, S.V., and Kulkarni, P.E. (1985). *The use of polyethylene tube with rubber balloon in open-teat surgery in goat.* Ind. J. vet. Surg. 6(2): 131-133.

INDEX